Psychiatry Rounds:
Practical Solutions
to Clinical Challenges

D1518962

Nutan Atre Vaidya, M.D.
Michael Alan Taylor, M.D.

ISBN #0-940780-67-4

Made in the United States of America

Published by
MedMaster Inc
P.O. Box 640028
Miami FL 33164

To

Our Parents

**(Ramchandra and Suman Atre
and
Eddie and Classie Taylor)**

and

Our Mentors

Acknowledgment

Michael Schrift, DO, read an earlier version of this book and gave a helpful critique. Several of our residents enthusiastically read this book and found it helpful and let us know. Georgette Pfeiffer tirelessly and meticulously prepared several drafts, created the layout, and helped with references. Both of us are grateful for her dedication. Anshuman Vaidya, Avinash Vaidya, and Ellen Taylor were always there when we needed them.

About the Authors

Nutan Atre Vaidya, MD, is Associate Professor and Chair of Department of Psychiatry and Behavioral Sciences, at Rosalind Franklin University of Medicine and Science, North Chicago, Illinois. Michael Alan Taylor, MD, is Professor Emeritus of Department of Psychiatry and Behavioral Sciences at Rosalind Franklin University of Medicine and Science, and Adjunct Clinical Professor of Psychiatry, University of Michigan School of Medicine, Ann Arbor, Michigan. Balasubramania Sarma, MD, is Associate Professor and Director of Child Psychiatry at Rosalind Franklin University of Medicine and Science.

Foreword

So many books, so little time. This would be our sentiment if we were again starting our training in psychiatry. So, why add another book? Part of the answer lies in the nature of textbooks: They may offer a wealth of information, but they rarely synthesize this information into a practical fabric readily worn by novice clinicians caring for patients. Standard textbooks cannot approximate the teaching of the art of medicine that is initially learned from experienced clinician teachers.

Unfortunately, current medical practice also limits the needed time and freedom to be with experienced clinical supervisors for extended periods. Trainees are lucky to get one or two hours of clinical teaching weekly. In psychiatry, supervision is often an office experience and rarely done with the patient present. Opportunities to learn the art of psychiatry and to synthesize it with the science of the brain are limited.

So much to know, yet so few chances to learn it, has led us to this book. We have tried to approximate the bedside teaching experience by describing patients as they appear in clinics and hospitals. We then guide the reader through the steps of diagnosis and management, the way a supervisor would on rounds. Thus, by its nature, this is not a data-dense, comprehensive textbook. We focus on what we know best and what we practice: neuropsychiatry. However, nature has not divided patients as neatly as does the DSM.[1] Patients with depression and seizure disorder often experience anxiety, and may also present with eating disorders. We discuss these conditions, particularly in how they co-occur with so many other conditions.

We also offer our clinical conclusions about psychiatric syndromes and their treatments that reflect our experience and biases. Others may disagree with some of them. But, like good supervisors should, we explain our reasoning. When we differ from standard viewpoints, we say so and explain the "why" of our position. Because our intended readers are trainees or clinicians new to the constructs of neuropsychiatry, we have deliberately chosen review articles and chapters over original articles as references. We believe that this strategy will make it easier for trainees to assimilate the database.

We want this book to be as close to an apprenticeship experience as possible. Thus, we describe many patients to illustrate common clinical experiences. We "cover the ground" unevenly, but offer principles

---

[1] DSM: *Diagnostic Statistical Manual. The official guide to the classification of psychiatric disorders.*

that can be generalized to many clinical situations. We have pitched our discussion to the trainee: psychiatric residents, residents in specialties that are often called upon to care for patients with behavioral syndromes, and medical students whose interest in psychiatry goes beyond the board review book. Recognizing our readers' special needs, however, we include clinical challenges likely to be encountered on national examinations.

Good teaching is often vivid in language, metaphor and illustration. We have styled our writing this way. We have also adopted a format to make learning easier: We present information, ask questions, expect thoughtful answers, and then offer our explanations and conclusions. We highlight principles rather than simply enumerate detail. this is not a psychopharmacology book. We assume a general knowledge of psychiatric drugs. For the novice reader, we have included a glossary and psychopharmacology table to help the reader better understand this book.

Nutan Atre Vaidya, M.D.   *Michael Alan Taylor, M.D.*

North Chicago, 2004

Table of Contents

Chapter 1

Principles of Diagnosis
and Treatment

Patient 1-1: Feathers and Frauds

It's Saturday night in a busy urban emergency room. A man enters. He is unsteady on his feet. His speech is slurred and his eyes bloodshot. You smell alcohol on his breath.

What is the most likely explanation for this patient's condition?

Patient 1-1's behavior suggests simple alcohol intoxication to most readers. The Duck Principle is based on the realization that most diseases, most of the time, produce the same pattern of signs and symptoms. Diseases have signature clinical features. You see a patient, you recognize the pattern, you make that diagnosis. Most of the time you will be right, as long as you learn the typical pattern for the disorders you are likely to see in your practice. Clinical medicine is full of patterns with signature features. Signature features represent the duck. *Table 1.1* displays some common examples.

Table 1.1 Some Ducks	
Signature Features	**The Duck**
23-year-old well-nourished woman who has missed two periods	Pregnancy
Purplish, itchy, raised skin areas at pressure points and along the hairline	Psoriasis
Cough, fever, malaise, purulent sputum, rales and dullness to percussion in left, lower chest	Pneumonia
64-year-old man in otherwise good health who needs to urinate 3-4 times nightly	Prostatic hypertrophy

What are other important conditions to think about and what do you do to find out about these conditions?

"Most diseases" also means that sometimes the obvious duck can be a decoy, a fraud. For example, Patient 1-1 could be a diabetic with hypoglycemia and the alcohol on his breath a "red herring." He could have been in a bar drinking, got into a fight and was hit on the head, resulting in a concussion or subdural hematoma. He might be an epileptic who stopped for a drink, then had a seizure on the way home, and is now in a post-ictal state. You always start with the Duck Principle, but thoroughness requires additional investigation: a careful history and physical examination.

Discussion

The first step in diagnosis is looking for the Duck. Looking for decoys adds to the differential diagnosis. For Patient 1-1 the differential could be: *simple alcohol intoxication, diabetes with hypoglycemia, post-concussion syndrome, subdural hematoma, epilepsy, post-ictal state* or *nonconvulsive status epilepticus.*

There are other possibilities, but you need to start somewhere, and the list above has the obvious suspects. The next step is screening for each "suspect" until you catch the culprit. For example, a blood alcohol level will take care of the first choice. There is no post-concussion syndrome without a head injury. Subdural hematoma is unlikely without a head injury or bleeding disorder. Checking the patient's head for injury, eyes for unequal pupils, and memory for any such injury should solve this part of the diagnostic mystery. Questions about diabetes and a blood sugar level should resolve the next mystery, and questions about a seizure disorder will solve another.

> Always get a barbiturate level when you get an alcohol blood level in a patient with suspected intoxication, because occasionally patients use both alcohol and barbiturates and the combination can lead to respiratory depression and death.

Patient 1-2: Does It Have Stripes On It?

A 58-year-old woman is hospitalized because of a dramatic loss in function over the past year. She can no longer work or care for herself at home. She is dirty and disheveled, has lost 40 pounds during the past year and looks emaciated. She is agitated. She is disoriented to date and day, but her level of arousal is not reduced (i.e., she is not delirious). She is fearful, and has paucity of speech. When she does speak, she says she is confused, frightened, and dead. She says she has not slept for six months. She performs poorly on numerous bedside cognitive tests and scores within the demented range. Her admitting diagnosis is dementia.

> **Principle of Diagnosis**
>
> Willy Sutton was a US bank robber in the early 1950's. When interviewed on TV after his capture, he was asked, "Willy, how come you robbed so many banks?" Sutton, incredulous, answered "Because that's where the money is!" has become known as "Sutton's Law": Go with the probabilities. Thus, the most common condition given clinical circumstances is most likely the correct diagnosis.

What is your first step in diagnosing Patient 1-2's condition? In fact, what is the first step in trying to diagnose anything?

Find the duck! In Patient 1-2 the big picture is: a middle-aged woman with a one year dramatic decline in functioning.[1] Many things can cause this. But she is apprehensive, fearful, and agitated. She has experienced severe weight loss, sleeps poorly, and has diffuse and substantial cognitive impairment in clear consciousness. Some would say the duck is dementia. Others would say the duck is depression. Still others would say both. Because she appears to have elements of both, we're stuck with an odd duck. When the duck principle leads to ambiguity, use Sutton's Law.

What is Patient 1-2's differential diagnosis, and what does Sutton's Law tell you about the odds for each choice?

Once you identify the syndrome, next determine etiology. *Table 1.2* shows likely possibilities and what we would do to solve these diagnostic mysteries. We are sure you can think of other choices, but given Patient 1-2's depression/dementia picture and her age, Sutton's Law leads us to our list.

Sutton's Law puts the possibilities in *Table 1.2* in order of most to least common in persons between 40 and 60 years of age.

Table 1.2 Differential Diagnosis for Patient 1-2's Condition		
Possibility	**Reasoning**	**What to do**
Drug reaction	Many medications can cause a dementia, and drug-induced dementia is the largest single *cause* of reversible dementia.	Careful history from collaterals, and previous treating physicians about general medical health and treatments Look for signs of other side effects (e.g., antipsychotic extrapyramidal features, anticholinergic peripheral signs)
Depression	A decline in function characterized by apprehension and agitation, weight loss, insomnia and feeling dead. Depression is the most common single *condition* producing reversible dementia.	Look for other features of a depression (other delusional ideas, hallucinations) History from collaterals and previous treating physicians about previous mood disorder, family history of mood disorder
Thyroid, parathyroid disease	Thyroid disease (hypo- but also hyper-) accounts for about 1% of all reversible dementias, but will be more common than that in this age group. Hyperparathyroidism can cause dementia with depressive features.	TSH is the best single test, although T_3/T_4 levels are usually also done at this time Calcium levels; history of renal stones
Inflammatory disease, such as lupus	More common in women of childbearing age. Associated with cognitive deficits and depression.	Presence of autoantibodies confirm diagnosis History of rheumatological problems, earlier presence of arthralgia

Table 1.2	Differential Diagnosis for Patient 1-2's Condition (cont'd)	
Possibility	*Reasoning*	*What to do*
Early form of Alzheimer's disease	In a woman, Alzheimer's disease represents 50% of all dementias.	Early onset Alzheimer's disease is associated with a strong family history; these patients may have rigidity or aphasia early on, so look for it
		On brain metabolic studies (SPECT, PET) Alzheimer's disease shows an early bilateral temporoparietal pattern of hypometabolism, whereas depression shows frontal or generalized hypometabolism.
Vascular dementia	Vascular dementia represents about 15% of all dementias.	Look for cardiovascular disease below the neck and in the eyes, or hypertension;
		get an MRI of the brain with contrast.
Paraneoplastic effect or metastasis	Dementia with large weight loss in a middle-aged woman.	Evaluate for breast, lung, pancreatic, ovarian tumor.
		MRI with contrast of the brain.
		Paraneoplastic antibodies

Discussion

Sutton's Law dramatically changes how you think about a patient. Although Alzheimer's disease accounts for 50% of all dementias, it is actually rare before age 75. Depression is four times as common as is Alzheimer's disease in persons 60 to 75 years of age.

There are of course other conditions we could have thought about, but are zebras, i.e., they are not common, for example, Creutzfeldt-Jakob disease, Pick's disease, Lewy body dementia.

Patient 1-2 was ultimately diagnosed as having a depression. She received electroconvulsive therapy (ECT) (see Chapter 3) and had an almost full recovery with minor residual cognitive problems attributed to her large and rapid weight loss.

Patient 1-3: In Unity There Is Strength

A 34-year-old man is hospitalized with an irritable depression. Other than speaking as if he "has marbles in his mouth," which he says is typical for him since a young man, his general medical and neurologic examinations are initially unremarkable. Tests of liver, thyroid, kidney and heart function are normal. Blood studies reveal an anemia with reduced and distorted red blood cells. The patient's history is unremarkable except for an untreated obsessive compulsive disorder (OCD) that began in his mid-teens and that has waxed and waned until the present. His OCD symptoms only minimally affect his functioning, and include checking, ordering and ritualistic behaviors that take hours daily to complete. For a period in his teens he repeatedly stole unneeded and inexpensive objects from stores, and was once arrested for shoplifting.

The patient received ECT for his irritable depression and it resolved, but as it did his gait became awkward: occasional subtle hesitancies were observed as if he had been struck in the chest by a strong wind, and as he walked he fully extended his fingers, like a "fork" in a motor overflow movement. A week later, he developed mild choreiform movements.

> **Principle of Diagnosis**
>
> Always try to reduce the patient's signs and symptoms to as few pathophysiologic processes as possible, one being the best. The *Rule of Parsimony* helps simplify treatment.

How many syndromal diagnoses could Patient 1-3 receive?

Major depression (a DSM Axis I mood disorder)
Obsessive compulsive disorder (a DSM Axis I anxiety disorder)
Kleptomania (a DSM Axis I impulse control disorder)
Normochromic anemia (A DSM Axis III disorder)
Possible Huntington's disease (a DSM Axis I and III disorder)

DSM or Diagnostic and Statistical Manual (the official nomenclature and criteria-based diagnostic system of the American Psychiatric Association, now in version IV) is organized into axes. *Axis I* includes states of psychiatric illness like mood disorders, *Axis II* includes personality disorders (*see Chapter 8, Table 8.13*). *Axis III* represents general medical and neurologic conditions. *Axis IV* defines temporally related stressful life events and situations. *Axis V* is a rating of the patient's overall functioning. Diagnostic criteria are specific in Axis I and II. Each syndrome has specific diagnostic criteria. If the patient meets the criteria that is the syndromal diagnosis. If the patient "comes close" or there is other diagnostic ambiguity, the diagnosis is the most likely category plus NOS (not otherwise specified, e.g., psychosis, NOS).

Applying the Rule of Parsimony, how many pathophysiologic processes are needed to explain his syndromal diagnoses?

Basal ganglia disease can cause depression, motor syndromes, and OCD. Kleptomania is best thought of as a variant of OCD (an obsession with a compulsion to take things). A Huntington's disease-like disorder will also likely involve the basal ganglia. The only diagnosis that does not seem to fit basal ganglia disease is this patient's anemia, but that too can be linked to his other conditions, because acanthocytosis, an autosomal recessive gene produces a Huntington's-like syndrome, basal ganglia degeneration, and an anemia due to reduced and distorted red blood cells.[2] Thus, one pathophysiologic process accounts for all five of Patient 1-3's diagnostic labels.

Discussion

Familial chorea with acanthocytes (spiny red blood cells) is a rare condition characterized by mouth and tongue tic-like dyskinesias, vocalizations, mild cognitive decline in frontal lobe functions, and later on, seizures, peripheral neuropathy and muscle atrophy. Parkinsonian features are sometimes present. Beta-lipoprotein concentration in the blood is normal, unlike other disorders with acanthocytes.[3]

The rule of parsimony shapes treatment by getting you to focus on the big problem, thereby hopefully avoiding polypharmacy or dealing with side issues that complicate management or fail to treat the fundamental problem. For example, Patient 1-2, in an earlier vignette, had a depression that was so severe it resulted in a dementia syndrome. There are many causes of dementia and depression is only one. But not recognizing that cause would lead to a failure to treat the depression and also the dementia.

Patient 1-3 might do best on one drug for his depression, OCD, and kleptomania, such as an antidepressant with serotonin reuptake inhibition, but with little dopaminergic activity so as not to exacerbate his movement problems. If his choreiform movements become worse, low doses of a dopamine-blocking drug (e.g., risperidone) might be needed.[4]

Patient 1-4: Spin Doctor

A 44 year old man is treated for a moderately severe depression that developed following the death of his father. Although he does not quite fit any specific DSM personality disorder label, he describes himself as somewhat shy with low energy levels, and as a worrier. He has held a steady job for 20 years and should be able to quickly return to work. He has never married, but has had several relationships with women and presently is dating. He has one sister with whom he is close. He is estimated to have an average IQ,[5] and no long-term cognitive problems are anticipated from his depression. Because he had two previous depressions, the treatment plan is to continue antidepressant treatment indefinitely. He has mild hypertension treated with a beta-blocker.

> **Principle of Management**
>
> Treat the patient, not the disease. These are high idealized words, but unfortunately, are rarely put into practice. It can be done, however, and the DSM gives you the structure to do it – the multiaxis format. Thus, take a spin on each axis. Be a spin doctor.

List the DSM axes, their names and implications. What is Patient 4's assessment on each axis?

	Table 1.3 DSM Axes and Their Uses		
Axis	**Use**	**Treatment implication**	**Patient 4's Assessment**
I	These are states of illness, i.e., diseases of the brain	Choice of medication and determining prognosis and long-term management. A patient can simultaneously have more than several Axis I conditions (Patient 1-3 had four)	Major depression, recurrent, requiring medication treatment indefinitely
II	Personality disorders, i.e., combinations of long-standing maladaptive traits	Often co-occurring with Axis I conditions and complicating treatment. When occurring alone, remain difficult to treat	No DSM personality disorder, but appears to have several anxious fearful traits. These may affect his tolerance to medication side effects and how he deals with stress in his life.

		Table 1.3 DSM Axes and Their Uses (cont'd)		
Axis	Use	Treatment implication	Patient 4's Assessment
III	General medical and neurologic conditions	Sometimes these conditions cause the Axis I condition (then termed secondary to the Axis III problem). When present, even if not causative, these conditions always complicate management	Mild hypertension that needs to be watched because, among many things, it puts Patient 4 at greater risk for vascular brain problems later in life. It also may make it risky to use any antidepressant that can cause hypertension (e.g., venlafaxine in high doses)
IV	Environmental and social strengths and weaknesses	Illness that occurs following stress is common. If the stressors can be minimized or the patient can learn to deal with them better, some episodes of illness may be avoided. Social strengths (job, family) and weaknesses (homeless) always affect treatment.	Depression followed the death of his father. Other present or potential stressors in his life need to be identified so he and you can help him avoid or deal with them.
V	Global function (0-100)	Often ignored, but very helpful in getting you to detail the patient's strengths and weaknesses	Having to take medication indefinitely for both hypertension and to avoid future depressions and having some anxious-fearful traits might get Patient 4 ten points off. Not being married with a family of his own, another 10 points off. But he also gets 80 points for his recovery, good cognitive function, steady job, and supportive sister.

Discussion

To take care of patients well, you need to know their strengths and weaknesses. The DSM multi-axis system gives you a structure to thoroughly assess patients and then develop your management plan. Patient 1-4 does not need help with his job. He will not need cognitive rehabilitation. He can be adequately educated about his illness and his treatments. His sister will help, if needed. His present girlfriend may also help, but you cannot count on her without more information. Because of his anxious-fearful personality traits, he may be prone to stress. Changing his personality is unlikely, but stress can be avoided and response to stress ameliorated.

The key to Patient 1-4's minimal recurrence of depressions will be his continued compliance with medication. Behavioral techniques such as systematic desensitization and autogenic relaxation may also help.[6] Group therapy may with his avoidant traits, by having him experience (learn) how to socialize better.

Patient 1-5: Treatment Is a Three-Legged Stool

A 36 year old woman is hospitalized with a psychotic depression. She had a depression when she was 23 following the break up of a love affair, and a second depression at age 30 following the birth of her daughter. Her present depression developed without any precipitating event. Her general medical health is good, and the depression is primary.

> **Principle of Management**
>
> Decisions about treating the acute condition must also consider the long-term interactions between the illness and treatments. Treatment is a three-legged stool: 1) acute management, 2) continuation, and 3) maintenance.

What are the three legs of treatment and their goals?

Acute treatment. The goal of acute treatment is to achieve the best possible response, remission whenever possible. Acute treatment usually takes 6-12 weeks, depending on the illness.

Continuation. The goal of continuation is to preserve the best possible acute treatment response and prevent relapse of the acute episode. Preserving a "so-so" response to acute management is not adequate treatment. Virtually all patients with an Axis I condition need continuation as well as acute treatment. Continuation treatment, if successful, lasts 6-12 months.

Maintenance. The goal of maintenance is to prevent future episodes. Maintenance can last for several years to a lifetime.

How do you go about setting and monitoring these goals?

Acute treatment. Predicting outcome is difficult, but possible in most situations. *First,* know the numbers – what is the response rate of disease X to treatment Y? We will discuss these rates and how to specifically use them in subsequent sections. *Second,* know the variables that have been found helpful in predicting outcome, and match them to your patient. Predictors of recovery have been established for patients with traumatic brain injury and stroke, and these also work fairly well for psychiatric patients. Specific forms of psychopathology also predict response. *Table 1.4* displays the variables you need to consider for each patient. We will repeatedly come back to them. Psychotic features do not predict outcome. Nor does the presence of severe depression or mania. If patients with these conditions have many of the good prognostic features displayed in *Table 1.4,* they can have a full recovery. Always be a therapeutic optimist.

     Continuation treatment. Continuation treatment is almost always needed to preserve remission and to prevent relapse of the acute episode. The 12 months following the *end* of the episode is the critical period during which relapse is most likely to occur. The pharmacotherapy that worked for the acute episode is the choice for continuation and usually at the same dose. *Maintenance treatment* depends on many factors, which we will discuss in detail in subsequent sections.

Table 1.4 Predictors of Recovery [7]

Pre-episode Good Prognostic Features

The better the functioning, the better the episode outcome. Specifically assess a) level of self-sufficiency in activities of daily living, b) level of social skills, c) level of motor behavior, and d) level of cognition.

No change in personality traits after earlier episodes

No inter-episode a) avolition, b) circumstantiality in speech, c) loss of libido, d) newly developed religiosity that disrupts social and interpersonal functioning, e) temporal lobe psychosensory features or frontal lobe signs[8]

> Formal thought disorder refers to disorganized, aphasic-like speech. It is most commonly observed in schizophrenics and patients with secondary behavioral syndromes, thus, its association with a poorer outcome.

Acute Episode Good Prognostic Features

No loss of emotional expression or volition

No formal thought disorder

No basal ganglia or cerebellar motor signs

Immediate Post-episode Good Prognostic Features

Volitional

Normal emotional expression

Normal motor behavior

Good cognitive function, specifically in the following areas: attention and concentration, serial verbal new learning (e.g., learning a list of unrelated words) and executive functioning (e.g., problem-solving and thinking, flexibility in problem-solving)

Patient 1-6: Don't Use an Elephant Gun to Kill a Mouse

A 21 year old man is brought to an ER because of an acute onset psychosis. He is disheveled, dirty and mildly dehydrated. He is extremely fearful, his eyes darting around the examining room as if looking for danger. He is agitated and cannot sit still. He says objects in the room look "sharp-edged" and are pointing at his eyes and that people are whispering to him from outside the room. He refuses further examination and suddenly runs into the hallway, shouting to people to stop whispering at him. He is given haloperidol 10 mg IM to control his agitation. Thirty minutes later he develops a painful spasm, cramping his tongue and mouth so he cannot speak. Diphenhydramine 50 mg IV is given, which immediately relieves his cramping. Benztropine 1 mg PO BID is prescribed for the next several days to prevent further cramping. No further antipsychotics are given.

> **Principle of Pharmacotherapy**
>
> Control agitation with a sedative. Use antipsychotics to treat psychosis, but use them sparingly.

What happened to Patient 1-6 in the ER?

Patient 1-6 developed an oral-buccal dystonia. Young male patients and older women patients with neurologic disease are at greatest risk. High-potency typical antipsychotics are most likely to cause it.[9]

What other medications could have been used to control Patient 1-6's agitation?

Sedation for acute agitation, even for patients in restraints, can be achieved fast and safely with benzodiazepines. Lorazepam and oxazepam are good intermediate-length half-life benzodiazepines for this. They can be given slowly, IV with follow-up IM or oral doses. Diphenhydramine can also be used because of its sedating properties.[10]

Why was diphenhydramine chosen to stop his cramping?

First, because it works immediately when given IV. Benztropine is also used, but it has substantial anticholinergic properties. Diphenhydramine IV will also produce sleep for an hour or all night for some patients. Patient 1-6's condition suggested he would sleep and might be much better upon wakening.

Why was benztropine given for several days?

Haloperidol's half-life is over 24 hours. The dystonia could recur unless the haloperidol is covered for the next day or two. Benztropine is an anticholinergic drug which is used to treat extrapyramidal side effects of acute psychosis. It has a half-life of 6-8 hours and so is given BID or TID for several days to match the half-life of the offending antipsychotic. It is also less sedating at that point than diphenhydramine, and too much sedation after the first day may interfere with management. Elimination half-life refers to the time it takes for 50% of a given dose of a drug to be eliminated from the body.

> The big picture of a drug-induced psychosis (an intoxication state): acute onset, lots of emotion, hallucinations, often in several sensory modalities, and hyperarousal.

Why were no further antipsychotics given?

Automatically giving an antipsychotic to every psychotic patient will eventually lead to disaster – death or severe morbidity. Deadly etiology might be missed (a form of status epilepticus). Persons prone to dystonia can get other movement disorders. Some psychotic patients in drug induced states need control of their agitation, a safe place, and some sleep to resolve their psychosis. This is particularly true for acute drug-related psychoses. In a young person with an acute onset psychosis with lots of emotionality and several different kinds of perceptual disturbances, a drug intoxication is a good diagnostic bet. Patient 1-6 woke the next morning without any psychotic features. He had had mescaline at a party a few hours before his admission.

Which life-threatening condition was Patient 1-6 at risk for?

The use of high-potency antipsychotics in excited patients can induce a malignant form of catatonia that has been called neuroleptic malignant syndrome (NMS). About 1-15% of patients with NMS will die from it. We will discuss NMS later on.

Discussion

Antipsychotics are big guns. Like big guns, they are needed for big game, but they can be dangerous if misused. They can cause tardive dyskinesia (TD), an irreversible syndrome that includes many disfiguring and socially disrupting motor features plus frontal lobe cognitive loss.[11] Atypical antipsychotics are less likely to cause the acute and chronic motor abnormalities associated with antipsychotic drugs and have become first-line treatments. Clozapine is reserved for chronic patients because it can cause agranulocytosis and has substantial side effects. It is a powerful anticholinergic drug, and 3-6% of exposed patients will develop seizures. Risperidone is not yet available in IM form. The doses needed to control acute agitation in acutely psychotic patients cause all the extrapyramidal effects of the typical agents. Olanzapine is without IM form and can induce excitement in some patients. However, it is available in a form that is absorbed sublingually. If an antipsychotic is needed and the patient is willing to take an oral dose, 5 mg held in the mouth can calm many patients. Quetiapine and ziprasidone are also atypical antipsychotics, but are not used if rapid results are needed. See the section *Psychopharmacology at a Glance* for a summary of some of the basic pharmacokinetic and dynamic information about atypical antipsychotics.

The therapeutic choices are more limited than it would appear. *Table 1.6* displays the therapeutic uses and limitations of these agents. Also keep in mind that NMS has been reported with each of these agents, and one of us has treated patients with NMS who were exposed to each of these agents, except quetiapine.

Table 1.6 Atypical Antipsychotics: Therapeutic Uses and Limitations

Drug	Indications	Concerns and Limitations
Clozapine	Treatment-resistant psychoses (billed as "the schizophrenia drug," but may be most helpful for patients with psychotic mood disorder), so not a first-line drug	Agranulocytosis risk mostly during first six months of treatment As powerful an anticholinergic as the tertiary TCAs, so not a good choice for older patients or patients with cardiac disease Seizure inducing
Quetiapine	A compromise choice between what works and what makes psychotic patients worse; may be helpful in demented psychotic patients	Tolerated well by most patients, but many clinicians doubt its effectiveness as an antipsychotic
Olanzapine	First choice for many psychotic disorders; may have mood stabilizing properties	Anticholinergic properties may be a problem for some patients Weight gain almost always a problem Can cause increased blood glucose levels
Risperidone	First choice for many psychotic disorders as it acts like a typical antipsychotic	In doses < 6 mg, its lower EPS advantages over typical antipsychotics disappears
Ziprasidone	Another compromise between what works and what makes patients worse	Tolerated well by most patients, but many clinicians doubt its effectiveness as an antipsychotic

Patient 1-7: If One is Good, Two Is Usually Worse

A 36 year old man is hospitalized for agitation, irritability, and being verbally abusive to family members and strangers on the street. He is considered psychotic and a potential danger to others. In the ER he is given haloperidol 10 mg IM and then 10 mg PRN PO or IM BID for his abusive behavior. He is delusional, has auditory hallucinations, is agitated (pacing), irritable, and speaks fast with press of speech. His general medical health is good, except that he is mildly dehydrated. His clothes appear loose, suggesting recent weight loss. He has not eaten for several days.

Once hospitalized, he is also given lorazepam 1 mg PO or IM QID for agitation. Olanzapine 10 mg PO BID is also prescribed, but this is not the fast absorption form. Benztropine 1 mg BID is prescribed to avoid any extrapyramidal side effects from the haloperidol. Because he has not been sleeping during the acute phase of his illness, lorazepam 1 mg po qhs is added.

Principles of management

- Unless an emergency, do not do two things at once. If something good or bad results, you cannot be sure which thing accounts for it.

- Treating target symptoms (anxiety, agitation, insomnia, hallucinations) rather than disease processes (mania, depression, panic disorder) typically leads to polypharmacy. Automatic polypharmacy is doing two things at once. In only rare instances does research support the efficacy of two drugs over one in the initial treatment of most psychiatric disorders. Polypharmacy increases the risk for side effects, adverse effects, and problematic drug-drug interactions. Polypharmacy automatically reduces your options (you give two drugs simultaneously, the patient does not respond, you want to switch to another drug in a different pharmacodynamic class, but you have already given two. Ergo, your options are down by two rather than one).

What would have been a better pharmacologic strategy for Patient 1-7?

The semi-trick here is to try and make a diagnosis first before treating. The examination revealed Patient 1-7 to have no immediate life threatening conditions once in the safety of the hospital. Using modest doses of lorazepam or oxazepam for the first day or so until making a diagnosis would have been a better strategy. Many clinicians think that they cannot afford the luxury of doing this because the patient's insurance or other pressures will not permit a longer hospital stay. Unfortunately, precipitous treatment, particularly with several drugs, increases the likelihood of side and adverse effects, a stormy hospital course, and a longer not shorter stay. A day or two up-front to figure things out can save a week or more of turmoil later on.

What are the danger signals in Patient 1-7's situation? What life-threatening condition do they predispose him to?

The danger signals are psychotic excitement, exposure to two antipsychotics simultaneously, agitation that might result in exhaustion, dehydration and possible nutritional imbalance, and the use of two strong anticholinergic drugs. The life-threatening condition is neuroleptic malignant condition (NMS).

> Despite vigorous treatments about 10% of patients with NMS die from it.

Discussion

Sometimes you cannot avoid doing two things at once. For example, if Patient 1-7 developed NMS, you would 1) stop all antipsychotics and 2) treat the NMS. But, for most patients, most of the time, start with one treatment. If a patient is on two or more drugs, do not increase or decrease doses simultaneously unless it is a critical situation. Do not add or subtract two drugs simultaneously, unless you suspect drug toxicity (then stop!).   Never automatically give an antiparkinsonian drug to avoid possible antipsychotic induced extrapyramidal side effects.[12] A third of patients even on oral high potency typical antipsychotics never need these agents. Never give two antipsychotics simultaneously. The notion that using two antipsychotics simultaneously provides some synergistic or broad spectrum effect is unproven, whereas their simultaneous use substantially increases their risks.

Patient 1-8: Will the Real Patient Please Stand Up?

A 44 year old man with a history of alcohol abuse and bipolar mood disorder is hospitalized because of increasing agitation and irritability. One resident wants to give him haloperidol 10 mg IM and then 10 mg PO BID PRN for agitation. A second resident wants to give him lorazepam 2 mg Q4-6h PRN as needed for agitation.

> ### Principles of Management
>
> - Control agitation with sedatives; reserve antipsychotics for definitive treatment.
> - The more PRN medications used, the less unit staff observes the patient behaviors and the more unsure the doctors.

What are the problems with resident one's choice?

Resident one wants to give an antipsychotic to control agitation. That is a "no-no" unless you are sure the agitation is the direct result of a psychosis and the antipsychotic is the best treatment for that psychosis. Some psychotic agitation is better definitively treated with lithium, valproic acid or ECT. In Patient 1-8's situation the agitation could be alcohol related and not the result of the bipolar disorder. A sedative drug would be safer, until a definitive diagnosis can be made. *But* maybe Patient 1-8's agitation requires only hospitalization, a firm caring staff, a safe place, and a good night's sleep. Resident one ordered medication that might not be needed. PRN medication is often ordered for the convenience of the physician or the unit staff. *But* that is not a goal of treatment. The goal of treatment is what is best for the patient.

What are the problems with resident two's choice?

Resident two at least starts with a sedative-type drug, and lorazepam or oxazepam are commonly used to control agitation. *But* like resident one, the order is automatically given and the patient may not need any sedation. *Admission to a well run psychiatric unit with well trained staff is active treatment* and by itself can calm many patients. Many "out of control" or "assaultive" elderly nursing home patients are transferred every day to psychiatric inpatient units where good care and structure immediately calms them. Sometimes no further treatment is needed.

Resident two makes another mistake. Lorazepam is an intermediate-length half-life benzodiazepine. Two mg q4-6h could quickly result in an oversedated patient, masking symptoms and making diagnosis impossible. In elderly patients benzodiazepines can lead to falls. In all patients they can produce memory problems. If given too long, they can be addicting and withdrawal is difficult. If Patient 1-8 needed sedation to control most causes of agitation, a benzodiazepine would have been appropriate, but in lower doses and less frequently. PRN is used only to titrate doses during the initial 24-48 hours of use to determine what the total daily dose of a drug should be. For example, you start a manic patient on valproic acid and order lorazepam 1 mg PO or IM q6h PRN. The patient gets 750 mg of valproic acid BID for several days, but PRN lorazepam is needed 2-3 times each day. That tells you that you will probably have to raise the valproic acid dose. If your first-choice medication is working, PRNs should quickly become unnecessary.

What is the problem with our answers to the above questions?

Only 5% or so of persons dependent on alcohol go into severe withdrawal, or delirium tremens (DTs), when denied alcohol. Those going into DTs typically are debilitated by their drinking.

Because Patient 1-8 has bipolar mood disorder, we have assumed that his agitation and irritability are due to mania. If true, we are all set. *But*, Patient 1-8 is also an alcoholic. So is his acute episode due to alcohol intoxication, or worse, alcohol withdrawal?

Intoxication, when severe enough to produce substantial agitation, usually requires one dose of a benzodiazepine to sedate because the patient already has reduced cortical arousal from the alcohol intoxication. Intoxication can be handled in an ER holding bed, and 12 hours of rest is usually sufficient. However, when withdrawal from alcohol results in substantial agitation, the patient is in DTs, which is a potentially lethal condition requiring hospitalization. Then the use of antipsychotics rather than a benzodiazepine borders on malpractice. If you determine Patient 1-8 is in alcohol withdrawal (see *Table 1.7*), follow the basic steps in

Altered sensorium with agitation and disorientation is called delirium. Deliria are associated with diffuse slowing on EEG, with the exception of DTs which is characterized by diffuse fast activity.

management: 1) *Protect* the patient from self-harm and from hurting others (restraints), 2) *Maintain* homeostasis (IV normal saline, control blood pressure and balance electrolytes), 3) *Sedate* with Intermediate or long-acting benzodiazepine initially given to the point of sedation, and 4) *Withdraw* by first sedating for 24 hours and then slowly tapering the drug over 5-10 days when the drug is then discontinued. Anticonvulsants are not automatically given and, if needed, are also tapered and stopped once the withdrawal period is over, 5) Do not give glucose to an alcoholic as thiamine is a co-factor in glucose metabolism. A sudden glucose load can reduce already depleted thiamine levels, and precipitate a Wernicke's encephalopathy in the genetically susceptible alcoholic, and 6) do not over-hydrate. Many patients in DTs consume lots of fluids in an attempt to feel more comfortable.

Table 1.7 Clinical Features of Alcohol Withdrawal
Altered sensorium (when severe, delirium)
Anxiety (when severe, terror)
Agitation (when severe, requires restraints)
Perceptual disturbances (frightening visual and auditory hallucinations)
Central nervous system excitation (hyperreflexia, tremor, myoclonus, sympathomimetic instability from hypothalamic dysregulation, seizures)

Patient 1-9: Liar, Liar, Pants on Fire

A 38 year old woman is hospitalized for acute mania. She became increasingly verbally abusive and threatening to her family, was walking around her house semi-nude to the embarrassment of her teenage children, husband, and sister who lives with them. She was recently arrested for speeding and reckless driving, was verbally abusive toward the police officer and eventually was brought to the hospital where she was convinced to voluntarily sign herself in for "a day or so" to "get some rest."

Principles of Hospital Management

- For patients barely in control or who are out of control, voluntary hospitalization is like "the road to hell." Both are paved with good intentions. When admitting a patient, the decision regarding voluntary vs. involuntary admission is determined by the patient's *ability* to give an *informed* consent, not just their agreement.

- Lying or minimizing, or otherwise being misleading with a patient is only acceptable if you are in physical danger. Otherwise, it will result in a stormy acute treatment period and a bad doctor-patient relationship.

How were the above management principles violated with Patient 1-9?

Patient 1-9 was verbally abusive and threatening. She was arrested for reckless driving. These facts indicate an increased degree of imminent danger to herself and others. If you were Patient 1-9's doctor and concluded she would sign herself into the hospital and stay for treatment because she recognized the seriousness of her situation, then voluntary admission would be best. However, if she has little recognition of her illness (anosognosia) and its severity, she will likely want to leave after a few days. Then, you will be faced with letting a potentially dangerous patient leave, or having to change her to involuntary status. Also, if she is voluntary and then refuses treatment, she cannot be treated. If involuntary, she can at least receive limited treatment to prevent self-injury or injury to others.

Telling a patient who clearly needs to be hospitalized for severe psychiatric illness that she will just be in for a day or so for a rest is *lying*. Once on the unit, she will quickly find out the truth. Better she knows beforehand and can make an informed decision. Most patients who are involuntarily admitted and then well treated, later appreciate the efforts made in their behalf. Patients who are lied to stay angry and mistrustful and are less likely to continue in treatment or seek help later in life.[13]

What could have been done to better serve Patient 1-9?

Given the information we have about Patient 1-9, admission is mandatory. Getting the family to be your ally is the best strategy. Explain to them your findings and what you want to do: hospitalize, medications, likely length of stay, what will likely need to be done after discharge. Get their consent for hospitalization, even if the patient is involuntarily admitted. Then explain all this to the patient and try to convince the patient of the need for hospitalization and treatment. If the patient concurs, great. If not, admit even if it has to be involuntarily.

Discussion

Families are typically relieved when something definitive is done to help a relative, particularly when they are clearly aware of the problem as is the family of Patient 1-9. Your relationship with them is second in importance only to that with the patient. The family can be an extension of your hands. They can be your eyes and ears. They can persuade patients and courts. Involuntary hospitalization and going to court to keep the patient in the hospital are annoying and inconvenient, but in the long run these efforts can be life saving.

Relating to the patient's family can strain the patient's right to confidentiality. Technically, if a patient forbids you to contact the family, even during the involuntary hospitalization you cannot break the confidentiality. However, if we think that contacting the family is necessary to save the patient's life or someone else's, we will contact the family after informing the patient that we are doing so. If we act in good faith and to save the patient's life, then in the worst case scenario the potential jury will be more sympathetic to the psychiatrist who broke the confidentiality and saved the patient than the one who kept the confidentiality but lost the patient. Defense attorneys always prefer to defend a physician with a live rather than with a dead patient.

Patient 1-10: Stop! Look! Listen!

A 50 year old man is hospitalized for a recurrence of psychosis. In the past, he has been diagnosed as having "schizophrenia" or an "atypical psychosis, NOS."[14] Patient 1-10 is a known noncomplier with medication, so on admission he is given 50 mg of fluphenazine decanoate IM, a long-acting form of a high-potency typical antipsychotic and benztropine 1 mg PO BID. The next day he becomes agitated, and disoriented to time of day and place. His speech is rapid, but intermittent, and his speech makes no sense. His temperature elevates to 101°F. His pulse is 100. His mouth is dry and his pupils are dilated. His skin feels dry and his face is flushed. Getting out of bed that night, he falls and cuts his head, requiring six stitches.

What principles of management of an acute psychosis were violated?

1. *Diagnose before you treat.* Patient 1-10 had been diagnosed as having an atypical or psychosis NOS. This implies clinical uncertainty. Whenever a patient has an atypical behavioral syndrome, consider it secondary until proven otherwise. A diagnostic work-up should precede definitive treatment and may lead to more specific treatment (e.g., an anticonvulsant for epilepsy).

2. *Never use a long-acting antipsychotic to treat an acute condition.* Long-acting forms of antipsychotics are for the continuation and maintenance phases of treatment, and only for patients for whom you have not been successful in getting to comply with treatment. Long-acting forms have half-lives of weeks. Once in the body and something goes wrong, you and the patient are stuck. Long-acting forms should only be used in patients who are behaviorally stable. This management approach is often violated.

3. *Doing two things at once.* It is usually not a good idea to do two things at once. If something goes wrong, which action or drug caused it? If something goes right, again which action or drug helped?

What happened to Patient 1-10?

Fluphenazine and benztropine each have substantial anticholinergic properties. Patient 1-10 got an anticholinergic overdose and became delirious. Hallmarks of anticholinergic delirium are summarized in *Table 1.9*. The classic quip describing this syndrome is "dry as a bone, red as a beet, blind as a bat, and mad as a hatter."

What could have been done to stop what happened and perhaps avoid the patient's fall?

1. Do not give long-acting antipsychotics to acutely ill patients.
2. Do not load a patient with anticholinergic drugs.
3. Once delirium occurs, recognize it.
4. Anticholinergic delirium can be treated with physostigmine 1-2 mg subcutaneously Q2h up to 8 mg in a 24-hour period or until the delirium has resolved.[15] After the first dose, heart rate and blood pressure are monitored, and if clinically meaningful drops *do not occur,* subsequent doses can be given. Because of the long half-life of antipsychotics, the decanoate form in particular, physostigmine with a shorter half-life will be needed for several days.

Table 1.9 Anticholinergic Delirium	
Delirium	Agitation, anxiety, disorientation with an altered sensorium, disorganized speech
Fever	Flushed skin in pale-skinned persons
Tachycardia	
Dry mouth and skin	
Dilated pupils	

Discussion

Managed care's drive to get patients out of the hospital quickly, and clinicians' desires to get the patient better fast can sometimes do more harm than good. Emergency treatments are always begun immediately, but most psychiatric clinical situations are not of that acuity: Stop and observe. Look and do a good assessment. Listen to what the patient is saying. Then treat.

Patient 1-11: Let's Change into Something More Comfortable

A 28-year-old man with a long history of drug abuse (hallucinogens and marijuana, now phencyclidine) is brought to the emergency room in an agitated, hostile state. He is delusional and has flight of ideas with paraphasic utterances and episodes of driveling speech. His chart indicates he has been receiving valproic acid 3000 mg and haloperidol 20 mg daily. He is admitted on this regime. Once in the hospital, he becomes increasingly angry, pulls a small knife, and stabs an aide in the arm. The crisis team is called. During the struggle he bites a security guard. Haloperidol 10 mg IM is given. Once in restraints he calms down and accepts his oral medications. The next morning he has an oral buccal dystonia and coarse tremors.

> A paraphasia is an approximate word by meaning (e.g., "this writer" rather than "this pen"), by mix up of sound (e.g., band instead of hand), or by association (e.g., "this mechanism of muscle," rather than "this pen" as in the pen is mightier than the sword). Driveling speech refers to speech that is empty of meaning like double talk (e.g., He didn't it to the other thing that what can he do). Flight of ideas is speech that jumps from topic to topic so you can follow it (often with difficulty), but it never gets to the point, so the big picture meaning is lost.

What principles of inpatient management were violated?

1. *Safety first for all concerned (and that includes you).* Once you make the decision to admit a patient to an acute treatment psychiatric unit, it is generally best to have all patients unknown to you and any patient with any indications of violence or violent tendencies change into hospital pajamas in the emergency room admitting area or clinic where security personnel are present, rather than waiting until the patient gets to the unit. During the change, the patient's personal belongings are recorded and stored safely, and his clothes subtly searched for weapons. Do not be fooled by gender. Although male outpatients are more likely to injure mental health workers, women inpatients are more likely to do so.

> The first three days of hospitalization is the period of greatest risk. Women inpatients injure staff more often than do male inpatients. The lower the socioeconomic background of the patient, the greater the risk.[16]

2. *Get urine for a drug screen as soon as possible.* All patients with a history of drug abuse or suspected of being in a drug-induced stated should have a drug screen before admission.
3. *Get blood levels of recently prescribed psychotropics on all newly admitted patients.* All patients with a history of recent treatment with a psychotropic drug should have blood immediately taken for drug levels, and you should not automatically restart these medications until the blood levels are known.

This is important for two reasons: 1) If the patient is taking the drugs and the blood level indicates compliance, then you know the patient relapsed despite treatment, and may need additional or different medication, or 2) if blood levels are very low, you know there has been noncompliance, and then you can start the patient back on the same prescribed dose. Although haloperidol levels are not routinely ordered, in this patient valproic acid levels could have been ordered.

What are the implications of Patient 1-11's psychopathology and drug history?

Although we will discuss patients with drug problems later, recognizing psychopathology and its diagnostic and treatment implications is always important. Patient 1-11 was psychotic, hostile and agitated with flight of ideas, and formal thought disorder (paraphasic and driveling speech),[17] and recently used phencyclidine. All this suggests the patient may be in an acute phencyclidine intoxication. Violence is to be expected with phencyclidine, and prevention of violence is the best treatment.

What would be a better plan for managing such patients?

1. Always systematically assess a patient's violence risk prior to admission.
2. Patients who are violent or actually violent should always be placed in hospital clothes. Violent patients should never be admitted to an inpatient unit in their street clothes.
3. Under a show of force, by sedating the patient if necessary, get blood work and urine while the patient is in the admitting area. Do a screening physical exam while the patient is in the admitting area.
4. Consider the likely need for sedation, and prescribe accordingly. Hold definitive treatment until lab tests are back and you have made a reasonable diagnostic assessment.

What should be done now to "clean up" this clinical mess?[18]

1. Treat the dystonia immediately with IV diphenhydramine 50 mg. Benztropine 1 mg BID or TID may be needed for several more days.
2. Stop the IM and PO haloperidol and reevaluate the need for an antipsychotic. Some PCP psychoses end quickly once most of the PCP is excreted in the urine.
3. Cover any agitation and anxiety with low doses of lorazepam.
4. Because the patient is in restraints, he is also in hospital pajamas, and should stay in pajamas until he is no longer considered dangerous.

> PCP is a dissociative anesthetic and can also induce features of catatonia. Sedating with lorazepam is also somewhat protective, reducing the likelihood of catatonia.[19]

5. Watch for high blood pressure and other sympathomimetic problems from PCP and manage these.
6. Meet with the staff to try to resolve their anger toward the patient so they can maintain their therapeutic roles. They should recognize that the patient's actions, although harmful, resulted from illness not criminality.
7. Review the need for restraints and remove them as soon as possible. Having a "quiet room" on the unit that can be used to calm patients without locking them up or restraining them adds flexibility to acute care programming.

Patient 1-12: Go to Sleep, You're Interfering With My Work

A 44-year-old man is hospitalized for depression.[20]   Although his sleep problems have recently worsened, he says he has had insomnia for years and often has difficulty getting to sleep and is tired during the day. On his first night in the hospital, despite nortriptyline 75 mg HS and temazepam, 15 mg PO qhs, he cannot fall asleep. He goes to the nurses' station at 11:30 p.m. and asks to sit in the lounge to watch TV. The night nurse bluntly tells him he will disturb other patients and he should go to bed. He asks to sit up in the dayroom and read. Again he is told he has to sleep.

What should be the response to hospitalized patients with insomnia?

Patients never interfere with the work of hospital staff. They *are* "the work." Any other attitude is unprofessional and nontherapeutic.

Many hospitalized patients have sleep problems. Permitting a patient to quietly watch TV, listen to a radio or music (earphones can keep the sound to a minimal), and having books and magazines to read can help pass the time without getting into a power struggle. Encourage the night staff to chat with patients who are awake. Do not make "a federal case out of it." The only restriction is that other patients should not be disturbed. The sleepless patient should not be made to feel he has done something wrong.

What can you do to relieve insomnia, particularly long-standing insomnia?

Treating the acute condition that led to hospitalization often treats the insomnia. *Table 1.10* displays some medication strategies that can help during the early days before definitive treatment response is substantial. Some clinicians use sedating atypical antipsychotics like quetiapine as if it were a hypnotic. We prefer not to do this for reasons previously discussed.

Long-standing insomnia should be regarded as a sleep disorder. Like all disorders, assessment is needed to determine etiology and plan management. Drug side effects are expected results due to the pharmacodynamics of the drug. Although most noncompliance with medication is due to poor tolerance of side effects, side effects also have some therapeutic benefits. Mild expected side effects tell you the drug is being metabolized and getting to the organ you know it should. Some side effects, such as sedation, can be used during early treatment. In Patient 1-12's situation, a sedating antidepressant given at night helped his insomnia.

Table 1.10   *Medication Strategies for Acute Insomnia of the Hospitalized Psychiatric Patient*

If insomnia is due to primary psychiatric disorder, e.g., depression:

1. Use a sedating antidepressant to control the primary disorder.
2. Prescribe the medication at bedtime.
3. If the first two steps do not relieve insomnia, then use a nonbenzodiazepine hypnotic, such as diphenhydramine 50 mg PO qhs or 5 mg qhs.
4. If step 3 is not helpful, then a short-acting benzodiazepine hypnotic, such as temazepam 15-30 mg or nonbenzodiazepine, zolpidem 5 mg may help.

If insomnia is not due to a primary psychiatric disorder and is transient, then use steps 3 and 4.

Long-acting benzodiazepines cause residual daytime sleepiness, whereas ultra-short-acting benzodiazepine can cause anterograde amnesia.[21]

Patient 1-13: Just Say "No"

A 56-year-old man is hospitalized because of a recurrence of mania following the discontinuation of valproic acid because of chronic liver problems. Because he has cardiac conduction problems, he cannot take lithium. Electroconvulsive therapy (ECT) is recommended, but he and his wife say "no," despite being told of the limits on pharmacotherapy from his liver and heart disease, and that ECT works about as well for mania as any medication. Gabapentin, another anticonvulsant with some mood stabilizing properties that is not metabolized in the liver, is tried without success. The man's wife wants him to get an antipsychotic, although he is not presently psychotic.

What should be done?

If you thought the addition of an antipsychotic with gabapentin might help or some other multiple drug combination might help, you might acquiesce to the wife's preference. Olanzapine is approved as a mood stabilizing antipsychotic and so might be an option. But what if you thought the antipsychotic would not work, or was dangerous for the patient? What if all possibilities acceptable to you had been tried? What then?

Just say "no."

When you treat a patient, you are more than a cab driver taking a fare where he or she wants to go. Your professional *opinions* and your care are what you are providing. They cannot be separated into you have me as your doctor, but you do not need to follow what I think must be done. Thus, if you decide ECT is the only appropriate treatment for Patient 1-13, and he and his wife still refuse, you would tell them a) you are sorry they do not agree with your opinion, but ECT is the only treatment you are prepared to give now, and b) they should get a second opinion if they think that will help, and you can arrange that, and c) you will try to find them another physician in whom they have more confidence. Most patients and their families in this situation will recognize your strong commitment to your treatment choice and will then really listen to you as you educate them about the treatment. Then, they usually agree. Some, however, will need referral.[22]

Patient 1-14: One Size Does Not Fit All

A 20 year old woman comes to see you because of a depression. She has had two other episodes. As a child she was repeatedly sexually fondled by an older stepbrother. Her father was an irritable alcoholic who physically abused her mother. The father also frequently hit her, but not to the point of abuse. He died of a heart attack during her seventh birthday party. She now lives with her mother. Although she is going to college, she feels she is not doing well and has no goals or prospects. She says she has let her mother down. She is begun on an antidepressant.

Principles of Management

- Medication alone is never as good as medication combined with some form of psychotherapy.

- Like all treatment modalities, psychotherapy comes in different forms and can be given at different doses for different periods of time. The goals of different psychotherapies also vary. One size does not fit all.

- All treatments can be planned with the three-legged stool in mind: acute, continuation, maintenance phases. Psychotherapy is no exception.

- All your encounters with a patient will either be therapeutic or not. Chance meetings in public places count. There are no data that show that a therapeutic encounter has to be of a specific length of time (e.g., 50 minutes) or in a specific setting (e.g., your office).

- Therapeutic encounters do not require you speaking in psychobabble: "I wonder why you did that?.....I understand your issues .....Can you see you are an enabler .....You're hearing but you are not listening to me .....Unless we work on the issues of your past, we will not be able to achieve your full potential."

- A therapeutic encounter has the following characteristics:
  1. You let the patient talk about what he thinks is important, not just listen to what you think is important.
  2. You are empathic and demonstrate it verbally and nonverbally.
  3. You are courteous and respectful.
  4. You are realistically optimistic.
  5. You help educate the patient to his illness and treatments and you help clarify his present life concerns.

What should be the psychotherapy goals for the acute, continuation and maintenance phases of Patient 1-16's treatment?

Acute phase:

1. Reassure the patient that the depression will resolve and she will likely return to her normal self.
2. Help her understand about her illness: that it is not her fault, that her feelings of self-blame and worthlessness are part of the illness and are the results of the chemical imbalance in her brain, and not her reality.
3. Help her understand about her pharmacotherapy, and that mild side effects are to be expected and indicate that the medicine has started working.
4. Reinforce any early symptomatic improvement, no matter how modest.
5. As the depression improves, clarify what feelings, attitudes, and reactions are normal and what are still the results of the depression.
6. As the depression improves, help her decide what she is going to tell friends and family about her illness and treatments.
7. Help her clarify what she feels about having such an illness and what is the reality of such an illness.
8. Start discussing goals for the continuation phase of treatment.

Continuation phase:

1. Continue discussions about medication and side effects.
2. As she increasingly resumes more and more of a normal life and is exposed to normal life stresses, help her deal with these stresses. Reinforce that normal ("mild to moderate") upset to stress is not depression relapse.
3. Begin to discuss longer-term goals: school, job, independent living, need for lifetime medication and PRN psychotherapy after the continuation phase is over (about 12 months from time of remission).
4. Education about early detection of future episodes, need for compliance, potential stressors, likelihood of otherwise normal life.
5. After 6-8 months of successful continuation begin discussing termination. Reinforce progress that has been made.

Maintenance phase:

1. Psychotherapy PRN
2. Dealing with childhood problems with stepbrother and father only if raised by the patient, or if her feelings about that period in her life is affecting some present life situation.

Try to organize the above goals into a flow chart so you have a template you can use.

Table 1.11 Psychotherapy Flow Chart Goals		
Acute Phase	*Continuation Phase*	*Maintenance Phase**
Comprehensive assessment	Resolve any short-term goals	Psychotherapy PRN
Short term acute phase goals based on assessment	Deal with problems and opportunities likely to arise during the next 12 months	
	After 6-8 months begin discussing termination and prophylaxis phase	

*Because she has had two previous depressions, her risk for relapse is high unless she is on prophylactic antidepressant medication indefinitely

Discussion

The most important aspect of the above psychotherapy plan is not to engage the depressed patient in a stressful exploration of her traumatic childhood. Such an exercise will cause the depression to become worse or last longer. An ongoing multicenter study of depression and acute heart disease has demonstrated that psychotherapy during the acute phase of illness will be detrimental for some patients, both for their depression and cardiac morbidity.[23] During the continuation phase, when a depressed patient remains highly vulnerable to relapse, intensive, analytic psychotherapy can actually increase the relapse rate. In contrast, there is some evidence that some forms of reality-oriented psychotherapy during the continuation period improves compliance and reduces relapse rates.[24] Goals for acute and maintenance phases always focus on the here and now. They deal with present problems and weaknesses and use present strengths and resources. This is a *rehabilitation model of psychotherapy.*[25]

The most important part of this model (just like any other) of psychotherapy is the doctor-patient relationship. The rehabilitation model of psychotherapy begins with assessment of current problems without focusing on early childhood conflicts. All the areas are assessed so that you can establish treatment goals and start comprehensive management. As part of the rehabilitation model of psychotherapy, the assessment itself becomes an early goal: "We need to find out the following because . . . ." Thus, even obtaining laboratory tests becomes an early goal, and ideally the patient should want the tests done as much as you do. The assessment can educate and clarify problems for the patient as much as it can reveal the diagnosis. Once assessment is complete, you and the patient can establish long-term goals and work on them.

Like all treatment, psychotherapy is finite. Inpatients get better and are discharged. Outpatients no longer need continuing treatment. Patients and physicians move to different towns. The last phase of any psychotherapy is saying "good-bye." Next to a good doctor-patient relationship, a good "good-bye" is the most important phase because it establishes closure on the condition and problems being treated, ends the therapeutic relationship positively so that what has been achieved is not tarnished by bad feelings, and sets a good foundation for any future treatment. Saying "good-bye" to the patient takes time and should not come as a surprise to the patient. The biggest goal of treatment is to end it. The focus of this treatment is not to change the past or the patient's personality, but to help him live with and adjust to his deficit.

Patient 1-15: Getting on Two Horses at Once Can Be Bad for Your Patient's Health

A 42-year-old man has a history of recurrent depressions and anxiety disorder both secondary to a seizure disorder. He is being treated with carbamazepine 1200 mg (blood level of 10 ug/ul) and clonazepam 2 mg daily. On his next office visit the patient reports an exacerbation in depressive symptoms and anxiety following a recent seizure. His physician responds by increasing carbamazepine to 1400 mg daily and also starts nefazodone 100 mg BID (an antidepressant with both serotonergic and noradrenergic properties). Within a week the patient is lethargic, disoriented, has spotty amnesia, and is ataxic. The carbamazepine level at that time is 14 ug/ul.

What therapeutic principles did Patient 1-15's physician violate?

1. Assess before you treat.
2. Do no harm.
3. Do not do two things at once, unless the situation is critical and it cannot be avoided. It is like riding two horses at once; if they go a couple of steps away from each other, you are in deep trouble, giving new meaning to the word "crotchety."

What now has to be done?

1. Hospitalize to protect the patient.
2. Hold the nefazodone; need for an antidepressant has not been established.
3. Repeat carbamazepine levels in 4 days. Nefazodone has been reported to increase carbamazepine levels. Once you have discontinued the nefazodone, carbamazepine levels will drop.
4. If carbamazepine levels are still elevated, consider reducing the carbamazepine back to 1200 mg.
5. Assess what happened prior to the most recent seizure to determine precipitating factors for seizure.

Discussion

The patient described the exacerbation of depression and anxiety following his most recent seizure, suggesting a causal relationship.

Better seizure control might be all that Patient 1-15 needs, not the addition of another medication. Seizures can be triggered by stress, fatigue, general medical ill health (e.g., the flu), among other things.[26] Assessing for these factors and trying to resolve them might work better than increasing carbamazepine.

Assessing first could have led to management that would have done no harm. If the evaluation suggested more carbamazepine was needed, then that should have been the next step rather than doing that plus adding nefazodone. Nefazodone interferes with carbamazepine liver metabolism, thus leading to increased blood levels and toxicity.

For every drug you give a patient, you need to know several important things. *Table 1.12* displays these.

Table 1.12 *Things to Know About Each Drug You Order*
Spectrum of indications
Absorption, metabolic site, protein binding, excretion site
Half-life (time required for a drug concentration to decline by 50% after a single dose administration)
3-4 most common side effects and how to minimize their occurrence and manage them if they occur
All dangerous adverse reactions
Important drug-drug interactions

Patient 1-16: What's Worth Doing is Worth Doing Until It's Done

A 43-year-old woman becomes depressed and is started on nortriptyline 100 mg daily. Three days later her blood level is 45 ng/l (accepted range is 50-150). Nortriptyline is increased to 150. After three days with no response, it is increased again to 200 mg. The patient becomes confused, her vision is blurred, and severe muscle twitching develops.

What happened?

Nortriptyline was started at too high a dose (usual starting dose is about 50 mg), and it was increased too rapidly. The patient became toxic and developed a delirium with myoclonus.

Why did this happen?

Dosing is based on the *pharmacokinetics* of the drug (what the body does to it) and the pharmacokinetic "health" of the patient. A critical variable is *steady state,* that point in treatment when the amount of drug being taken equals the amount being excreted. Usually a steady state is achieved in a time equal to 4-5 times half-life. Each drug dose has its own steady state, and blood levels are drawn during steady state, not before it occurs. In the case of Patient 1-16 the blood level was taken after 3 days, but the steady state for any given dose of nortriptyline is about 4 to 5 times its *half-life* (the time it takes to eliminate 50% of a given dose), and its half-life is 24 hours plus. Steady state for the initial 100 mg could be 5-6 days or more later, not 3 days. Thus, the blood level of 45 was a low reading. Had the clinician waited the 6 days or so, the blood level would have been higher, perhaps discouraging the dose increase. Of course, steady state should not be confused with onset of action for that drug. For example, for lorazepam it takes about 30-100 hours (half-life 6-20 hours) to reach steady state level, but onset of anxiolytic effect is less than an hour. For nortriptyline, the onset of antidepressant action may take several weeks. Onset of action is dependent on minimum effective concentration. If the selected dose does not produce high enough concentrations and rises above minimum effective concentration, then despite being in steady state, the drug may not be effective.

Discussion

Drugs need time to work. If you pick a drug that you think is the best choice for a patient you need to know what is a reasonable therapeutic trial for that drug. The length of a therapeutic trial will vary with different illnesses. For example, most depressions respond to adequate doses of an antidepressant in 6-8 weeks. Obsessive compulsive disorder using the same antidepressant may take, on average, 12 weeks or more to substantially respond. Patient 16's doses were increased too rapidly, outdistancing its pharmacokinetics.

You also need to keep in mind the other side of this therapeutic coin. Keeping a patient on a dose that is not working for longer than necessary is also poor therapeutics. Some guidelines for using half-life and steady state are listed in *Table 1.13*.

Table 1.13 Guidelines for Using Steady State and Half-Life [27]
Drugs with a half-life of 18 or more hours can be given once daily.
A therapeutic trial with a psychotropic begins when the drug is at a therapeutic dose that is in steady state.
For most conditions an adequate initial phase of treatment is two times the steady state figure. Thus, if a drug dose reaches steady state in 4 days, the initial phase is the *next* 8 days.
At the end of the initial phase of treatment, reassess and adjust (increase dose, enhance, etc.).

Quick Rounds

1. A 28-year-old man is admitted for mania with psychosis and is begun on valproic acid and haloperidol oral tablets. His initial response is erratic, and valproic acid blood levels widely fluctuate, despite the nurses insisting he is taking his pills. What is wrong with this picture?

2. A 32-year-old woman is admitted for mania and is given lithium 1200 mg daily. A week later her lithium blood level is 0.3 meq/L, and she is only marginally better. What do you do now?

3. A 38-year-old woman is treated for an anxiety disorder with desipramine. At 50 mg daily, she says she is worried about the medication because it makes her sleepy and makes her mouth dry. What do you do?

4. A 22-year-old man is admitted with an acute psychosis and agitation requiring four-point restraints. What do you do if you agree restraints are needed?

5. A 50-year-old man with a long history of mood disorder comes to you for refilling his prescriptions. He has been taking nortriptyline 150 mg po qhs and chlorpromazine 300 mg po qhs for the last 15 years. The patient has been stable for the last 10 years. His chlorpromazine was increased from 250 to 300 at that time. There is no history of psychosis. What should you do?

6. A 35-year-old woman with mania is started on lithium carbonate 600 BID and haloperidol 10 mg po BID. A few days later the patient is no longer psychotic but reports severe anxiety and restlessness. Nurses note that the patient is becoming agitated. You increase the haloperidol dose a few days later, but the patient becomes even more restless and agitated. What do you do?

7. A 31-year-old woman comes to you for treatment of her major depression. As you are writing her a prescription of fluoxetine, she casually informs you that she has been taking St. John's Wort and kava kava. Should you be concerned?

8. A 78-year-old man with a long history of chronic depression is finally stable on sertraline 200 mg po qd. However, the patient's only side effect is difficulty in maintaining an erection. There is no other cause for this erectile dysfunction. The patient also has a history of two myocardial infarctions and wishes to stop or switch the antidepressant. What do you do?

9. A 36-year-old woman with a history of bipolar mood disorder and an Axis II personality disorder (dramatic-emotional) comes to the clinic requesting admission because she recently broke up with her boyfriend and feels she is again getting depressed. The patient has a history of multiple psychiatric admissions for both mania and depression. During each admission, once her symptoms are stabilized, the patient often has difficulty getting along with the staff and usually wants to stay in the hospital much longer than her physician's recommendation. What should you do?

10. A 72-year-old man with history of recurrent depression comes to you because his medication will not be reimbursed by his insurance unless it is prescribed by one of their approved doctors (you). The patient was being followed by his private generalist physician for 20 years and is very happy with him. He requests that you write the medications that are prescribed by his private physician whom he will continue to see as his doctor. What do you do?

11. A 35-year-old man with a history of nonmelancholic major depression is stable on fluoxetine 20 mg po qhs. He wants to stop smoking, so his primary care physician asks you if he can start on Zyban (generic name, Wellbutrin, a drug used for smoking cessation, also used as an antidepressant). What do you do?

12. A 76-year-old man was diagnosed as having Alzheimer's disease 6 years ago. Over the last 3 years the patient has been continuously deteriorating. The patient was prescribed donepezil 10 mg 6 years ago as a cholinergic enhancing drug, and he still takes this. During one office visit his wife requests that you discontinue donepezil because it does not seem to help at all and is very expensive. Should you oblige?

Quick Rounds Answers

1. For acute inpatients, using the tablet form of medication typically results in inadequate or inconsistent absorption with erratic results. "Cheeking" and regurgitating of medication is also easy with the tablet form of medication. Whenever possible, specifically order concentrates, but pay attention to any incompatible interactions between concentrate forms. You can always ask the hospital pharmacist for the latest information.

2. If lithium is given on a full stomach, absorption will likely be good. Because it is not metabolized in the liver and it is not protein bound, the low blood level is either due to excretion (she is flushing it out because of a kidney problem, such as diabetes insipidus, unlikely so early in treatment) or because she is not complying and cheeking pills or regurgitating concentrate. For the next several days, have her sit in the nurses' station or assign a nurse to her for 20 minutes after her dosing and then repeat the level. Also observe for too much fluid intake.

3. All medicines have side effects. Common side effects are expected and tell you that the patient is taking the medicine and the medicine is doing what it should be doing. Good education prior to prescribing can better prepare patients to tolerate side effects. Reassurance about side effects (many are transient), going more slowly with increases, telling the patient that the side effects are signs the medication is doing what it was designed to do, and ultimately managing the side effects are the best responses. Nighttime dosing typically resolves problems with sedation. The use of sugar-free breath mints or hard candy commonly resolves mouth dryness.

4. Patients in restraints are involuntarily hospitalized. The reasons for the restraints must be documented. Because most agitated, restrained patients fight their restraints, sedation is usually needed until definitive treatment can be given. (If you know the definitive treatment, give it.) Patients in restraints need frequent observation (at least every 15 minutes) and periodic review of the need for restraints (every 4-6 hours). Restraints are used to help a patient from harming himself or others, never as punishment or for staff convenience.

5. The pharmacology literature tells us that this patient most likely does not need to be on chlorpromazine, and that it can be discontinued. However, stopping any medication suddenly is not a good idea

especially since the patient has been asymptomatic. One option would be to discuss your concerns with the patient and design a plan to gradually taper chlorpromazine. As chlorpromazine is an anticholinergic the patient may experience anxiety upon withdrawal, so go slow. A second option would be to also discuss your concerns (and chart them), but to do nothing now, following the scientific principle that "If it ain't broke, don't fix it."

6. The patient's anxiety and restlessness are not due to her illness, but are a side effect of her haloperidol (akathisia). The best way to treat her symptom is not increasing the haloperidol but treating the akathisia. The first step would be to decrease the haloperidol dose. If this does not help, then use a benzodiazepine such as clonazepam 5 mg po bid, as long as the patient is receiving haloperidol. If you need to increase the dose of a benzodiazepine frequently, then an alternative medication with a psychotropic less with EPS such as risperidone may be used. Olanzapine may have some mood-stabilizing properties, so it too might be a better choice than haloperidol for this patient.

7. Yes! Yes! Yes! Managing a patient is not just prescribing medication. Over the counter natural herbal supplements are not necessarily inactive. Both St. John's Wort and kava kava have psychoactive ingredients. St. John's Wort has serotonergic activity and is known to interact with fluoxetine. It may cause a serotonin syndrome which resembles NMS and can be deadly. The active ingredient kavapyrone in kava kava is anxiolytic in nature and is known to interact with benzodiazepines. So, before you prescribe any antidepressants you should ask the patient to taper off her herbal supplements.[28]

8. For those of you who thought "What's the big deal, he's 78 and not having sex anymore" – for shame. You are also under 40 and will have (hopefully) different thoughts when you have all gray or no hair. So, what to do. When a patient is doing well on a medication, rather than stopping the medication you always try first to treat the side effect. The most common medications used to treat erectile dysfunction secondary to an SSRI are 1) sildenafil, 2) bupropion (37.5-75 mg, or 3) neostigmine (15 mg). Before you decide on any medication, you need to consider the side effects and the risk of each. In view of the patient's cardiac status, one would be hesitant to use these choices as all three agents can cause cardiac arrhythmias. Skipping one or two doses a day before intercourse may help minimize sexual dysfunction due to SSRIs. If the patient is not having intercourse frequently, this strategy should be tried first.

9. One of the principles of management is that the patient should be treated in the least restrictive environment that best treats the illness. Based on her history, hospitalization is not the best venue to treat her. If she is not actively suicidal, she should not be hospitalized. For this patient, we also need to determine if she has any present evidence of mania or depression that would require hospitalization. If no, then she does not need to be in the hospital. However, because of the current crisis, she may need some additional support that can be provided by arranging brief outpatient visits or phone contacts.

10. The patient can see more than one person if he chooses. However, for treatment to be cohesive and effective, only one person can manage the medication and be in charge. Whoever is writing the prescription should make the decision of what should be prescribed. All other treaters can make recommendations, but cannot dictate the medication management. No physician should agree to see patients under these conditions (the only exception is a trainee/supervisor team). You should respectfully explain the situation to the patient and agree to see the patient if you alone are his physician prescribing medication.

11. Zyban is a trade name for bupropion which is a dopaminergic antidepressant. Bupropion can be safely used with fluoxetine. In fact, bupropion is often used to treat sexual side effects caused by SSRIs. Once the patient is on bupropion, you might consider discontinuing the fluoxetine.

12. Yes! The patient is no longer in the early stages of Alzheimer's. A cholinergic enhancing drug, such as donepezil, only slows the cognitive decline early on. At this time it is probably no longer effective.

Chapter 2

Behavior and the Brain

Brain Organization

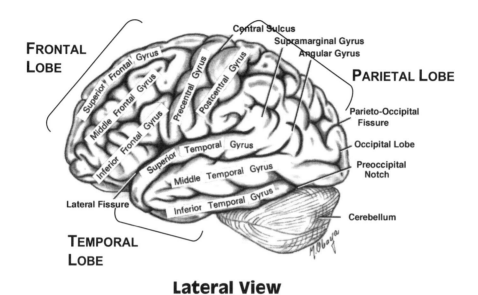

FRONTAL LOBE

Central Sulcus
Supramarginal Gyrus
Angular Gyrus

PARIETAL LOBE

Superior Frontal Gyrus
Middle Frontal Gyrus
Inferior Frontal Gyrus
Precentral Gyrus
Postcentral Gyrus

Parieto-Occipital Fissure
Occipital Lobe
Preoccipital Notch

Superior Temporal Gyrus
Middle Temporal Gyrus
Inferior Temporal Gyrus

Lateral Fissure

Cerebellum

TEMPORAL LOBE

Lateral View

Midsagittal View

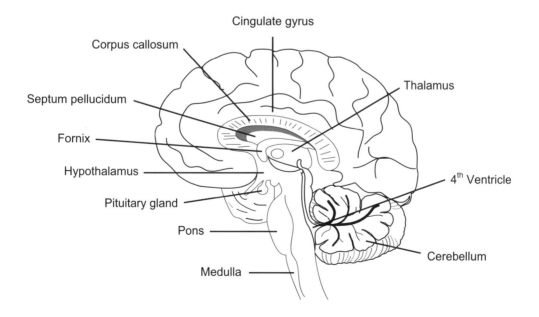

Cingulate gyrus

Corpus callosum

Thalamus

Septum pellucidum

Fornix

Hypothalamus

4th Ventricle

Pituitary gland

Pons

Cerebellum

Medulla

Patient 2-1: Cherry Pie Was Good for Her Health

A psychiatrist is finishing his lunch in the hospital cafeteria when he gets a page to come to the inpatient unit. His patient, a 63-year-old woman, is angrily shouting at the nurses, accusing them of hiding her bedroom. She had gone to the unit dining room, but could not find her way back to her bedroom. The physician says he will be right there to examine her and prescribe an antipsychotic, but he delays to finish a slice of fresh cherry pie. While eating, he tells this story.

The woman, in previously good general medical health, stopped answering her phone a few days ago. Her daughter who spoke with her daily became concerned and went to her mother's home. Her mother refused to let her in, yelling through the door that aliens were trying to control her mind by beaming rays into her house, forcing out her thoughts, and replacing them with alien thoughts. She did not want to open the door but finally relented. Upon doing so, she pointed to her daughter and said, "You're one of them. You're not my daughter. You're an imposter." She went on to say that the aliens had taken over her neighborhood, removed it to a different place with all of her neighbors, and replaced the houses and people with alien houses and alien neighbors.

Recognizing the mother was psychotic, the family finally was able to bring the mother to the hospital, where she was admitted to psychiatry with the diagnosis of late-onset schizophrenia.[2] She had no previous psychiatric illness and her general neurologic exam was unremarkable.

Principles of Brain Organization[1]

- Ninety-eight percent of humans have language organized primarily in their left cerebral hemisphere (termed the "dominant hemisphere").

- The dominant hemisphere best processes high-frequency information (dense, and detailed), and language-related information is typically in high-frequency form.

- Lesions in the dominant hemisphere can produce aphasias and other speech and language problems, such as neologisms (making up new words) in schizophrenia, reading and writing difficulties, and psychopathology, such as auditory hallucinations, avolition, excessive or reduced speech, verbal reasoning problems.

- The nondominant hemisphere (usually the right) best processes big patterns, shapes and contours, and visuospatial information.

- Lesions in the nondominant hemisphere can produce problems with facial recognition, awareness of surrounding space (particularly the left side of space termed spatial neglect), poor recognition of one's illness or symptoms (termed anosognosia), poor recognition of visuospatial information.

Listening to the story, a colleague says,

1. Do not give the antipsychotic; mildly sedate or have the staff redirect her attention.
2. She will likely fully recover in a week or so with no other treatment.
3. After asking one question, he tells the cherry pie lover to order one laboratory test that will show a specific lesion in a specific part of the brain.

What happened to Patient 2-1?

Successful diagnosis often depends on being able to reduce clinical details to a big-picture statement. Look for the forest, not at the trees. Thus, what is the most likely explanation for a woman in her 60s, in apparent good general medical health and previously good psychiatric health, to suddenly have a dramatic behavioral change? Since this behavioral change must reflect some change in brain function (even if you think stress induced the change, stress works on the brain), what is the likely cause of a sudden brain change in her age group? The answer is stroke.

> Stroke is the third leading cause of death in industrial countries, causes 10-12% of all deaths mostly in persons over age 65. In the US women are at slightly greater risk of stroke than men.

Which side of the brain is likely affected?

Patient 2-1 had no obvious speech and language or related problems and was not hearing voices. If her stroke were cortical (we will worry about subcortical strokes later on), it is unlikely that it would be in the dominant hemisphere. On the other hand, she was not able to find her way around the inpatient unit and did not quite recognize her daughter, saying she was an imposter (the memory of the face didn't match the perception of the face). She also did not seem to recognize her neighborhood or her neighbors. All this suggests the stroke could be in the nondominant hemisphere. Nonrecognition often occurs as a result of parietal lobe dysfunction. Parietal lobe disturbances cause various syndromes indistinguishable from the psychiatric syndromes described in the Patient 2-1. *Prosopagnosia* is an inability to recognize faces and can occur as a result of bilateral, as well as unilateral, lesions. Brain areas other than parietal lobe, such as the superior temporal sulcus, temporal cortex, and prefrontal cortex are also involved in causing prosopagnosia.[3]

What additional information did the colleague ask for?

There is lots of important information still needed to properly treat Patient 2-1, but to enhance the localization of a stroke or any suspected localization lesion, it helps to know the patient's hand preference. Patient 2-1 was a pure right-hander, indicating her dominant hemisphere was her left.

Handedness roughly correlates with cerebral organization, and almost all pure right-handers, particularly men, are left cerebral dominant for language. Women are less lateralized than men. Left-handers (about 10% of the population) are less lateralized than right-handed women. Less lateralized means some language and some visuospatial abilities may be in both hemispheres. Eye and foot preference do not predict the cerebral hemisphere organized for language.

Surprisingly, some persons cannot tell you clearly which hand they use for different tasks. Thus, you must have them show you. When a person shows you a learned motor task, they are demonstrating what? If you do not know, recheck Patient 2-1. *Table 2.1* displays the questions you should ask for assessing handedness. Ask the patient to show you, not tell you. Most persons will use their preferred hand to write, pour, brush, cut, and hold the thread.[4]

Table 2.1 Tests for Handedness
Writing a sentence
Pouring liquid into a glass
Brushing one's teeth
Cutting bread with a knife
Threading a needle

What lab test did the colleague suggest be done?

Brain imaging is helpful in identifying stroke, and CT scanning is done first to identify any hemorrhagic lesion. After 7-10 days an MRI will pick up even small strokes and will show the extent of the stroke.[5] A CT scan was done, and it showed a wedge-shaped ischemic stroke in Patient 2-1's right parietal lobe near the temporoparietal junction.

Why did the colleague say not to give an antipsychotic to a clearly psychotic patient?

Sedatives and antipsychotics can mask emerging stroke symptoms and can make the cognition worse, delaying recovery.[6] Further, if spontaneous recovery is likely (and with no speech or motor problems, recovery from stroke is usually good), prescribing an antipsychotic would have given the false impression that it worked. Thus encourage her doctor to keep her on it indefinitely, which may lead to tardive dyskinesia or some other side effect.

What psychopathology does she show?

In addition to the visuospatial "flavor" of her symptoms and no speech and language problems, Patient 2-1 had specific features suggesting nondominant temporoparietal dysfunction. These included *experiences of control and of alienation* (in her case literally) that some outside force was trying to control her and take over her brain. In the 1950s, McDonald Critchley, a famous British neurologist, first described patients with parietal lobe strokes with such symptoms.[7] Patient 2-1 also had *anosognosia*, or unawareness of her illness. She had *delusional ideas*. She believed her neighborhood and neighbors had been moved or replicated, a symptom termed *reduplicative paramnesia* (the delusion of doubles). She thought her daughter was an imposter. A delusion that familiar persons are imposters (possibly due, in part, to an impaired aspect of facial recognition of familiar persons) is termed *Capgras syndrome*. A related delusion that unfamiliar persons are familiar, often famous persons, is termed *Fregoli syndrome*. On the inpatient unit, she could not find her way back to her room. She got lost, suggesting *topographic disorientation*, which is inability to remember places and direction. All of these psychopathological features suggest nondominant hemisphere dysfunction.

> Dominant parietal lobe lesions are characterized by problems with naming, reading and writing, and calculating. Gerstmann's syndrome due to lesions in the dominant angular gyrus is characterized by dysgraphia (problems writing), dyscalculia (problems calculating), trouble recognizing or naming one's fingers (finger agnosia or anomia), and right-left disorientation (trouble putting hands on contralateral body parts).

Discussion

Diagnostic principles are discussed in the Chapter 1. Looking for the big picture is just one of these principles. Patient 2-1's big picture suggests a recent sudden process that dramatically changed her behavior. Because of her age and the pattern of behavior seemingly lateralized to one hemisphere, stroke is a good bet. The colleague also predicted it would be in the temporoparietal junction and parietal lobe above it rather than in the frontal or anterior temporal lobe because her psychopathology and her other behaviors appeared intact.

Localizing brain lesions incorporates both the important positive and important negative findings. Patient 2-1 had no obvious dominant hemisphere signs. She has lots of nondominant hemisphere signs. Her traditional neurologic exam is unremarkable, which means her cranial nerves were intact, and her motor exam was normal. It was another good bet that her stroke was on the right side in the temporoparietal regions.

Patient 2-2: The Fender Benderer

A 74-year-old right-handed widower is brought to see you by his daughter who is concerned because her father recently has had several minor auto accidents. He says, "Traffic is bad nowadays." She says he is not properly judging distances and space between cars. She thinks it is too dangerous for him to drive, and they have been arguing about his giving up his car and living with her. She also says he has become forgetful. Although he remains active as a volunteer at the afternoon recreation center, he has been making mistakes: forgetting to turn off an oven, incorrectly giving out color-coded locker keys, bringing out the wrong equipment for after school programs.

On examination he is friendly but denies any problems, even when you point out his difficulty in naming the objects you show him and his difficulty in remembering the details of a single paragraph story you read to him. He also has trouble copying geometric shapes and remembering the shapes he was asked to copy.

Principles of Brain Organization

- One view of brain organization is to consider left versus right as you did for Patient 2-2. This left-right cerebral lateralization of function is superimposed upon two brain systems: an action brain and a perceptual-integrating brain. Figure 2.1 displays components of the action brain and perceptual brain. *Tables 2.2* and *2.3* display the functions of the action and perceptual-integrating brain systems. The perceptual-integrating brain takes in stimuli from the external world, organizes it, makes sense of it and stores this information as memory. The action brain uses this information.

- The neuroanatomical areas of the action and perceptual-integrating brains are listed in *Table 2.4*. The thalamus connects the action brain's frontal circuit (prefrontal cortex, basal ganglia, thalamus) with the posterior, cerebellar-pons, component. The thalamus is also one of the connections between the action brain and the perceptual-integrating brain.

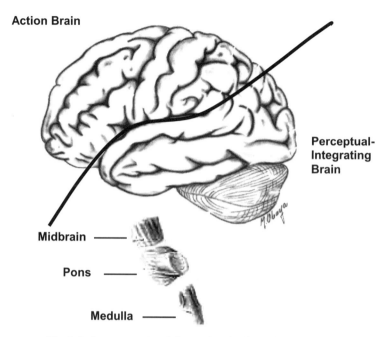

Action Brain

Perceptual-
Integrating
Brain

Midbrain ———

Pons ———

Medulla ———

Fig. 2.1 Components of the action brain and perceptual brain

Table 2.2 Functions of the Action Brain
Generates ideas
Executive functions: planning, initiating action (motor behaviors and speech), monitoring actions and self-correcting, verifying the planned action is being done correctly, and *terminating* the action when completed, problem-solving
Emotional expression
Recall of declarative and procedural memory
Motor behavior

Table 2.3 Functions of the Perceptual-Integrating Brain
Organizes perceptions and makes sense of the external world
Stores external world information as memory
Recognizes boundary between oneself and external world

Table 2.4 Action Brain and Perceptual-Integrating Brain Anatomy	
Action Brain	*Perceptual-Integrating Brain*
Prefrontal cortex Basal ganglia Thalamus Anterior hippocampus, amygdala, and hypothalamus Cerebellum and pons	Temporal, parietal, occipital lobe 1^0, 2^0, 3^0 cortices Thalamus Posterior hippocampus

Does Patient 2-2 primarily have problems in the action or perceptual-integrating brain?

Look at the functions listed in *Tables 2.2 and 2.3,* and match them with Patient 2-2's behavior.

Patient 2-2's pattern

1. Not properly judging distances between cars (chief complaint) (parietal) (perceptual-integrating brain [PI] brain)
2. Forgetfulness (chief complaint) (post-hippocampus) (PI brain)
3. Not recognizing or understanding which equipment goes with which activity (chief complaint) (parietal lobe) (PI brain)
4. Having difficulty putting names to objects (temporal lobe) (PI brain)
5. Having trouble remembering new information and details (tested) (temporal lobe) (PI brain)
6. Poor copying of shapes (tested) (parietal lobe) (PI brain)
7. Poor remembering of shapes (tested) (parietal lobe) (PI brain)
8. Not recognizing his symptoms (examination finding) (parietal lobe) (PI brain)
9. Eager to do things (history) (intact action brain)

Putting names to objects is tested by asking the patient to name things you show him, e.g., a key, a watch, a pen, a wall socket, the corner of a table. The patient is also asked to find things, e.g., show me a button, cuff, shoe, door knob.

Remembering new information can be tested by reading a paragraph story and asking the patient to tell you the details of what you read, or by giving the patient things to remember, rehearsing the list and then testing recall 5 or 10 minutes later. A list might be a yellow bicycle, a football, an elm tree, a leather jacket.

Copying and remembering shapes might include the following:

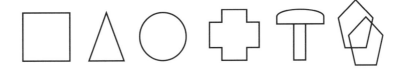

Thus, the above is primarily the pattern of perceptual-integrating brain dysfunction.

What is the term for his not recognizing his symptoms?

If you did not remember, anosognosia. Also review Patient 2-1.

Is his dysfunction in the left or right cerebral hemisphere, or is it bilateral?

Again, consider his problems listed above and divide them into language vs. visuospatial behaviors. Then look at the number key that follows.

The left-sided language naming and memory items listed above are numbers 2, 3, 4, and 5.

The right hemisphere neglect and visuospatial items are numbers 1, 2, 3, 6, 7, and 8.

So his dysfunction is bilateral.

Do you know of any disorder that early on affects elderly persons this way?

Alzheimer's disease typically starts with bilateral problems in the perceptual-integrating brain.[8]

Discussion

You have begun to learn two ways of thinking about how the brain is organized: 1) left-right, 2) action and perceptual-integrating systems. The brain is like the digestive tract in that it is comprised of units (e.g., stomach, liver, gut) each affected by different disorders and each component with its signature symptoms: liver and bowel diseases have different etiologies and pathophysiologies, and different symptom patterns. The action brain and the perceptual-integrating brain are affected by different conditions and also have different signature symptoms.

In *Table 2.4,* you will see that the perceptual-integrating brain includes 1^0, 2^0, 3^0 cortices.

1. *Primary cortex* is where sensory input is initially cortically accepted and organized into some usable form (sensory

representation). It is analogous to a computer file being transferred to a disc.

2. *Secondary cortex* is associational cortex, but only for the specific sensory modality involved. It elaborates the sensory representation and relates it to other perceptions in that modality. This cortex is thus also termed *unimodal*.

3. *Tertiary cortex* is associational cortex that links two or more unimodal cortices. It can handle more than one sensory modality and is thus also termed *heteromodal*.

> The amyloid plaques and neurofibrillary tangles deposited in the brains of patients with Alzheimer's disease typically are first seen in the olfactory bulb, tract, and entorhinal cortex. Patients with these lesions can still detect odors, but they misidentify them. So always test the 1st cranial nerve (olfactory) which often is not tested. [9]

Patient 2-3: The Words But Not the Music

A 68-year-old man is brought to the clinic by his daughter who says his family physician has been treating him for the past 6 months for depression (present medication sertraline 100 mg), but he is no better.

She says he has been depressed for at least two years and that he has stopped his hobbies, interests, and being with friends. She says he does not eat as he usually did, but is not losing weight. He denies sleep problems, says he is always tired and has no energy. She further says he has become forgetful, irritable, and unkempt.

On examination he moves and speaks slowly, but the remainder of the traditional neurologic examination is unremarkable. He is somewhat unkempt and has several food stains on his shirt, but he shows no signs of tearfulness, sadness, or apprehension. On one occasion, he makes a coarse joke at his daughter's expense. He perseverates his ideas.

> **Principles of Brain Organization**
>
> - The perceptual-integrating brain organizes and recognizes external world information and stores it. The action brain takes this information and uses it to solve problems and make plans. The action brain, thus, must be able to generate ideas, be flexible, recall the information (stored as memory), put "2 and 2" together.
> - When the action brain is dysfunctional, a person may seem slow in movement and thought. Abilities to deal with real life situations and the challenges of cognitive testing will be impaired, consistent with functions listed for Patient 2-2 in *Table 2.2*.
> - When the perceptual-integrating brain is dysfunctional, a person may have symptoms of perceptual distortion, psychosis, agnosias (not recognizing), and inability to learn new information.

When asked to name as many animals as he can think of as fast as he can, Patient 2-3 names 7 in one minute, repeating some several times (norm is 13 or more). He does poorly on a test of his ability to shift from one set of things to another (connecting circles in which numbers and letters alternate from 1 to 13, and A to L). He rehearses a list of 5 words, but can only remember 1 until shown a list that includes the words, and then he identifies 3 others. His copying of shapes is good, as is his language other than some mild word-finding problems. He does poorly on similarities (e.g., how are a bicycle and a plane alike?).

> Moving and speaking slowly form the psychiatric concept of psychomotor retardation. The neurologic terms are *bradykinesia* (moving slowly) and *bradyphrenia* (thinking slowly). They are classic signs of action brain dysfunction.

Does Patient 2-3 have an action or perceptual-integrating problem?

Movement difficulties mostly indicate an action brain problem. Patient 2-3 moves and speaks slowly. He also stopped doing things he liked and became avolitional, another signature feature of action brain disease. His perseverativeness and failure to keep up his personal hygiene are also action brain signs. Perseveration indicates poor self-monitoring, i.e., not recognizing it is time to stop. Some older persons perseverate the same stories because they too have had some decline in their ability to self-monitor.

> The best way to test for volition is to ask the patient about his typical day and what he does to keep busy. Avolitional persons do little, without any obvious explanation.

Why does Patient 2-3 have "the words," but not "the music" of depression?

Patient 2-3 has some features of depression. He has lost interest in his hobbies and in being with friends. He is not eating well. He is tired and irritable. He speaks slowly. But depression is a mood disorder, and it is typically characterized by substantial apprehension or sadness. Patient 2-3 has some irritability, but he shows no signs of a depressed mood. The depressed mood is "the music." It is missing in Patient 2-3, although he expresses some of the words associated with depression: loss of interest, not eating well, being tired and slowed down.

Discussion

Action brain function is extremely sensitive to mood and arousal.[10] Thus, action brain function is disrupted by conditions that decrease arousal (sedative-hypnotic drugs, brain stem and midbrain lesions) or increase arousal (stimulant drugs, strong emotion), or that produce sustained or intense emotional states (e.g., depression, mania, anxiety disorder). Compared to the action brain, the perceptual-integrating brain is much less sensitive to these factors. Patient 2-3 has normal arousal, and his emotional state during the exam is normal, despite the incorrect interpretation of his avolition as a depression.

Hypertension resulting in small white matter strokes in the frontal circuits, strokes elsewhere in the action brain, basal ganglia disease (e.g., Parkinson's), demyelinating disease, and many other processes can cause an action brain syndrome. Patient 2-3 had a small lacuna stroke in the head of the left caudate.

Always remember that primary (those without any medical or neurologic etiology) depressions must be associated with a morbidly sad or apprehensive mood ("the music"). Apathy alone is not depression.

Patient 2-4: Cosmo Kramer (of Seinfeld)

A 50-year-old man has a change in personality that leads his family to bring him to you. The man, a CPA, is described as a previously hard working, reliable person, who spent his leisure time with his family. He was even-tempered, active in community affairs, and, although not a leader, always a principle participant in work, community, and family activities. Over the past year, however, all this changed.

Principles of Brain Organization[11]

- Each frontal lobe has 5 parallel circuits. Each circuit begins in a particular part of the frontal cortex, has neuronal connections with specific nuclei in the basal ganglia, which in turn send fibers to specific nuclei in the thalamus that then completes the circuit by sending feedback connections to the originating part of the frontal cortex.

- The five circuits on each side develop independently and are arranged vertically, like old computer boards. They are named for the prefrontal cortex from which they originate. Damage in any part of a given circuit can produce that circuit's characteristic syndrome. *Table 2.5* displays these circuits and their syndromes.

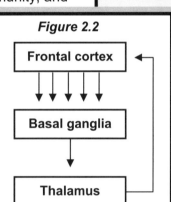

Figure 2.2

Frontal cortex → Basal ganglia → Thalamus

Table 2.5   Frontal-Basal Ganglia-Thalamic Parallel Circuits and Their Syndromes[12]

Circuit	Syndrome
Premotor and supplementary motor area cortex	Catatonia, akinetic mutism, other motor signs
Oculomotor cortex	Deficits in eye tracking
Dorsolateral prefrontal cortex	Avolitional syndrome (loss of drive and ambition, loss of interests and energy, perseverativeness of ideas, reduced ideas, speech and action), atypical depression, perseverations of movement and speech
Lateral orbitofrontal cortex	Dysinhibited syndrome (easily distracted, impulsive, hyperactive, lability of mood, loss of social graces, coarsening of personality)
Anterior cingulate cortex	Akinetic mutism, stupor, generalized analgesia, intense fear

The family says the man is now impulsively beginning new projects, many of them foolish, and most left unfinished. He has neglected his work and was forced to take a leave of absence or be fired. He is now boisterous, loud, intrusive, and outspoken. His friends no longer speak to him, and he was asked not to participate in a recent community picnic because of his socially inappropriate outspokenness.

On examination, he is overly friendly and frequently makes silly or coarse jokes. He asks you where you got such ugly clothes and chuckles at what he perceives to be his cleverness. His speech is mildly rapid, and he is easily distracted by minor points in the conversation resulting in many parenthetical comments. His speech is often circumstantial.

The remainder of the behavioral examination and traditional neurologic examination is negative except for a clear loss of smell in his left nostril, for which there is no peripheral explanation.

Which circuit is likely affected in Patient 2-4? (Hint: Use Table 2.5 for help.)

Patient 2-4 has a classic dysinhibited syndrome resulting from dysfunction in the lateral orbitofrontal circuit.[13]

What accounts for his unilateral loss of smell?

Olfactory pathways leave the nose, run along the orbital surface of the frontal lobe and then into the forebrain and temporal lobes. Trauma, space-occupying lesions, and occasionally other diseases of the frontal lobe can result in damage to these pathways and loss of smell (anosmia). Anytime you suspect frontal lobe dysfunction, test olfaction.

What might have caused such a specific syndrome?

When a patient has a specific frontal lobe syndrome, rather than a combination of them, the reason is usually a lesion affecting the specific cortical area or, less commonly, a very small lesion in the circuits, basal ganglia, or thalamic nuclei. A mixture of syndromes usually results from a large cortical process or a subcortical lesion (e.g., stroke) that knocks out several circuits simultaneously. This happens because from the widespread cortical areas, the circuits have to converge into the relatively cramped space of the basal ganglia and thalamus.

Because of the duration of onset over a 12-month period and the involvement of one olfactory pathway, a tumor impinging on the lateral orbital cortex is the most likely explanation for Patient 2-4's problems. He had a meningioma.

Discussion

Personality is pretty much fully developed by late adolescence or early adulthood. After that it does not change much. Dramatic changes in personality after the mid-thirties almost always results from brain dysfunction (e.g., substance abuse, chronic psychiatric disorder, strokes, tumors). These changes may include exaggeration of basic personality traits due to lack of cortical regulation or a complete change in personality due to a lesion. For example, a lesion in the dorsolateral surface of the frontal lobe can change the personality of a person from outgoing to apathetic.[14] The neurologic substrates of personality overlap with the action brain. Action brain disease often leads to personality change early on, whereas perceptual-integrating brain disease affects personality in later stages. Vascular dementia often affects personality early, whereas in Alzheimer's disease, personality changes typically occur several years after the diagnosis.[15]

Patient 2-5: New Wine in an Old Bottle

A 72-year-old pure right-handed retired construction worker has progressive speech problems over 18 months. He also becomes inactive, losing interest in his hobbies and in seeing friends at a local social club.

On examination his speech is mildly dysarthric, almost scanning, but spontaneous. In conversation he is circumstantial and he sometimes missounds words resulting in neologisms (new words). Thus, rather than saying "I never was in a hospital," he says, "phosphatal" (termed a phonemic [sound] paraphasia [approximate word]). He also omits words from his speech – usually verbs – so when looking at a picture of a boy toppling from a stool while reaching for a cookie jar on a high shelf, Patient 2-5 describes it as, "Boy on a stool, stool fall." His naming is adequate, auditory comprehension is good, but impaired for complex sentences (he can repeat the sentence, but misses some of the meaning). Reading aloud is adequate.

> **Principles of Brain Organization**
>
> - The motor system can be used to triangulate suspected lesions just as you can use the left-right action perceptual-integrating concepts of brain function to do this.
> - The motor system is contralaterally organized so, for example, when a person has a stroke and cannot move his left arm and leg, you can say with some assurance that the stroke is on the right side of his brain.
> - The motor system has a front and back. The front is the frontal circuits; the back is the cerebellum-pons unit of the action brain.
> - The motor system has a top and a bottom. The bottom is the basal ganglia. The top is the cortex: frontal and parietal. *Table 2.6* displays motor features categorized by this system.

His mood is slightly elevated and he tries to make a joke about each task the examiner asks him to do and about his own variable performance. His gait is slightly wide-based, tandem walking is poor and rapid alternating movement ability is marginal. His smooth eye pursuit is jerky with slight horizontal nystagmus.

Table 2.6 Motor Features Grouped to Facilitate Localization of Brain Lesions

Perspective	Clinical Features and Implications
Left and right	Features are contralateral from the lesion, so always test for asymmetry in motor function. Signs include paralysis and paresis, upper motor neuron reflexes, dyspraxias, tremor.
Front and Back	Frontal motor signs include bradykinesia (slow movement), flexed posture, floppy (cortical) or increased (basal ganglia) muscle tone, resting tremor, poor sequencing of movement (frontal dorsolateral circuit), adventitious motor overflow (chorea), motor impersistence or perseveration, dysarthria.[16] Back and motor signs include: intention tremor, past pointing, dysmetria, poor alternating movements, dysarthria, poor coordination, poor tandem gait.
Top and bottom	*Top:* frontal motor signs described above; parietal motor signs including ideomotor, kinesthetic and dressing apraxias (see discussion). *Bottom:* basal ganglia signs

Does Patient 2-5 have an action or perceptual-integrating brain problem?

Patient 2-5 has no perceptual-integrating brain problems. He has many problems with actions, including being inactive and losing interest in hobbies and friends. He has motor speech difficulties, inappropriate jocularity (self-monitoring problem), gait, eye, and other movement problems. Movement problems almost always mean the action brain is involved.

> The cerebellar vermis, a very old structure of the brain, is the only part of the motor system that relates ipsilaterally to motor behavior. The cerebellar neocortices relate contralaterally.

Does his motor symptoms localize his disease?

Patient 2-5 is exhibiting poor alternating movement, wide-based gait, and abnormal eye movements with nystagmus in absence of any other motor features. This pattern indicates that he has cerebellar disease.

Based on the conclusion that Patient 2-5 has a cerebellar-pontine problem, can that be related to his behavioral problems?

If you remember that the action brain includes an anterior and a posterior component, then it should be possible for a patient to have an action brain behavioral syndrome even though the lesion is only in the posterior (back) component of that system. See the discussion for an explanation of this.

Discussion

Patient 2-5 seems to have conflicting signs and symptoms. He has a mild frontal lobe behavioral syndrome combining some aspects of the avolitional syndrome and the disinhibited syndrome. This mixed picture tells you that the dysfunction is probably not in a discrete area of the prefrontal cortex. No mention was made of his praxic function (ability to do commonly learned motor tasks), but he had no problems with these, so again, not cortical. You test praxic function in several ways. Asking a patient to put on a bathrobe tests for *dressing apraxia* (often associated with nondominant parietal lobe lesions). Asking a patient to demonstrate the use of a key or hammer tests for *ideomotor apraxia* (often associated with dominant parietal lobe disease). Some tests of handedness also test praxic function. Asking the patient to mimic your movements is a test for *kinesthetic apraxia.* Asking the patient to mimic with one hand a posture you create in his other hand while his eyes are closed is a test of interhemispheric transfer of information. Copying geometric shapes (a square, a Greek cross, intersecting pentagons) are tests for *constructional apraxia*.

The conflict with Patient 2-5's signs and symptoms is that he has motor symptoms *and* some speech and language problems, but the motor symptoms indicate cerebellar dysfunction – back, not front. His MRI shows mild vermal atrophy and small cerebellar neocortical infarcts, which explains his motor problems. But what about his speech problems and frontal lobe features?

The solution to the apparent conflict in Patient 2-5's symptoms is in understanding that the action brain functions as a unit. The frontal circuits interact with the cerebellum-pons via the thalamus to produce the action.

Additionally, the cerebellum-pons is one of those brain areas that has taken on new function in humans. *Table 2.7* displays the functions of the cerebellum. The old cerebellum has learned new tricks and mixing metaphors: new wine in an old bottle.

Table 2.7 Cerebellar Functions [17]
Motor coordination and balance
Modulation of the limbic system
Coordination of thinking
New motor learning (procedural memory)
Motor planning
Speech and language

Patients with cerebellar disease (e.g., multiple sclerosis, alcohol related and familial degeneration, stroke), can, therefore, have symptoms beyond cerebellar motor features. These include mild frontal lobe syndromes, irritability and explosive behavior (particularly if the person also has some limbic problem), poor motor learning and motor memory, and word fluency and word finding problems, particularly for action verbs.[18]

Patient 2-6: The 3M Company

A 78-year-old pure right-handed man complains of depression of two years duration. His complaints center around loss of energy and not enjoying previously enjoyable activities, and his feeling that his life is over. He has little appetite, but his weight is unchanged. He sleeps well, often napping during the day. Antidepressant medication has not helped.

Examination shows him to be alert, pleasant, and without signs of present morbid sadness or apprehension. He has no other behavioral symptoms. Except for a right hand resting tremor, his traditional neurologic exam is unremarkable. He has slight word finding problems during conversation and is slightly circumstantial in his answers, but otherwise he has no signs of a speech or language disorder. He is able to properly demonstrate how to use familiar objects, can name objects by challenge (What is this?) and by asking him to find an object in the room (Can you show me a telephone?). His ability to recall a list of rehearsed words is poor, but he can recall them when shown a word list which includes them.

General medical evaluation reveals him to have an artificial mitral valve (10 years post-operation) and to have a steady-beat pacemaker (8 years post-operation). The remainder of the general medical exam is unremarkable.

Principles of Brain Organization [19]

- Human brain structures that are also present in other species may have acquired functions during our evolution additional to their original purposes. Thus, the thalamus, a sensory integrating structure in all vertebrates, also functions in humans in conversational speech. To fully understand human brain-behavior relationships, the phylogenetic view of the brain needs to be added to the left-right and action-perceptual-integrating perspectives of brain organization.

- The human brain can phylogenetically be divided into three systems: 1) the oldest central core structures from brain stem to primitive forebrain, similar to the brains of reptiles, i.e., the reptilian brain, 2) the elaborated limbic system seen in social mammals, i.e., the paleomammalian brain, and 3) the elaboration of the neocortex seen in primates and most enlarged in humans in the prefrontal, tertiary parietal and cerebellar neocortices, i.e., the neomammalian brain. See Figure 2.3.

- The left-right lateralization of cognition works best for the neomammalian brain. Although primary emotions (anger, fear, happiness, sadness) are bilaterally generated from the limbic system, social emotions (guilt, shame, disgust, nostalgia) with their social learning attributes seem influenced more by left than by right-sided structures.

- Although each part of the phylogenetic brain has a cortex, we can at this point oversimplify and say that the reptilian and paleomammalian systems are mostly subcortical, whereas the neomammalian system is neocortical.

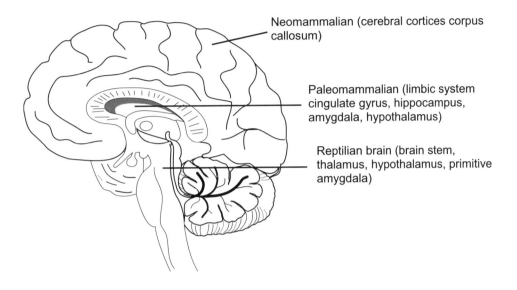

Fig. 2.3 Triune Brain

Neomammalian (cerebral cortices corpus callosum)

Paleomammalian (limbic system cingulate gyrus, hippocampus, amygdala, hypothalamus)

Reptilian brain (brain stem, thalamus, hypothalamus, primitive amygdala)

Does Patient 2-6 have an action or perceptual-integrating brain problem?

Patient 2-6 complains of loss of interest and energy, and not doing or enjoying past interests. These complaints are almost always signs of action brain disease. Patient 2-6 also has a right-hand resting tremor, and motor features express action brain problems. Patient 2-6 also needs cueing to recall, has some trouble generating words in conversation. He shows no perceptual-integrating problems.

Action brain and anterior hippocampal disease can result in the pattern of being able to learn new information, but not being able to adequately recall it. Cueing helps. Patients with vascular dementia often have this pattern. Depressed patients also benefit from cueing. Patients with perceptual-integrating brain disease (e.g., Alzheimer's disease) often have posterior hippocampal dysfunction and cannot store the new information, so cueing does not help.[20]

Does Patient 2-6 have a left- or right-sided lesion or both?

The only indications of a lateralized lesion are Patient 2-6's right hand tremor, word finding problem, and vague depressive features of avolition. Each of these is consistent with a left-sided lesion.

Does Patient 2-6 have an intrinsic cortical or subcortical lesion?

A resting tremor usually indicates a basal ganglia problem. As Patient 2-6 has no aphasia, dyspraxias, or agnosias; he speaks and understands well; he can do simple tasks; he recognizes objects (all cortical features); he likely has a subcortical, left basal ganglia lesion.

Discussion

Patient 2-6 was taking coumadin to prevent embolus formation from his artificial mitral valve. Patient 2-6 occasionally missed several days' doses, probably leading to an embolic stroke, which was seen in his left caudate nucleus on MRI. However, some patients develop emboli anyway, because anticoagulants only reduce the risks. Lesions in the left caudate commonly produce mood symptoms, and basal ganglia disease commonly results in varying degrees of cognitive problems: reduced working memory[21] and new learning, visuospatial difficulties. Think of the basal ganglia as the 3M company of the brain, typically producing *M*otor, *M*ood, and *M*emory problems.

Patient 2-7: The Pentium Chip

A 77-year-old pure right-handed former lawyer is referred for evaluation for a depression. He says he has no drive or energy, that he cannot do anything anymore, and that he is "stupid." He has no sleep or appetite disturbances but has sudden brief episodes of weepiness. These episodes (1-2 minutes) occur even in happy situations. Sometimes he is taken by surprise by the weepiness because subjectively he is not sad. He denies gloominess, dread, or apprehension. Fifteen years before, during a divorce, he was depressed and at that time would have "welcomed death." But he had no suicidal plans then and does not feel that way now. He was not treated then. He says his present problems began two years ago following a stroke during which left him with left-sided weakness, and difficulty walking, and word finding problems.

Principles of Brain Organization

- In addition to cortico-cortical connections, the action and perceptual-integrating brains are linked through the thalamus. The thalamus also links the two components of the action brain. Thalamic lesions can disrupt the coordination between these components, resulting in balance and positioning problems.
- The thalamus also collates perceptions from different sensory modalities so that you experience the world as an integrated whole. In addition to the traditional thalamic nuclei and the pulvinar, some neuroscientists include the medial and lateral geniculate bodies as part of a thalamic complex so that all somatosensory, visual and auditory perception is understood as collated by the thalamus. These integrated perceptions are stored as episodic memory in a specialized cortex in the anterior temporal lobe. Thalamic disease has also been associated with psychoses such as schizophrenia.
- The thalamus receives input from the reticular activating system (RAS). It transfers arousal input from the RAS to the frontal circuits and, thus, provides tone to that system. Thalamic lesions can produce avolitional, low energy syndromes.
- The thalamus is part of the action brain's frontal circuits. Thalamic lesions can produce frontal lobe syndromes.
- The thalamus is integrated with the parietal lobes. Some neuroscientists have described the heteromodal parietal lobe cortex as the tertiary cortex of the thalamus. Thalamic lesions can result in parietal lobe syndromes.
- The thalamus is involved in conversational speech. It is part of a self-monitoring system that checks on the accuracy of the phonemic strings (a series of sounds) we utter as speech. The self-monitoring system also checks on the appropriateness of the sounds to the thoughts. In conversational speech, the thalamus "asks" the temporo-parietal cortex if the sounds are okay and then lets the frontal circuits know the results of the "check," so it can self-correct. During this time the basal ganglia puts the speech "on hold" until told to release it. All of this, obviously, takes place in milliseconds. Thalamic lesions can produce speech and language problems, and the formal thought disorder of schizophrenia has been likened to aphasias seen with thalamic strokes.
- The thalamus acts as a relay station, so thalamic lesions can cause a variety of syndromes.[22]

Up until the stroke he played racquetball, socialized regularly, continued to work as a tax accountant, wrote a novel, wrote music, was "always on the go" and over the years was married three times to women 20-30 years his junior. Now he has a woman friend, but sex is minimal. He plays pinochle twice weekly (and wins), but does nothing else. He used to be a "voracious reader," but now he cannot concentrate on reading.

On examination he is neat and well groomed, somewhat overweight, cooperative and alert. He looks tired, sighs as if exhausted and is modestly slow in movement, speech and thought. He looks concerned and has three episodes of sudden and brief crying during the 40-minute exam, but he denies being depressed and can share a joke. He has word finding problems that he describes as "not being able to bring my thoughts down to my lips." His speech is spontaneous and fluent. He is not dysarthric. Except for the brief crying episodes he has no present psychopathology. He has trouble recalling the names of some familiar places, but cueing helps him. He says he has balance problems, and when sitting straight, arms extended forward, he can maintain his posture, but when he closes his eyes he has truncal ataxia and says he is "dizzy."

He thinks he is going to "fall backwards." His episodic and biographic memory are good. He has problems with working memory, trouble with serial 7's, and concentrating on a left-right orientation task. His handwriting is poorly formed though he says prior to the stroke it was extremely precise and neat. He has trouble with some calculations. Finger agnosia is not present. He cannot correctly point to the east when north is said to be behind or in front of him.

Does Patient 2-7 have a clinical depression that requires antidepressant treatment?

Patient 2-7 does not have a typical depression. He has no trouble sleeping or eating, he says he is not depressed, and his mood differs from typical depression (see *Chapter 3*). At best you might try to force this square peg into the round DSM hole of depression NOS (not otherwise specified). But the category should always suggest secondary syndromes, and Patient 2-7 had a stroke. An antidepressant might not work for a secondary depression that is so atypical and without a sustained sad mood. (See *Chapter 3* for alternative treatments for secondary depressions). However, the answer to the question below plays the trick.

What do you make of Patient 2-7's sudden bursts of weepiness during which he is sometimes not sad?

This phenomenon is termed *emotional incontinence* (the bursts of exaggerated or socially inappropriate emotion along with the subjective mood), and *pathological crying* (the outward emotional display disconnected from the subjective emotional experience). These phenomena, although not depression, can be treated with low to moderate doses of broad spectrum antidepressants: the trick. So, Patient 2-7 will benefit from an antidepressant, but at doses lower than those needed to treat a typical depressive syndrome.

Could all of Patient 2-7's present problems be explained by a thalamic lesion?

Yes, and *Table 2.8* shows why.

Table 2.8	
Thalamic Functioning	*Patient 2-7's Problems*
Feedback loop in frontal parallel circuits	Problems with concentration and working memory
Provides tone from the RAS to the frontal circuits	Loss of energy and drive, depressive-like features
Self-monitoring of speech	Word finding problems
Integration with parietal lobe	Problems with directions, right and left orientation, writing and calculations
Linking anterior and posterior action brain units	Balance and positioning problems

Discussion

The thalamus is centrally located in the brain. It has input and output from almost all other brain systems and collates the perceptual-integrating brain, holds the action brain together, and integrates these two systems. It is the pentium chip of our brain computer.

The thalamus consists of several nuclei, each with its own interconnections.[23]

Basal Ganglia and Thalamus

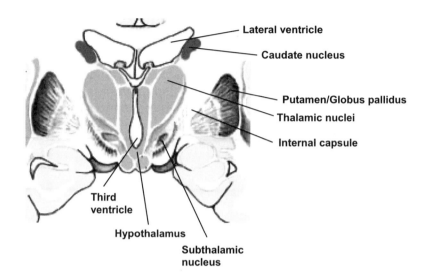

Patient 2-7's MRI confirms that he has a right-sided thalamic stroke. This led to his initial left-sided weakness and difficulty walking. Since the thalamus connects the contralateral cerebellar neocortex with the prefrontal cortex, the right thalamus is involved in some language functions. The matching of symptoms with the various roles of the thalamus in *Table 2.8* explains Patient 2-7's other symptoms. His emotional incontinence and pathological crying was controlled with low doses of nortriptyline, and his loss of energy with low doses of methylphenidate.

Patient 2-8: The Champion Knitter

A 50-year-old man is sent to you by his doctors to determine if he is depressed or is suffering from posttraumatic stress disorder (PTSD). A year ago he was in a fire that destroyed his trailer home and all his belongings. He was not burned and suffered only minor smoke inhalation. Since the fire, he has had no energy and no interest in his previous hobbies: playing the guitar and knitting. He was a prolific knitter for family and friends and won prizes for his efforts. Since the fire, however, he has stopped his hobbies and he now does little. He was treated with an antidepressant for his complaints, but with no benefit.

On examination he is mildly slow in his movements and subdued in mood, but not sad or apprehensive. He is friendly and low-keyed, and at times even humorous. However, he says he is now a useless person and does not have much of a life. He says he sleeps too much and enjoys nothing. He is not experiencing features of PTSD (no nightmares, no ruminations about the fire, or flashbacks). He says he stopped playing the guitar and knitting, because "the notes and stitches are no longer in my hands. I can't make the needles work smoothly."

Other than flame and smoke, What can happen in a fire that can affect the brain?

Carbon monoxide is often released in fires and can cause brain damage. Carbon monoxide has great affinity for hemoglobin. When a person is exposed to carbon monoxide, its brain damaging effects tend to localize in brain areas that were working hard (needing more blood and oxygen) at the time of exposure. The characteristic pathology is bilateral necrosis of the globus pallidus, implying specific affinity for the basal ganglia.[24] The basal ganglia were affected.

> Although MRI provides greater resolution than a CT scan, CT is better at identifying new hemorrhagic lesions, bone pathology and calcifications.

When the damage results in bilateral basal ganglia calcifications, it is referred to as *Fahr's disease*, which is what Patient 2-8 had.

Can loss of interest and change in behavior (becoming a couch potato) reflect problems in the action brain?

Disease in the frontal circuits typically causes behavior change. Because of their important involvement in this circuitry, basal ganglia lesions can cause frontal lobe syndromes including loss of interest and lost skills. One syndrome is characterized by avolition (lack of interest and drive, low energy, indifference).[25]

What is the explanation for the champion knitter's no longer being able to knit?

Procedural memory is memory of motor skills and patterns that must be demonstrated. For example, you could describe how you would ride a bicycle, but the only way anyone would know you had the motor memory for bike riding, would be for you to do it. Your daily life is loaded with procedural memories. Some examples are dressing, preparing a meal, driving, doing a physical examination, knitting, and playing a musical instrument. The champion knitter lost the ability to use his procedural memory for bimanual, highly skilled motor sequences: knitting and playing the guitar. The basal ganglia are involved in initiating procedural motor sequences.[26] When symbols or language are highly integrated into these bimanual tasks, the motor programs seem to be stored more often in the dominant (usually the left) than the nondominant hemisphere. The cerebellum and pons are also involved in new procedural learning. Although this patient is unlikely to fully regain his lost abilities, he might be able to relearn some of it, and some new procedures.

How can a person have some features of depression and not have a sad mood? How would you treat such a syndrome?

Frontal circuit disease often produces a depressive-like picture, particularly when dominant structures (usually) are affected.[27] Patient 2-8 has some features of depression, but not the sad mood. "He has the words, but not the music." When you see a patient with this atypical picture, think of a depression that is secondary to an identifiable neurologic or general medical cause.

Avolitional depressive-like frontal lobe syndromes may not respond well to typical antidepressant medications. However, because a main neurotransmitter in the frontal circuitry is dopamine, dopaminergic medications may substantially help.[28] In our experience bromocriptine or pramipexole works well when the patient also has Parkinsonism or other "positive" motor features. Methylphenidate works well when the patient does not have motor abnormalities other than slowing and loss of procedural memory. Modafinil, a stimulant-like drug used for treating narcolepsy, may also have some value. However, there are no studies or reports demonstrating its efficacy in avolitional syndromes. Patient 2-8 was given methylphenidate 10 mg BID. He had a substantial improvement in his energy and interest level and concentration, but was unable to regain his champion knitting skills.

Quick Rounds

1. A 48-year-old woman is hospitalized for a sudden onset psychosis. She is intensely frightened and continuously cries. She states the police are going to kill her and her food is poisoned. Prior to becoming psychotic, she had a spasm in her right hand that forced it into a posture. She was unable to speak and had reduced responsivity. Then as the spasm resolved, she repeatedly uttered several phrases in a robotic manner. Where in the brain is the lesion?

2. A 26-year-old man developed severe pain over much of the left half of his body following a car accident during which he was thrown into the windshield. An MRI within hours of the accident was read as normal. In addition to the pain for which no specific cause could be established, and which inexplicably ended at the midline, he was unsteady when he walked and occasionally fell backwards. He was diagnosed as having hysteria, and a psychiatric consult requested. What happened to this man? Where did it happen, and why did it happen? What was the problem with the initial evaluation?

3. An 81-year-old man comes to a psychiatric clinic for evaluation. He gives a history of crying at inappropriate times, even when he is not sad. For example, he could not control his tears when he was watching the movie "Enemy of the State." He also complains of memory problems. On a test of general cognitive function, he scores as moderately impaired. He has no sleep or appetite problems. His mood is otherwise normal, and he is nonpsychotic. What has happened to this man?

4. A 72-year-old man gives a history of crying at inappropriate times, even when he is not sad. He has no sleep or appetite problems. His mood is otherwise normal and he is nonpsychotic. His neurologic examination is normal except increased sensitivity to a light touch. He reports that he feels pain when you touch him. Where is the lesion? Don't jump to conclusions because this patient *seems* similar to Patient 2-2. What are the differences between them?

5. A 32-year-old college student has a history of traumatic brain injury that resulted in the loss of consciousness and coma for 10 days. According to the family, the patient underwent extensive rehabilitation. Ever since that accident, the patient has aggressive episodes that are often triggered by trivial stimuli. He suddenly becomes angry, verbally abusive, and, occasionally, he throws furniture. After these episodes, he is full of remorse and apologetic.

Which brain system is involved? The patient has no history of aggressive behavior before the head injury. He is functioning normally between these episodes.

Quick Rounds Answers

1. This patient has problems with mood and motor behavior (her hand spasm and her speech). The motor behavior is lateralizing to the right, suggesting a left lesion. Her speech problem ("forced" speech) also suggests left. Both are actions as is emotional expression. So she has a left anterior (assuming no cerebellar signs) lesion. If she shows no aphasia, apraxia, anomia (she did not), she likely has a subcortical lesion, as these are typical cortical signs. In her case a vascular malformation involved frontal-temporal tissue, producing seizures with post-ictal psychosis.

2. Car accidents that result in sudden acceleration and then deceleration of the head can cause axon shearing (and a dementia) or hemorrhagic lesions throughout the brain even with a closed head injury. When the thalamus is involved, pain syndromes and balance problems can occur. Although dermatomes go beyond the midline sensory field, representations in the thalamus do not. The man had a right thalamic contusion, leading to left-sided pain and balance problems. Hysterical neurologic features are more common on the left than on the right. Why this is true is unknown. The MRI was done too quickly to reveal the lesion. A CT scan may have been better early on, and the MRI done (with contrast) 7-10 days later.

3. Inappropriate crying in a nonpsychotic, nonmood-disordered patient suggests emotional incontinence. (Emotional incontinence or pathological crying or laughing occurs due to degeneration of corticobulbar pathways, which causes the patient to cry when he is not sad and to laugh when he is not happy). The most common cause of pathological crying along with cognitive deficits in an 81-year-old man is vascular disease. Selective serotonin uptake inhibitors, such as sertraline, are useful in controlling pathological crying. The patient also needs further evaluation and treatment of vascular disease, which could be treated with antihypertensive agents to control blood pressure, and antiplatelet agents, such as aspirin or anticoagulants, to prevent further strokes, depending upon the etiology.

4. Inappropriate or pathological crying is often due to disruption in corticobulbar tracts. However, absence of any motor sign and presence of pain suggest that the lesion is not in the basal ganglia, but probably in the thalamus. Although serotonergic agents can be tried and may help, an anticonvulsant, such as gabapentin or

carbamazepine that can reduce thalamic excitability and help both lability and pain may be a better choice.

5. The limbic system is responsible for the generation of emotion. However, socially appropriate emotional expression is regulated by frontal and temporal cortices. The amygdala are often involved in giving emotional meaning to a stimulus. The fact that this man's aggressive episodes are triggered by trivial stimuli suggests some degree of amygdala discharge or lack of adequate frontal inhibition. However, his near-normal function between episodes and the presence of remorse, suggest the dysfunction is less likely to be due to structural frontal changes. The most likely explanation of his symptoms is that angry emotion is generated by amygdala dysfunction that overrides frontal lobe inhibition. A mood stabilizer such as carbamazepine would help control his aggressive episodes.

Chapter 3

Depression

Patient 3-1: Da Funk, Da Blues, Da Blahs, Da-pression

A 26-year-old woman complains of having no energy or interest in doing the things she usually likes doing (going to restaurants, movies, and museums with her boyfriend). She says she does not enjoy life, is occasionally tearful, eats and sleeps too much, and is feeling mildly anxious, which makes it difficult for her to breathe. Sometimes her boyfriend can cheer her up, and during the examination she smiles and becomes animated. For the most part, however, she is subdued. Although she has been feeling worse over the past two months, she says she has felt this way on and off since high school.

Does Patient 3-1 have a depression? If so, is it melancholia?

Dysthymia is the most common depression of adolescence, and adult patients with it say they have been depressed "since high school" or all of their lives. Dysthymia is a low grade chronic depression and its lifetime prevalence in the general population is about 6%. In all age groups, females are 2-3 times likely to be dysthymic than males.[1]

Any time a patient describes symptoms that make you think of depression, always ask *yourself,* "Am I seeing a clinical depression, or demoralization or the low points everyone occasionally experiences?" If the patient has a clinical depression, regardless of life circumstances, the patient has a disease: some biochemical or pathophysiologic brain change that will require biologic intervention. Demoralization, funks, blahs, the blues are best treated by the caring of family and friends, and sometimes with counseling. There is no pill for the blahs. On the other hand, clinical depression always requires treatment. So, is Patient 3-1 depressed? No energy, anxiety, general anhedonia (but with some reactivity), tearfulness with disturbances in appetite and sleep is a duck: depression. It is just not the duck of melancholia. Melancholic depression is not just a severe form of nonmelancholic depression, but is a distinct subtype (see endnote 20 in Chapter 1 for more details). *Table 3.1*[2] displays the key variables distinguishing melancholia from nonmelancholic depression. This distinction is important because treatments are different for patients with a "major depression with melancholic features," the DSM phrase for melancholia. These patients respond better to ECT or to antidepressant drugs with broad pharmacodynamic properties, such as venlafaxine.

Table 3.1 Melancholia versus Nonmelancholic Depression	
Melancholia	**Nonmelancholic depression**
Autonomous (nonreactive) unremitting mood	Mood reactive to some situations (they can temporarily forget their worries)
Mood typically apprehensive, terrible worry and insecurity, despondency, inability to cry	Mood typically anxious or irritable, tearful
Hypothalamic pituitary end organ axes in "overdrive," circadian rhythms disturbed, sleep architecture disturbed (little stage 3 or 4), poor sleep (early morning awakening) and appetite, loss of libido	Have sleep and appetite disturbances; often oversleeping or overeating, but may also have poor sleep and appetite
Psychomotor retardation (bradykinesia, bradyphrenia) or agitation or both	Subdued but minimal psychomotor retardation, agitation directly correlates with level of anxiety
Associated more often with psychosis, stupor, catatonia, completed suicide	Associated more often with anxious-fearful personality disorder, sedative-hypnotic drug abuse. May be associated with suicidal ideation.

Patient 3-1 has a nonmelancholic depression. Although DSM describes several types of nonmelancholic depression, that separation is rarely clinically helpful. *Table 3.2* characterizes these types.

Two or more episodes of adjustment disorder with depressive features = mood disorder[3]

Would you treat Patient 3-1? If "yes, " what factors must you consider in planning her treatment?

Anyone who is clinically depressed needs treatment. Because Patient 3-1 has a long history of depression, she will likely need treatment indefinitely. Assuming a primary depression (we will discuss secondary depressions later on) your treatment planning includes the three phases of acute, continuation, and maintenance management.

Table 3.2 DSM Nonmelancholic Depressions	
Major depression without melancholic features	An episode of moodiness, irritability, or loss of both interest and energy (sleep and appetite disturbances)
Dysthymia	Chronic low grade nonmelancholic features: some good days, lots of bad days, some exacerbations that develop into a major nonmelancholic depression
Abnormal bereavement	A major clinical depression precipitated by the death of a loved one. Treat for depression.
Adjustment disorder: depressed type (not in the DSM mood disorder category)	A transient, low-grade depressive-like episode triggered by mild to moderate stress that eventually resolves. Cannot meet DSM criteria for melancholia or major depression. Typically seen in younger patients, this is often the first episode or an early episode of a recurrent major depressive illness.
Atypical depression	An odd duck (the ugly duckling), and like the fable, look for something other than the duck of depression.

A loved one dying is bad and stressful. Most bereavements are normal and the person feels lousy, but after a week or so continues with his or her responsibilities. Prolonged dysfunction (>2-3 months), melancholic features, psychosis, and suicide attempts indicate a clinical depression requiring treatment.[4]

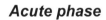

Acute phase

Always look for comorbidities. Persons with nonmelancholic depression also often 1) abuse alcohol, sedative-hypnotic drugs, or benzodiazepines, 2) have associated anxiety disorders or eating disorders, especially in a young woman, and 3) have a personality disorder, often an anxious-fearful pattern that makes them shy. They are worriers with increased anxiety levels.

Always assess general medical health even if you are sure the depression is primary. This is critical because it will influence your choice of antidepressant by its side effect profile and drug-drug interactions.

Always look for suicide risk. Although melancholics are more likely to kill themselves, patients with nonmelancholic depressions also have an increased risk and make attempts. Asking about suicidal thoughts or impulses does not make patients suicidal; it helps prevent suicide.

> Before active treatments were invented, half of severe depressions spontaneously remitted after about 9 months, which is why today some patients tell you about a past episode that got better without treatment. But prolonged depression is prolonged suffering and a potential suicide. Some bacterial pneumonias also got better before the antibiotic era, but no one would deny treatment for such conditions today. Pneumonia and depression are both potentially fatal diseases. Prolonged depression also can adversely and permanently affect brain structure and function, leading to hippocampal volume loss and cognitive deficits.

Always assess strengths and weaknesses, and particularly for depressed patients, their family and other social supports. In Patient 3-1's case, how reliable and helpful will her boyfriend be in her treatment? Does she have friends or family members she can count on? What is her general level of education and intelligence that you will use to guide you in teaching her about her illness and treatment?

Always try to match your antidepressant choice to the patient. But be warned! The pharmaceutical industry will want you to use every new psychotropic on the market. Don't be sucked in. Using too many different agents dilutes your experience and, therefore, your expertise. You need to learn the subtleties of how patients respond and the rare, as well as

> Among women of childbearing age, endocrine function must be stabilized if treatment of any depression is to be successful. Irregular menses, for example, need to be regulated. High-dose estrogen birth control agents are likely to exacerbate depression.[5]

common, side effects. Thus, knowing a few antidepressants very well is better than knowing all of them superficially. However, using just one antidepressant is too restrictive – one size does not fit all. So! What do you do?

The literature on antidepressant drug treatment offers the following conclusions: 1) all antidepressants have about the same efficacy, 2) new agents have fewer side effects than old agents, 3) new agents are safer because in overdose there is less likelihood of death than from older tricyclics (TCAs). Close examination of this literature, however, indicates a somewhat different story. We conclude: 1) the broader pharmacodynamic agents are better for melancholia, and 2) pure serotonin reuptake inhibitors are too anxiety/agitation provoking.

Our experience and reading has led to the following recommendations because our goal is to get people better, not just to avoid side effects.

1. Our first-line antidepressants for most patients with major depressions are venlafaxine, and nortriptyline.
2. Our second-line antidepressants are mirtazapine, higher-dose paroxetine.
3. In special situations MAOIs, lithium (as an add-on).

Although Patient 3-1 had a primary depression, you must always consider specific neurologic or general medical causes *before* treating. Some conditions to look for in depressed patients are listed in *Table 3.3.*

Table 3.3 *Some Causes of Secondary Depression in Adults*		
Age <30	*Age 31-65*	*Age >65*
Head trauma (men)	Endocrinopathies (women)	Antihypertensive and cardiac medications
Sedative drugs (including alcohol)	Basal ganglia disease (e.g., Huntington's, Fahr's disease)	Stroke (left anterior brain; right posterior brain)
Epilepsy	Carcinoma	Parkinson's disease
Vascular malformations	All items in *Age<30* column	Vascular dementia; dementia of Alzheimer type
Fragile X		Lymphoma, and other neoplasms
		All items in the other two columns

Patient 3-2: How Long Has This Been Going On?

A 37-year-old man has been coming to your clinic for the past 10 years for treatment of a nonmelancholic depression. You see him during a regular scheduled visit, and he tells you that he wants to take his own life. He would rather die than live the way he is living.

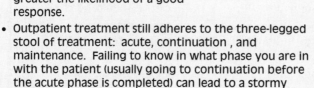

Some Guidelines for Treating Depressed Outpatients

- Suicide risk remains high during the year of the depression; repeatedly assess for it.
- Suicide risk is lowered when 1) you pay attention to and facilitate family and social supports, 2) you reduce access to weapons, and 3) you help ameliorate social stressors.
- Depressed patients are at greater risk (morbidity and mortality higher) for infection (lowered immune system activity) and cardiovascular disease. Particularly pay attention to these possibilities in older patients who are by their age at risk for these conditions.

The brain's lateralized functioning differentially relates to the heart (more innervation from the right hemisphere). Sudden emotion can cause fatal arrhythmias, whereas chronic anxiety and an abnormal mood can lead to arrhythmia, infarction and hypertension.[6]

- The greater the attention paid to preventing or managing side effects, the better the compliance. The better the compliance, the greater the likelihood of a good response.
- Outpatient treatment still adheres to the three-legged stool of treatment: acute, continuation , and maintenance. Failing to know in what phase you are in with the patient (usually going to continuation before the acute phase is completed) can lead to a stormy course.
- Having to hospitalize an outpatient is not admitting failure, it is recognizing a change in illness acuity that now requires different management. Psychiatric hospitalization is in itself an active treatment.

What should you immediately do after Patient 3-2 tells you his suicidal thoughts (a semi-trick question)?

You first find out if his thoughts represent serious intent and the immediacy of that intent. Patient 3-3 has been depressed a long time. Are his suicidal statements new? Or, if they are not new, have they changed in some way? Does he have a plan, and does he have the means to carry out the plan? What does he mean by "not wanting to live the way he is now?" Is he currently agitated, despondent? Has something terrible recently happened to him? Has he been drinking? If the answers to these concerns reveal no other risk factors, then Patient 3-2 is not imminently suicidal. However, recent job loss and access to a gun might tip the scale toward too high a risk.

Assume Patient 3-2 is not likely to kill himself within the next 24-48 hours but is still at increased risk for suicide. You are now faced with the next question.

Under what circumstances would you hospitalize Patient 3-2?

Hospitalization does not totally reduce suicide risk, but it sure helps when needed. The decision is made on present, not past factors. Factors increasing risk include alcohol use, no social supports, a discomforting general medical problem, available lethal means, and a plan. Previous suicide attempts add to the risk because they indicate previous severe depressions and perhaps the impulsivity associated with high risk.

Suppose you do not find other risk factors, but two weeks later Patient 3-2 returns to the clinic and still has suicidal thoughts. Perhaps frequency has increased to 3-4 times daily, and he is now clearly depressed with melancholic features. Although he denies any specific plans, he seems agitated and reports that his wife of 12 years has left him and has asked for a divorce. His risk is now very high, and he needs to be in a hospital.

When would you admit Patient 3-2 involuntarily?

A depressed patient who has no support system at home and is at high risk for suicide needs hospitalization. If you are convinced about his risk, you are obligated to hospitalize. If the patient refuses, you legally can and should hospitalize. To legally hospitalize someone involuntarily, he either has to be a danger to himself at the time of hospitalization, or you are reasonably sure he is a danger to himself within the next several days. Patient 3-2 is now a danger to himself and can be involuntarily hospitalized if he refuses. Most successful lawsuits involving a suicidal patient result from lack of action by the treaters.[7]

Discussion

Table 3.4 summarizes clinically *important* risk factors in a depressed patient. Patients with recurrent depressions and other periods of hypomania (termed bipolar II) are at greatest risk for suicide. In the U.S., Euro-American males over 50 constitute the cohort of highest risk. Alcohol is found in the blood of 50% of suicide victims. Delusions about ill health, worthlessness or guilt spurs the suicidal person to act. Mild cognitive impairment in elderly depressed patients reduces their capacity to deal with stress. Debilitating general medical conditions make life less worth the effort for many. Inherited personality traits of impulsivity and high harm avoidance may underlie familial suicide in some, but mood disorder is the most likely cause.

Table 3.4 Clinically Important Risk Factors for Suicide in a Depressed Patient
Depression with anxiety and agitation
Psychotic depression
Co-occurring heavy alcohol use or abuse
Co-occurring chronic pain
Bipolarity (see Chapter 4)
Male (Euro-Americans over age 50, African-Americans under 30 and over 50)
Mild to moderate cognitive problems
Suicide in the family

National standardized exams require the memorization of other factors less helpful clinically, but needed to generate enough questions.[8] Table 3.5 lists high-low risk factors.

Table 3.5 Important Test-Related Risk Factors for Suicidality in the U.S.	
Increased Risk	**Decreased Risk**
Living in U.S. mountain states	Living in upper Midwest
Protestant	Catholic
Nonpregnant	Pregnant
Time of year (late fall)	Puerto Rican or Mexican descent
Day of week (Sunday)	

Patient 3-3: A Rose by Any Other Name

A 33-year-old man says he has not been himself for several months. He has become extremely anxious, apprehensive, and unsure of himself since the birth of his daughter. She has feeding difficulties and has been fitful, crying most of the day and night. He has been unable to sleep, even when going to a different room in the house. He has become afraid that he will hurt her, and is afraid to touch her or help with her care because of these fears. He ruminates about this and believes he is a terrible person for having such feelings. Nothing relieves his apprehension. He barely eats, and has lost 10 pounds since her birth. He needs constant reassurance. A family physician prescribes fluoxetine 20 mg daily for 30 days and makes a follow-up appointment in one month.

What best accounts for this man's problem?

Your first step in evaluating a patient is to get the big picture -- the duck. Patient 3-3 has recent onset of unremitting apprehension and anxiety. He also has insomnia, loss of appetite and weight, and guilty ruminations. Although Patient 3-3's symptoms fit the classic description of melancholia[9] when Patient 3-3 is described to them, many students and residents think about a "stress reaction" to the birth and difficult infancy of his daughter or of obsessive compulsive disorder (OCD), or some other anxiety disorder. Sutton's Law tells you, however, that the odds favor depression, which is eight times as common as OCD. Although anxiety disorders are very common, the rule of parsimony (one explanation is better than two) indicates that Patient 3-3's symptoms can all be explained by depression.

> About 40-60% of patients with OCD achieve a 50-60% improvement, about 60-70% of depressed patients obtain a 50-70% response to antidepressant drugs and of those 30-40% achieve remission. Ninety percent plus can remit to ECT.[10]

It is also better to consider Patient 3-3 as depressed rather than has having OCD: 1) depression is the condition with the better prognosis, 2) thinking of OCD may relax clinical concerns discussed in question 2 below, and 3) there are more and better treatments for depression than there are for OCD.

But why isn't Patient 3-3's problem just stress? The answer is that although stress is bad and can precipitate disease in persons prone to disease (e.g., hypertension, myocardial infarction, asthma, stroke, eczema, diabetic instability).[11] If stressful events raise a person's blood pressure and that person has a stroke, we say that the stroke was due to

The characteristic mood of melancholia is not the sadness we all feel from time to time, but rather an unrelenting, intense apprehension, anxiety and gloom. The world seems overwhelming.

contributing stress and treat the stroke and not call it stress. The same for psychiatric illness. If it walks, talks, and looks like a duck, it's a duck. Patient 3-3 has melancholia.

What should be your major concern about this man and what specific additional information do you need to best deal with this concern?

Suicide Risk. Every depressed patient is a potential suicide risk, and several factors increase that risk. The presence of melancholia is a big risk factor. An anxious mood with agitation further increases the risk. The regular use or abuse of alcohol increases the risk as does being male, being over 50, having a chronic or painful general medical problem and no family or social supports. Patient 3-3 is not a regular drinker, but he has an anxious melancholia, is male, and male depressives are more likely than women to kill themselves because of greater access to guns (1 bullet is worth 1000 pills). Men are also more likely to hang themselves and jump to their death. The use of a gun, however, is still the most common cause of suicide in women. The absence of a specific plan does not eliminate the suicide risk, although the presence of a definite plan increases the risk.

Guns and depression do not mix, and a depressed patient cannot be allowed to be in a house with a gun. One or the other has got to go! Always ask about guns.

What errors, if any, did the family physician make?

Oh, boy, we think he may have set a record!

1. By giving the patient a 30-day supply, he gave a potential overdose of a drug to a depressed patient. 600 mg of fluoxetine is toxic.[12]
2. He did not consider suicide or taking precautions. Patient 3-3's wife had a gun in the house.

It is pharmaceutical industry propaganda that the newer antidepressants are better or have fewer side effects than the older medications. Side effects are different, but occur with similar frequency. The partially specific reuptake inhibitors (e.g., desipramine, nortriptyline) have modest anticholinergic properties and may work better (we think so) for melancholia than specific SSRIs. Which would you think Patient 3-3 would choose when well again -- a mildly dry mouth (TCA) or inability to have sex? (SSRI)

92

3. He gave fluoxetine, which often causes initial agitation, to an already anxious, agitated patient[13]
4. He gave fluoxetine, a drug with a very long half-life and onset of action, to a patient who needs to get fast relief.
5. He gave a drug with substantial sexual side effects to a young, sexually active man.[14]
6. He did not make regular phone rounds during the first 2 weeks of treatment to provide reassurance, education about the illness and drug side effects, to catch and treat side effects that do occur, and to monitor response and any need for hospitalization.
7. He did not see the patient by the end of the first week to assess how things are going.
8. He did not take into account the stressor (the crying baby). In fact, the baby was an air swallower during breast feeding and required some antispasmodic and gas medication, and the mother required further breast feeding education).

Patient 3-4: A Sheep in Wolf's Clothing

For the past 3 months, a 33-year-old woman has been attending a group for patients diagnosed as having *borderline personality disorder.*[15] She has had recurrent suicidal feelings and made several "gestures" several years before. She attends group regularly, but rarely speaks. She sits quietly fidgeting and sighing. She avoids eye contact with other members and never smiles. One day she calls her group therapist and says she is experiencing increased anxiety and depression after receiving divorce papers from her husband. The therapist tells her to do relaxation and breathing exercises, and to call him in the morning. Patient 3-4 is found dead in her garage the next day, having inhaled carbon monoxide from her car.

What is wrong with Patient 3-4?

Patient 3-4 had a sustained sad mood. She has been withdrawn for the past three months. She has past suicidal behavior, and was worse following a recent stressful event. She said she was anxious. Using the duck principle, the most likely explanation for her condition is clinical depression. Persons with personality disorder diagnoses are at higher risk than the general population for depression.

What errors did the therapist make?

1. *The therapist focused on the label "borderline" and not on the patient's behavior.* Thus, did not evaluate Patient 3-4 thoroughly. He did not recognize that depressed patients often have suicidal thoughts that worsen when faced with interpersonal difficulties, and expected "borderline" patients to have uproars in their lives. Therefore, he sent the patient to a support group.

Almost 50% of patients labeled borderline meet all or most of the criteria for one of the DSM mood disorder labels. These patients have become "difficult patients," in part, because their mood disorder has gone unrecognized or has been given second billing to its consequences – a life of turmoil. Remember, if you intend to do no harm, when there is ambiguity in the diagnosis, start first with the diagnosis and treatment that has the best prognosis. Childhood onset bipolar disorder, is most likely to be misdiagnosed as borderline. It is typically of lower intensity and less episodic than the adult onset form, but nevertheless with emotional instability and storminess.[16]

2. *The therapist did not make a reassessment of suicidality even though the patient's situation and symptoms changed.* Past

94

Over a third of suicide victims go to a physician within three weeks prior to their death. How come these suicides are not prevented? Studies demonstrate the reasons: lack of recognition of the depression and suicide risk, inadequate pharmacotherapy, and not following the rules of outpatient management of a depressed patient. Thirty thousand suicides are reported each year in the US (in the top 10 of leading causes of death) and another 60,000 are estimated as occurring, but go unreported (bringing suicide into the top 6 causes of death). Suicide is preventable.

behavior is never as important in diagnosis and management as present behavior. Suicide is often an impulsive act that can occur when a patient becomes anxious and agitated. Patient 3-4 has four major risk factors for suicide: 1) major depression, 2) an acute stressor, 3) an anxious mood, and 4) lack of interpersonal support. Her death may have been avoided if her depression had been properly diagnosed and treated.

Discussion

Psychological autopsies are studies that trace the events over the weeks and months that precede a suicide.[17] These studies repeatedly demonstrate why so many persons (mostly with depression) needlessly kill themselves each year. *Table 3.6* displays these errors.

Not recognizing depression like Patient 3-4's therapist is common. In one study of suicide attempters, although all met DSM criteria for major depression and had the recent suicide attempt as a red flag, only 39% were diagnosed as depressed by a psychiatric consultant.[18] In the elderly, the poor sleep and appetite of depression is attributed to their general medical problems and their depressed mood to "being old."[19]

Table 3.6 Suicide Prevention Errors
Nonrecognition of depression
Attributing depressive symptoms to stress, not illness
Not adequately assessing suicide risk
Poor pharmacotherapy
Inadequate follow-up and monitoring of depressed outpatients
Failure to hospitalize or involuntarily commit
Failure to give ECT

Patient 3-5: Despite Galileo, a Heavy Mood Weighs More Than an Equally Heavy Psychosis

A 68-year-old man comes to your clinic and anxiously relates his fears that he is of no use to anyone and should die. He says that he is a terrible person whose brain waves have gotten "out of hand" and have killed people – well known persons in the news. Occasionally he can hear his victims shouting at him and screaming as they are injured. He says others are now trying to kill him in retribution. He says he cannot sleep and when he does, he has nightmares, then wakes, and "the whole thing is facing me again. . .I can't go on like this." He has lost 15 pounds since it all started three months ago. He says he is despondent, his life is over and that he would kill himself if he had the means, but he cannot formulate a plan on how to do it. He fidgets continuously as he describes his fears. He looks frightened, unsure, and his speech is hesitant. His recent medical examination was normal. He has no history of any medical or neurologic illness.

> **Principles**
>
> - All persons who hallucinate and are delusional are psychotic, but few psychotic persons are schizophrenic (see glossary).[20]
>
> - Most psychotic features reflect severity of an individual episode and none are pathognomonic of any one disorder.
>
> - Avoid treating targeted symptoms; treat diseases.

What's the Duck?

Get the big picture: A senior citizen has a 3-month history of anxiety, agitation, and despondency to the point of being suicidal. He is guilt-ridden, with sleep and appetite disturbances, who hears voices, and has delusions. This duck is melancholia, because the patient has no evidence of any cardiovascular disease.

> The content of the voices and delusions are rarely of diagnostic importance. The fact that someone is having perceptions without external stimuli (hallucinations) and fixed false beliefs (delusions) is much more important in your differential diagnosis.

Table 3.7 lists the characteristic features of melancholia.

Table 3.7 The Characteristic Features of Melancholia	
Dysfunction	**Feature**
Mood disturbance	Unremitting apprehension and gloom
Motor disturbance	Slowness that may progress to stupor, agitation increases with anxiety, fixed hollow and distant stare, stereotypies or perseveration, catatonia
Autonomic dysfunction	Decreased salivation, tears, intestinal secretions and motility (constipation), morning sweating
Midbrain and limbic dysregulation	Altered temperature and cortisol circadian rhythms (higher early in the morning), oligo and amenorrhea, loss of libido, anhedonia, anorexia with >5% body weight loss
Cognitive disturbance	Feelings of hopelessness, worthlessness, and guilt that may become delusional (guilt, sin, poverty, ill health, being dead), poor attention and concentration, poor new learning, bradyphrenia
Perceptual disturbances	Illusions, hallucinations, psychosensory features (dysmegalopsia [objects seem altered in size], dysmorphopsia [objects seem altered in shape])

What does Sutton's Law tell you about the likely explanations for Patient 3-5's condition?

Depression is very common and 10-15% or more of the general population has a lifetime risk for some depressive-like syndrome. Perhaps 6-8% of the population is at risk for primary depression, and of these 20-35% will be melancholic (less than 1% of the population gets schizophrenia).

Depression is increasing in incidence among persons born closer to the present (the period effect). First depressions are also occurring at an earlier age than they used to (the cohort effect).[21]

Table 3.8 lists common causes of secondary depression by age group. Check out Patient 3-5's list of suspects. In fact, he has a primary depression.

Table 3.8 *Common Causes of Secondary Depression by Age Group*				
Prepuberty	*Adolescence*	*Young Adult*	*Middle Age*	*Elderly*
• Prescription medications • Viral illness	• Street drugs • Traumatic brain injury • Epilepsy • Viral illness	• Street drugs • Traumatic brain injury • Epilepsy • Viral illness	• Prescribed drugs • Alcoholism • Cancer and its treatments • Endocrinopathies • Brain tumors • Metabolic disorders	• Prescribed drugs • Stroke • Parkinson's disease • Dementia • Metabolic disorders

What do you do first?

Patient 3-5 is a very high suicide risk: anxious-agitated melancholia, male, senior citizen (the risk goes up each decade after 40), and he expresses suicidal thoughts. You hospitalize him immediately. He does not "get to pass go," or go home for "a few things."

When told he was going to be hospitalized to prevent him from harming himself, Patient 3-5 was relieved.

> Fifteen percent of all depressed persons kill themselves. The risk for men and women goes up each decade after 40. Young immigrant women are at greater risk than men and no one knows why.[22]

What must you think about in shaping your treatment plan if you decide Patient 3-5's condition is primary?

1. Is this depression part of a bipolar or unipolar disorder (see glossary)? If the former, any antidepressant medication you give will require simultaneous coverage with a mood stabilizer (e.g., lithium, valproic acid, carbamazepine).

2. Does the patient have any comorbid general medical or neurologic conditions that, although they are not the cause of the depression, nevertheless, can interfere with treatment? Areas of concern include:

   a. Disorders affecting pharmacokinetics (e.g., liver disease)

b. Disorders affecting pharmacodynamics (e.g., competing or interacting drug-drug interactions such as an SSRI and an MAOI combination, potentially deadly leading to a serotonin syndrome)

c. Factors that make the use of an antipsychotic too risky (e.g., past or present catatonic features, dehydration, some tardive dyskinesia)

> The serotonin syndrome is like the neuroleptic malignant syndrome (confusion, autonomic instability, fever, muscle rigidity) plus GI problems. It occurs primarily due to serotonergic drug-drug interaction. Like NMS it can be treated with benzodiazepines or ECT.

3. The presence of factors that make antidepressant drug therapy too risky or unlikely to work

a. Pregnancy (not a problem for Patient 3-5, but in today's world, nothing is certain): ECT may be safer for the fetus than drug therapy (see Patient 3-9 for details).
b. Stupor or catatonia: ECT becomes the treatment of choice and life-saving in many instances where such patients (particularly elderly ones) become dehydrated and starve.
c. Psychosis: antidepressants do no better than placebo when given alone to psychotically depressed patients.[23] Your options are an antidepressant plus a mood stabilizer (our second choice), an antidepressant plus an antipsychotic (our last choice), or ECT (our first choice). In our opinion treating psychotic depression with antidepressants alone is malpractice.

Discussion

The effects of specific treatments on suicide rates have been studied for years.[24] Several conclusions are inescapable.

1. Antidepressant drugs have no clear effect on acute suicidality, but because they have some efficacy in reducing relapse and recurrence, and because 50-70% of suicides occur during a depression, they may have some long-term benefit.
2. Lithium, if taken at adequate doses over a sustained period of time, has a clinically meaningful long-term effect on lowering suicide rates, certainly for bipolar patients and maybe also for unipolar patients. It has no acute effect on suicide rate.

3. ECT is the treatment of choice for a suicidal depressed patient. Suicides during or shortly after ECT is virtually unheard of.
4. ECT has no clear long-term effect on suicide rates.
5. ECT has a dramatic short-term effect on suicide rates. Most recently, a multicenter trial of ECT found that among suicidal hospitalized depressed patients, suicidality virtually disappeared by the end of the second week of treatment (CORE ECT study group personal communication, M. Fink).
6. ECT is the treatment of choice for psychotic depression where suicide rates are very high. In the CORE study, the remission rate among psychotic depressed patients who received 12 or more bilateral ECTs was 96%! That is the best results in history for treating any group of depressed patients.

Patient 3-6: If at First You Don't Succeed

A 50-year-old man is referred to you by a colleague for a second opinion because the patient has been depressed for two years and has been given many medications in many combinations, without much response. The colleague wants a second opinion and treatment recommendation.

What are the steps in evaluating a patient with what appears to be a treatment-resistant depression?[25]

Step 1. Determine if the patient is truly treatment-resistant. Patients labeled "treatment-resistant" are often just inadequately treated (maybe 70% of such patients).[26] First, detail medication history including the class, dose, and duration of the trial for each medication. In our view, a depressed patient is not treatment resistant unless he has not responded to an adequate course of bilateral ECT.[27]

If the patient has received ECT, then you need to determine if the treatments were adequate. You need to know:

1. If the patient received unilateral or bilateral ECT. U.S. ECT machines cannot deliver the necessary currents for unilateral ECT to be effective (5 or more times seizure threshold), therefore, except for very young patients, those who received unilateral ECT may not have received adequate treatment
2. What was the duration of the seizures
3. Were the EEG seizures full and grand mal in pattern.
4. The total number of treatments
5. Was the patient simultaneously taking medications (i.e., anticonvulsants and benzodiazepines) that may have decreased the effectiveness of ECT

For a depressed patient to be considered ECT resistant, he should have received 12 or more bilateral ECTs with each seizure duration more than 25 seconds, and each seizure sustained and synchronized with high voltage slow waves and spikes. The actual quality of seizure is important (i.e., a typical pattern consisting of a buildup, spike and wave pattern followed by a clean end). Clinically, we have often observed poor seizure quality in "nonresponders."

Step 2. Look for the causes of treatment resistance. Untreated or undiagnosed comorbidities often account for treatment resistance.

1. *Alcohol and substance abuse.* Depression either due to, or complicated by alcohol and substance abuse is often resistant to standard antidepressant treatment. Noncompliance is the most likely reason for treatment resistance, followed by pharmacokinetic reasons.

> Depressed women who also abuse alcohol typically do so to self-medicate. If you can resolve the depressive illness and minimize relapse, the alcoholism is often treatable. In depressed men who are alcoholics successful treatment of the depression often leaves you with the difficult task of treating an alcoholic.[28]

2. *Stroke,* especially lacunar infarcts in the basal ganglia, is the second most common comorbidity that leads to treatment resistance. This is most likely in a patient with a history of coronary artery disease or hypertension.[29]
3. *Seizure disorder* is often associated with depression (40% of epileptics become depressed). Patients with undiagnosed and untreated seizure disorder may not respond to antidepressant medication unless seizures are first treated. The seizure form is most likely to be complex partial. Look for unexplained brief periods of memory loss, sudden intense olfactory or tactile hallucinations, sudden visuoperceptual or auditory perception changes.[30]
4. *Endocrine disease* can result in treatment resistance and, if unrecognized or untreated, most such depressed patients will not respond to the best antidepressant treatment plans. Look for subacute thyroid disease, hypothalamic-pituitary-gonadal dysregulation, and adrenal disease.[31]
5. *Personality disorder* is often comorbid with nonmelancholic depressions. If you do not consider the personality disorder in your acute and maintenance treatment planning, then poor response is likely.

What are the treatment options for treatment resistant patients? [32]

Option 1. If you identify a specific problem in step 2 above, correct that problem. Then retry the past treatment that gave the best response, and maximize the dose.

Option 2. If you do not find a specific problem from step 2 above, retry the past treatment that gave the best response and maximize the dose.

Option 3. If option 1 and 2 are not successful or do not apply (e.g., no past treatment stands out as successful), and the past treatment was not ECT, give a course of bilateral ECT. Often, after successful ECT, medications that previously did not work can then be of benefit, particularly as continuation or maintenance agents.[33]

Patient 3-7: Never Bet More Than You Can Afford to Lose

A 49-year-old attorney, is divorced by his wife of 25 years. He develops a major depression with vegetative features which he attributes to the divorce and its related financial problems. In addition to two previous depressive episodes, he has been hospitalized once for alcohol dependence. His father committed suicide when Patient 3-7 was 25 years old. His younger sister and older brother were also treated for depression. Patient 3-7 is started on fluoxetine 20 mg daily. One month later after a partial response, his dose is increased to 40 mg daily. After two weeks on the new dose, he reports increased anxiety, irritability, and fleeting feelings of wishing to go to sleep and not wake up. He also reports that he has resumed drinking to relieve stress.

What is the most important clinical problem you would face with Patient 3-7, and what should you do about it?

Patient 3-7 is a suicide risk. His risk factors include:

1. Dysphoric mood (depressed and anxious) and suicidal feelings
2. A clinical depression
3. Alcohol abuse
4. A middle-aged male
5. Financial problems and no evidence of adequate social or interpersonal support

Patient 3-7 needs to be in a hospital.

Unlike Patient 3-6, Patient 3-7 has gotten worse as his fluoxetine dose is increased. Further increase in the drug might not help. Fluoxetine, although helpful in nonmelancholic depression, is only modestly effective for many melancholic depressions and may make these patients more anxious and agitated.

What is the etiology of Patient 3-7's depression (a semi-trick question)?

The etiology of primary depression is unknown. We often tell patients it is due to a "chemical imbalance in the brain," but that oversimplifies. For Patient 3-7 depression is certainly familial and likely he has some genetic vulnerability. The heritability for depressive illness is about 40-50%. Early childhood stressors greatly influence the risk for later depressions. We also know that Patient 3-7's depression is not simply a reaction to the stress of his divorce and financial difficulties. This stress could certainly have precipitated his depression, but it is not the etiology. He is clinically depressed. He has had previous episodes when he was not in the middle of a divorce. We cannot overemphasize the fact that clinical depression is not merely a psychological reaction to stress that will resolve if the stress is removed or the patient "pulls himself together." Stress is bad and often precipitates disease in patients with disease vulnerabilities (e.g., hypertension, stroke, heart disease). Diseases of the brain are no exception. No one would say, "his blood pressure will get better on its own once he retires." The blood pressure problem is likely to improve without stress, but specific treatment is needed too. Same for depression. Also consider the fact that some depressions are associated with a long prodromal period during which the patient is moody and functioning below par, but not obviously depressed. The prodrome can cause environmental problems. Then the depression becomes obvious and it seems as if the environmental problems "cause it" when in fact the depressive prodrome caused the environmental difficulties.[34]

What would be the best treatments for Patient 3-7 if you could go back in time and start treatment over again for the episode?

1. The general rule for selecting an antidepressant medication for melancholia is to give the broadest pharmacodynamic spectrum drug that is most likely to be tolerated by the patient. When mild to modest anticholinergic side effects are unlikely to be a problem, nortriptyline is a good choice. When you need to avoid anticholinergic side effects, venlafaxine is a good choice. Selective serotonin reuptake inhibitors are not effective in melancholia.[35]
2. Remember that ECT is still the most rapid, most efficacious and safest antidepressant treatment.[36] Patient 3-7, in the hospital, might do best with ECT.

Discussion

There are so many statistics about suicide; *Table 3.9* lists some of them. Most are not relevant to practice. For example, although US Catholics are said to be at less risk than US Protestants, is that true or due to underreporting to spare the person and family of the taint of "sinning?" Hungary, over 90% Catholic, has the highest suicide rate in Europe. What counts is the patient in front of you.

Table 3.9 Suicide Variables	
Variable	**Clinical Meaningfulness**
Depression	Important
Melancholia with anxiety and agitation	Highest risk
Psychosis	Important if command hallucinations present
Mixed manic state	High risk
Alcohol use	Increases risk of impulsive suicide
Alcoholism	High risk when patient also depressed
Male	High risk when depressed because of access to lethal means (gun, hanging, jumping)
Age	Over 50
Social support	high risk when absent and person depressed
Chronic, painful or dysfunctional general medical illness	High risk when person also depressed
Unmarried or divorced	Important only as indicator of poor social support, and often the consequences of depression; being married, of itself, not protective
US Catholic	Less statistical risk than other US citizens, but of no clinical usefulness
Pregnancy	Least risk for psychiatric disorder during pregnancy and highest risk post-partum [37]

Patient 3-8: Don't Let These Gray Hairs Fool You, Buddy!

A 65-year-old man says he cannot work anymore because he thinks he is losing his mind. His wife reports that he has been having trouble with a new important work assignment, and he has been telling her he thinks he is being forced out of his job because his boss finally has concluded that he is incompetent (although, there is no evidence that this is true!). His wife says the situation has kept her husband awake most nights with worry. He has become short-tempered, and has not been eating. On examination, he looks frightened and fidgets in his chair. He says he would rather be dead than senile. Cognitive testing demonstrates poor performance on a wide variety of tasks, particularly with concentration and memory.

What are the three basic rules of diagnosis, and what do they tell you about Patient 3-8?

The Duck Principle: A 65-year-old man with decreased functioning, mood change characterized by severe apprehension, vegetative signs, cognitive problems and thoughts of death. The Duck is depression.

Sutton's Law: If you thought dementia, you are also correct. Anyone with a new onset of substantial diffuse cognitive impairment (particularly involving memory) who is also in clear consciousness is by definition demented. In persons under 70, depression is 4 times as common as nonreversible dementias such as Alzheimer's disease. Depression is the most common single condition causing reversible dementia (about 20-30% of reversible dementias).

> Reactions to over the counter and prescribed drugs are the single largest etiologic category among reversible dementias (30-40%).

The Rule of Parsimony: Explaining this man's dementia by, if possible, one pathophysiology would be best for management, and depression explains it all.

The term for this dementia is *pseudodementia*. Pseudodementia is a bad term because the patient is, in fact, demented. (*Pseudo-pseudodementia* would be more accurate.) This reversible dementia typically occurs in persons over 65 who have some cognitive decline from normal aging plus the superimposed cognitive deficits of depression which push them into the cognitively demented range.

What is the most likely misdiagnosis for Patient 3-8, and how can you tell it apart from what he has?

Because Alzheimer's disease represents about 50% of all dementias, patients like Patient 3-8 are usually misdiagnosed as having Alzheimer's disease and are treated for it. They usually get worse from this approach and about 25% of these missed depressed patients will be dead (suicide, infection, cardiovascular disease) within a year. *Table 3.10* displays some of the differences between pseudodementia (really pseudo-pseudodementia) and early Alzheimer's disease.

Table 3.10 Distinguishing Pseudo-Pseudodementia from Alzheimer's Disease	
Alzheimer's Disease	**Pseudo-Pseudodementia**
Typical onset after age 75	Onset variable but often before 75
Denies and minimizes problems (anosognosia)	Maximizes problems
Visuospatial and memory problems early on (getting lost, getting into auto accidents, not recognizing faces, poor new learning, and decaying old memories)	Symptoms of depression ; more likely to have melancholic features
Less likely to have prior mood disorder	More likely to have prior mood disorder
Family history of Alzheimer's disease, Down's syndrome, or myeloproliferative disease	Family history of mood disorder or suicide
Temporoparietal dysfunction on cognitive testing	Frontal dysfunction or bradyphrenia on cognitive testing
Temporoparietal hypometabolism on SPECT	Frontal hypometabolism on SPECT
MRI shows substantial cortical atrophy and ventricular enlargement and is most distinguishing when the patient is under 75	MRI normal or atrophy and ventricular enlargement modest and *reversible* because it results from increased cortisol levels that return to baseline when the depression resolves; some amygdala and hippocampal volume loss L>R can occur with melancholia

What should you do next for Patient 3-8?

Patient 3-8 is a 65-year-old man with an agitated melancholia, substantial cognitive impairment, who expresses thoughts of death. He needs to be in a hospital because his suicide risk is high.

Discussion

Up until this point, most clinicians would agree about what is wrong with Patient 3-8 and what should be done for him. Now the problem: Because he has a delusional mood, should he be treated with an antidepressant alone, an antidepressant plus enhancement with a mood stabilizer, such as lithium, an antidepressant and an antipsychotic, or ECT? Here's our thinking.

An antidepressant alone for a melancholic who is probably psychotic is unlikely to work, and studies indicate that for such patients an antidepressant alone is no better than a placebo. So, our choices are polypharmacy or ECT.[38]

If Patient 3-8 has no important comorbidities and is in reasonable general medical health and is bipolar, then an antidepressant plus a mood stabilizer would be a reasonable choice. However, this is not our first choice, because this approach will not change his short-term suicidality (the reason for admission), nor will it work as well or as fast as ECT. ECT is the treatment of choice for a suicidal, psychotic melancholic.

If Patient 3-8 is unipolar, then antidepressant enhancement with a mood stabilizer is less likely to work, and ECT is again clearly the best antidepressant, if "best" means fastest acting, safest, best efficacy. If Patient 3-8 has important comorbidities or problems with general medical health, then ECT again becomes the treatment of choice. Our first-choice acute treatment for Patient 3-8 is ECT, whether Patient 3-8 is bipolar or unipolar.

What role, if any, does an antipsychotic play in Patient 3-8's treatment? Very little. It would be our last resort treatment if Patient 3-8 became very psychotic and unresponsive to all other treatments. Why? Because why risk all the short- and long-term side effects when you do not have to? If we had to use an antipsychotic, we would pick an atypical for Patient 3-8.[39]

Patient 3-9: The Safety of the Womb

A 28-year-old, 5-month pregnant woman is brought to the emergency room by her husband because she was trying to jump off a balcony. Her husband says she told him that she does not want to live because she feels she is no good and will be a rotten mother. He also tells you that she is not sleeping and has lost 10 pounds since her last prenatal visit. For the last few weeks early every morning he finds her in the baby's room crying.

What is the best treatment for Patient 3-9?

> Five to 10% of pregnant women become clinically depressed. Depression during pregnancy is a risk factor for serious obstetrical problems and child development difficulties. It is worse for the fetus not to treat than to treat. Depression during pregnancy is the best predictor of a post-partum depression.[40]

Patient 3-9 is suicidal and needs to be hospitalized. She is morbidly sad, has lost weight, has poor sleep (early a.m. awakening), and may have delusions of worthlessness. She likely has a melancholic depression. To decide what would be the best treatment for Patient 3-9, you need to consider:

1. What will relieve her depression fast
2. What is the most effective treatment for psychotic depression
3. What can help her calm down and sleep
4. What treatment will be least intrusive or dangerous to her fetus
5. What treatment will also be the best for the continuation phase of treatment for this episode – a time frame likely to span the last few months of pregnancy and her child's first year

Of all the treatments that are used to treat depression, electroconvulsive treatment (ECT) fits all the above requirements and should be offered to Patient 3-9 as a first line treatment.

What special precautions do you need to take when treating Patient 3-9?

Giving ECT to a pregnant woman is automatically considered a high risk ECT procedure, even though ECT has little effect on the fetus. The following guidelines should be followed to reduce complications.

Choosing medications during ECT. The ultra-short-acting anesthetics, used routinely during ECT, readily cross the placenta and accumulate in the fetal liver. However, they are rapidly transferred back to the mother, thus limiting exposure to the fetal brain. Succinylcholine is the neuromuscular blocking agent used for inducing muscle paralysis during ECT. Pregnant women have low levels of pseudocholinesterase (PCE), a catabolic enzyme for succinylcholine. It is therefore best to check PCE levels in a pregnant woman and adjust the succinylcholine dose accordingly. The anticholinergic glycopyrrolate used to prevent vagal discharge and heart block and to reduce secretions does not cross the placenta as readily as atropine, and therefore is used in pregnancy. Once paralyzed with the muscle relaxant, the ECT patient is always ventilated by "bag" with pure oxygen. Oxygen saturation is typically 100% throughout the procedure. Fetal oxygen saturation will, thus, be 100%.[41]

Adjustments in the procedure. Because gastric emptying is extremely slow in late pregnancy, women in their second or third trimester are treated as if they have recently eaten. Endotracheal intubation is standard after 20 weeks. Anatomic changes in breast and chest diameter, and increased incidence of laryngeal and tongue edema can cause failed intubation, so pediatric size tubes are often used to prevent aspiration of stomach contents. An antacid such as sodium citrate is also given to neutralize gastric secretions. Fetal heart rate and maternal blood pressure are monitored. During ECT the patient in the second or third trimester is tilted to the left and supported with pillows to relieve uterine pressure on the aorta and inferior vena cava, so that cardiac flow is not obstructed. Uterine activity is recorded with an external tocodynamometer. The mother is monitored for premature contractions. A tocolytic agent, such as ritodrine, to prevent uterine contractions is on hand if needed. An obstetrician should attend the procedure to monitor maternal measurements.

What if Patient 3-9 or her family refuses your recommendations?

If either Patient 3-9 or her husband refuses ECT, you are faced with an ethical and moral issue. When you become a patient's physician she is not just getting a warm body; she is getting your experience, skills and opinions. When a patient disagrees with your opinion she cannot separate that opinion from you. It is a package deal. At that point you have to decide the risk benefits of your opinion versus those of the patient's preference. What you do should depend on how much better your idea is than the patient's. Some guidelines are:

1. If the difference between your idea and the patient's is minimal, agree to the patient's idea with the proviso that if that idea does not work, you will insist on yours.

111

2. If the difference between your idea and the patient's is substantial, you cannot treat the patient unless he comes up with a better idea that meets the first guideline or he agree to yours.
3. If you and the patient cannot agree, and if you are knowledgeable and experienced, the vast majority of patients will ultimately accept your opinion. Sometimes offering to get a second opinion resolves the patient's concerns. If the patient does not agree with you despite all your efforts, and in good conscience you cannot do what the patient wants, then you tell the patient that you will find him a physician in whom she will have greater confidence.

Discussion

Use of psychopharmacologic agents in pregnancy is not contraindicated, although strongly discouraged. Of the possible choices, current literature suggests that prenatal exposure to nonspecific reuptake inhibiting antidepressants is relatively safe. Treating a pregnant woman is not an easy task. You need to weigh the risks and benefits of each decision. You need to review all the data available, but remember, ultimately the decision is always about "this" patient and "her" baby.[42] However, numerous animal studies show behavioral abnormalities following in utero exposure to these drugs.[43] These abnormalities include low birth weight, delayed maturation, minimal social and environmental interaction. The incidence of teratogenicity is low. Selective serotonin reuptake inhibitors are also relatively safe, but their behavioral effects on the fetus are unknown. Data regarding fetal outcome for pregnant psychotic women are limited. Some studies show no effect, others show increased risk for congenital anomalies, especially during the first trimester. Although human data regarding neurobehavioral sequelae of fetal exposure show no adverse effects, there are behavioral consequences of antipsychotic exposure in nonhumans. If Patient 3-9 had a previous history of mania, some clinicians would consider lithium. Lithium, however, is a known teratogen (causes Ebstein's anomalies: abnormal tricuspid valve, right ventricular hypoplasia, patent foramen ovale) in the first trimester and therefore is contraindicated. Lithium is used to treat manic episodes during the second and third trimester. A floppy baby syndrome with paresis and increased muscle tonicity can occur. The use of anticonvulsants in pregnant epileptics also increases the risk of congenital anomalies during the first trimester (e.g., valproic acid may cause spina bifida), and may cause behavioral problems in infants exposed to them in utero. The risk of congenital anomalies from psychotropic exposure is low during the second trimester. However, the effect of the exposure to psychotropics on brain and behavior is unclear. So despite ECT being a relatively "high risk" procedure in pregnancy, it may be safer for the fetus than drugs.

Clinicians unfamiliar with ECT find it difficult, however, to reconcile the images from *One Flew Over the Cuckoo's Nest* and *The Snake Pit* with "safe and effective," let alone a treatment of choice. Some facts are:

1. The death rate from ECT is about 10% of the death rate of normal childbirth, or about 1/100,000 treatments.
2. The electrical current is delivered only to the head, and unlike cardioconversion you can safely hold a patient who is getting ECT. The electricity from ECT never effects the fetus who, therefore, does not have a seizure.[44]
3. The amount of anesthetic that crosses the blood-brain barrier each treatment (about 6-8 treatments are usual) is minimal and has no teratogenic or other adverse effects.
4. The depolarizing muscle relaxant used in ECT, succinylcholine may not even cross the placenta and the fetus is not breathing anyway. The mother's blood oxygen saturation will be higher during ECT than when she spontaneously breathes because during ECT she breathes 100% oxygen.
5. Pregnant epileptics having spontaneous grand mal seizures almost never have fetal problems (e.g., spontaneous abortion) directly related to seizure, and the convulsions with ECT are reduced to the point of minimal muscle activity.

On the other hand, a pregnant woman who is depressed and psychotic may need more than an antidepressant alone. Although the use of antidepressants in the second and third trimester is reasonably safe, the use of antipsychotics is less so. The combination also takes longer to work and has more side effects and potential adverse effects (e.g., agranulocytosis) than does ECT. Also, if Patient 3-9 plans to breastfeed, these medications will be secreted in breast milk and will be ingested by her baby. Continuation ECT during the 6 months post-acute treatment course is thus also safer for her baby.

The clinical challenge in treating a pregnant woman who is depressed is the balance between risk and benefit. In a nonpregnant depressed woman, particularly one with a severe depression, ECT is clearly the best antidepressant treatment in terms of efficacy and safety. In a woman over 20 weeks pregnant, ECT is considered a "high risk" procedure because of the likelihood that despite being NPO after midnight the patient will still have food in her stomach and might aspirate. Intubation also carries risk. So, under this circumstance, antidepressant medication may be safer for the mother, although ECT still has the better efficacy. The question is, "Is this increased risk of ECT to the mother *outweighed* by the risk of medication to the fetus, and how much better is ECT than drugs under the clinical circumstances at hand?" If we are guided by studies in nonhumans, we must conclude that the risks to the fetus exposed to medications is about the same as the risk to the fetus whose mother is getting ECT. ECT is clearly more effective. Therefore, ECT is the treatment of choice.

If we were to be guided by only studies in humans, we would conclude that other than lithium, anticonvulsants, and perhaps antipsychotics, the risk to the fetus is small enough to make the ECT risk to the mother too high, and that antidepressants become acceptable choices (see endnote 45 for a discussion of these studies). We have chosen to take into consideration nonhuman studies because Murphy's Law convinces us that whereas we can manage the risks to the mother, we cannot prevent the antidepressant drug entering the developing fetal brain, and Murphy's Law says "Bad things will happen in proportion to the importance for them not to happen." In the final analysis, if that fetus had our genes, we would not want it exposed to the drugs, and that is the guideline we use for patients.

Patient 3-10: To Treat or Not to Treat? That's the Trick Question

A 75-year-old man is referred to you by his internist. He told the internist that he was anxious and worried about his wife, who was recently diagnosed as having Alzheimer's disease. Patient 3-10 says because his own health is not what it once was, he is extremely concerned about who will care for his wife. His children live 1500 miles away and cannot help. He says he sometimes is so worried that he cannot sleep or eat. He denies depression. He does, however, feel lonely, because several of his friends have died and he has no one to talk to.

Is Patient 3-10 depressed, despite his statements to the contrary?

> Studies show that the elderly depressed respond to good treatment just as well as do younger patients.[45]

Patient 3-10 has no sustained clinical signs and symptoms of depression. His occasional problems with sleep and loneliness are most likely normal reactions to his stress. There is no duck here.

Does Patient 3-10 need treatment?

This is the trick of the question. Patient 3-10 does not need antidepressant medication -- but he is a patient who feels "out of sorts" and has come to a physician for help. He needs some help. When a physician helps a patient -- that's treatment!

Patient 3-10 needs reassurance that his symptoms are a normal reaction to what he is going through. He needs to be educated about Alzheimer's disease and what is in store for him and his wife in the future. Various support groups may also be helpful.

What is Patient 3-10's longer-term prognosis?

Patient 3-10 needs to be followed because the caregivers of Alzheimer's patients are at increased risk for depression. A kind word now and then is part of good medical care.

Patient 3-11: Bereaved, Bothered and Bewildered

A 45-year-old woman is admitted for depression following her mother's death from cancer 10 days before. Patient 3-11 says she not only lost her mother, but her best friend. She reports feeling sad and crying whenever she thinks of her mother, but can cheer up at other times. She says she has not slept well for the last 10 days, and does not feel like eating but eats to keep up her strength. She denies any suicidal ideation, and says she came to the hospital because she has no one to talk to. She has never married and quit her job as an accountant six months before to care for her ailing mother. She has no friends and is upset with her two brothers because they did not help their mother. She was hospitalized once for a week about three years ago with similar complaints following a quarrel with her roommate. She has no other psychiatric history, drug or alcohol problems, and she is in good general medical health.

Does Patient 3-11 have a clinical depression?

Patient 3-11 does not have a major depression. Her mood is cheerful when she does not think of her mother, and she recognizes that she is lonely and in mourning. She is neither suicidal nor psychotic, and it has only been 10 days since her mother's death. This duck is bereavement. *Table 3.11* displays some of the features of *abnormal bereavement*, which is a DSM way of saying clinical depression triggered by the death of a loved one.

Table 3.11 Abnormal Bereavement
Unable to resume all or most of daily responsibilities
A melancholic pattern in mood and vegetative signs
Suicide attempt
Psychosis
Continued poor functioning after 2 months

What is Patient 3-11's prognosis?

Although bereaved, Patient 3-11 has some red flags. Persons in mourning usually do not come to a hospital, so her response is at least excessive. Patient 3-11 might meet criteria for adjustment disorder (another DSM choice), and she has had a previous episode that sounds like it might have been an adjustment disorder. Persons with multiple adjustment disorders of a depressive pattern either have an underlying personality disorder or a mood disorder, or both. Patient 3-11 has led an isolated life with few friends, and her dependence on her mother suggests that she might have an anxious-fearful type of personality disorder. Patients with these traits are often at risk for developing nonmelancholic major depression. Patient 3-11's prognosis is guarded.

How can you help Patient 3-11?

Patient 3-11 should be discharged from the hospital as quickly as possible. The longer she is hospitalized, the more chronically dysfunctional she is likely to be. She will likely become dependent on the hospital and seek admission whenever under stress. She needs an empathic listener and follow-up to watch for changes in her sleep, eating, and weight. If she is mourning, her symptoms will improve. If she worsens, she will likely need an antidepressant. Once over the acute phase of her condition (whatever it is), her personality can be assessed and perhaps offered group therapy or cognitive behavior therapy.

Patient 3-12: Down in the Dumps and Shaking Like a Leaf

A 75-year-old former taxi driver is brought to your office by his daughter and son-in-law because he has become increasingly irritable and argumentative over the past several months. She has also found him in his bedroom with the lights out crying. He told her he is "depressed."

On examination Patient 3-12 walks stiffly into your office with small quick steps. He has no facial expression and does not gesture during conversation. He speaks slowly and without vocal tone or inflection. He has a bilateral resting hand tremor and increased muscle tension in all limbs. Cognitively he has problems with working memory (Digit Span backwards), sustained attention (serial 7's subtraction), and new learning (word lists and geometric shapes). He has some word finding problems during conversation and quantitatively performs just in the demented range.

> Whenever possible, greet the patient in the waiting area and walk with the patient to the examining room. During this seemingly informal introduction you can observe gait and other motor behaviors, alertness, language, mood and manner and much more.

Describe Patient 3-12's big picture (the pattern of his diagnostically important clinical features).

Patient 3-12 is a 75-year-old man who over a several month period has developed personality and mood changes (argumentative, irritable, says he is depressed), has motor abnormalities (expressionless face, slow speech, bilateral resting tremor, increased muscle tremor, and abnormal gait), and cognitive impairment.

Did you remember that the patient's gender, age, and type of illness onset are the three important initial diagnostic bits of information? They can dramatically affect the odds of your diagnostic choices.

Patient 3-12 has problems in several areas. Apply the Rule of Parsimony. Can you come up with a single pathophysiology to explain it all?

Apply the Rule of Parsimony. Disturbances in mood, memory and motor function (3M) implicate the 3M company of the brain -- the basal ganglia. So, what condition can do it all? Patient 3-12's clinical features fit the pattern of subcortical (slowing of speech and movement, but no aphasia, agnosia, or apraxia) action brain (motor problems plus problems with attention, working memory and new learning) disease. The most likely diagnosis is Parkinson's disease.

> Parkinson's disease effects 2% of the population and 20% of persons over age 65. Thirty percent of Parkinsonian patients become demented.

Although Patient 3-12 says he is depressed, and, in fact, he is (you would need to get more information to know this), his depression is part of his Parkinson's disease. Fifty percent or more of Parkinson's patients become depressed, and the depression is not correlated with the severity of the motor impairment. Knowing this is important for treatment.

> Depressed mood plus irritability is termed dysphoria.[46]

How can you best help Patient 3-14 and his family?

We phrased the question this way to reinforce the idea that patients do not appear alone before you, like Athena springing fully formed from the forehead of Zeus. Patients typically come with a family, and how you interact with the family is often the key to how well the patient does. In Patient 3-12's case, if his daughter and son-in-law are not satisfied, Patient 3-12 will not do well.

Things that need to be done for Patient 3-12 are:

1. Treat the motor features of Parkinson's disease. Levodopa/carbidopa is still the standard. Bromocriptine might also be added at some point.
2. If the levodopa/carbidopa does not ameliorate the depression, treat the depression. You have two choices here:

   a. *Pharmacotherapy*, applying the same rules of medication selection as previously discussed. In addition to the usual antidepressants, selegiline, an MAO type B inhibitor, which is an antiparkinsonian drug, in doses above 20 mg daily has some antidepressant properties. A transdermal 20 mg patch is preferred.[47]

   b. *ECT*. ECT works for depressions, primary or secondary, and it substantially ameliorates the symptoms of Parkinson's disease even in Parkinson's patients who are not depressed. Because of the combination of symptoms and Patient 3-12's age, ECT is our first choice.[48]

119

3. Educate the patient and his family about treatments and the progress of the disease. Help his daughter organize her household so Patient 3-12 will be able to go home and remain there (rather than a nursing home) as long as possible. We will discuss behavioral strategies for demented patients in Chapter 7 with neuropsychiatric syndromes.

Discussion

A typical response to hearing a story like that of Patient 3-12 is "well, of course he's depressed. Wouldn't anyone who had a debilitating brain disease?" Also, he is now living with his daughter's family, and perhaps his loss of independence and the death of his wife have made him gloomy. Perhaps he does not get along with his son-in-law, and that makes him irritable. All of this is true and can contribute to a patient's distress, BUT it does not change the implications of his clinical signs and symptoms. If a patient is clinically depressed, regardless of your interpretation as to why, he needs treatment. Check out Patient 3-13 for an example of what can happen if this principle is ignored.

Patient 3-13: War is Depressing

A 40-year-old ex-Naval chaplain during the Vietnam era is admitted for treatment of posttraumatic stress disorder (PTSD) of many years duration.[49] The treatment program is of several months' duration and consists of group and individual sessions that assume a psychological explanation for PTSD. The chaplain's friend (another ex-chaplain) feels his friend's condition is more serious and asks if a consultant will see him. The consultant finds the chaplain to be moderately slow in speech, subdued, and anxious. Patient 3-13 expresses feeling isolated and helpless. He says he often ruminates about sailors he should have helped. He blames himself for the bad things that happened to many of the sailors. He is unable to sleep because of his worries and has nightmares about what happened to people he was "responsible for." He has no appetite and over the past year has lost 20 pounds. He says the future is "not important" to him. His general medical health is good.

What is wrong with Patient 3-13?

Patient 3-13 is melancholic.

> About 2-4% of the population is at lifetime risk for melancholia (20% of all depressions). Untreated, 50% will slowly recover over 9 months, but 20% kill themselves. Half or more have more than one episode. Ten percent are bipolar.

What should the consultant do?

The consultant told Patient 3-13 that he was melancholic and that he needed to be treated. The consultant said he would speak with the PTSD treaters and arrange for a transfer to the psychiatric unit, where Patient 3-13 could get treated. He strongly recommended this. Patient 3-13 said he was committed to his PTSD treaters, and if they okayed the transfer, he would go, but otherwise he would stay on the PTSD unit. He said he did not "doubt" the consultant's opinion, but his present treaters were experts and said he had PTSD.

> With appropriate medication treatment and behavioral management, 60-70% of melancholics obtain a marked response or remission over 2 months. With appropriate ECT, 90% of melancholics obtain a marked response or remission with 6-8 treatments (2-3 weeks).

The consultant called the treaters, told them his opinion and urged them to transfer Patient 3-13 to the psychiatric unit, because he felt Patient 3-13 had a high suicide risk. The PTSD treaters declined, and Patient 3-13 went back to the PTSD program, where a week later he hanged himself and died.

Discussion

Treatment units dedicated to one diagnostic category (e.g., PTSD, epilepsy, mood disorder) can develop tunnel vision and only see "their thing." Sometimes, when a patient does not have "the thing," discharge quickly follows, not because the patient no longer needs hospitalization, but because the specialized program's interest is not in finding out what is wrong with the patient and then treating the patient for that condition, but rather in finding out if the patient has "the thing" they are interested in and treating that condition.

In Patient 3-13's situation, his depression was minimized and considered secondary to "the thing," in this case PTSD. But even so, his treaters violated the principle that a duck is a duck is a duck. For whatever reason, Patient 3-13 was depressed, and depressed patients sometimes kill themselves. Those indisputable facts should have guided treatment, not presumed etiology.

Patient 3-14: Getting Our Acts Together

A 58-year-old man complains of loss of energy and interest in his work over the past 3-4 months. He is fearful of losing his job because with his depression, he cannot function well at work and has become nonproductive. He says he cannot stay asleep. He has lost 15 pounds in the past two months. Although he was treated for a similar condition when he was 38, he attributes the present episode to his mother's death a year ago.

On examination, he appears anxious and mildly agitated. He constantly asks for reassurance. He feels that he is of no use to anyone and should just die. He says, however, that he has no plans of hurting himself.

What are the guidelines for evaluating Patient 3-14's depression as secondary?

Your evaluation for a secondary syndrome focuses on a) *typicality of presentation* (Patient 3-14's is typical); b) *typicality of course* (Patient 3-14 has had a typical course with a previous similar episode with apparently good interepisode function; c) *when other etiologically meaningful conditions co-occur* (e.g., drug abuse)*, which came first, those conditions or the syndrome* (Patient 3-14 has no co-occurring conditions); d) *family history (*looking for less ambiguous diagnostic patterns in first-degree relatives); e) *laboratory studies* (asking for specific etiologic suspects). *Table 3.12* displays the suspects you would think about for Patient 3-14, and *Table 3.13* displays the laboratory findings observed in primary melancholia. Patient 3-14 has no evidence of any secondary etiology, other than the possibility of normal bereavement. So why is bereavement not the diagnosis? It cannot be normal bereavement because Patient 3-14 is depressed now and his mother died a year ago -- the DSM cut-off is 2 months.

Table 3.12 Secondary Suspects for Patient 3-14's Depression

Suspect	Comments
Stroke	Cardiovascular disease below the neck predicts cardiovascular disease above the neck. Small basal ganglia strokes are relatively common and are often missed clinically.
Medication	Antihypertensives among many drugs can induce a depression that will occur shortly after the drug is introduced or dose raised to moderate to high levels.
Space occupying lesion	Subdural hematomas, vascular malformations, and neoplasms (incidence is rising in persons 40-60), particularly if frontal areas involved.
Seizure disorder	40% of epileptics develop clinical depression.
Endocrinopathy	Hypothyroidism and Cushing's disease most likely.
Autoimmune disease	Anything that can cause vasculitis can result in a mood disorder.

Table 3.13 Laboratory Findings Observed in Primary Melancholia [50]

Laboratory Measure	Findings
Brain imaging	Mildly enlarged ventricles and "atrophy" with smaller temporal lobes, caudate and putamen. Ventricular enlargement may return to normal with clinical improvement.
Brain metabolism	Decreased metabolism (hypoperfusion or decreased signal intensity) mostly frontally and in some patients L>R and in the caudate; returns to normal with clinical improvement.
Brain information processing	Increased latencies (slower) on evoked potential, some nonspecific slowing on EEG; both return to normal with clinical improvement
Sleep studies	Distorted architecture: shortened REM latency and reduced REM total time and density, loss of stages III and IV sleep.
Hypothalamic-pituitary function	The system is in "overdrive," so hormone releases are elevated, resulting in blunted growth hormone response to stimulants, nonsuppression of cortisone to dexamethasone, high TSH levels and blunted response to TRH.
Circadian rhythms	Phase shifted so that body temperature, cortisol release is higher rather than lower in dawn hours.
Cognition	Problems with attention and concentration; verbal and nonverbal new learning, slowed thinking (bradyphrenia) and poor problem solving in the pattern and range of a frontal lobe dementia.

What additional information do you need to know about Patient 3-14 to properly treat him?

1. *Comorbidities*

   a. *DSM States of illness (Axis I):* Alcohol and substance abuse (Patient 3-14 is not an abuser, although 40% of bipolar patients are); anxiety disorders (Patient 3-14 does not have anxiety disorder, although a substantial number of nonmelancholics may).
   b. *DSM personality disorders (Axis II):* Anxious-fearful personality disorder (Patient 3-14 did not have a personality disorder, although 40-60% of nonmelancholic [particularly dysthymics] do).
   c. *DSM general medical conditions (Axis III):* Any condition that can interfere with the pharmacokinetics of your planned treatment, or medications the patient takes that can cause adverse drug-drug interactions (Patient 3-14 is in good general medical health and not taking any medication regularly, except a daily baby aspirin).

2. *Psychosis or catatonia.* Melancholics are more likely to be psychotic (30%) or catatonic (5-10%) than are other depressed patients. These melancholics do not respond any better to a single antidepressant than to placebo, forcing polypharmacy. ECT works better for these patients.
3. *Bipolarity.* Melancholics are also more likely than nonmelancholic patients to be bipolar. They will need either ECT or a mood stabilizer along with an antidepressant. Patient 3-14 is unipolar.

What would be your general short- and long-term plans for treating Patient 3-14?

1. Because he has had two episodes, the last in late middle age, Patient 3-14 is likely to have more episodes unless acute and continuation treatment is followed by maintenance treatment. He needs all the legs of the three legged stool: acute treatment, maintenance of remission, and prophylaxis to prevent future episodes.
2. *Acute treatment goals.* Patient 3-14 is at high suicide risk: melancholic, older person, male, anxious and agitated, feels he should die. Hospitalization is the best choice followed by either vigorous drug treatment or ECT. The goal after suicide prevention is to get him *all* better.

Goals: Suicide prevention
        Full remission

3. *Continuation treatment.* To maintain the remission and
    prevent relapse, Patient 3-14 will need interpersonal support,
    and help to preserve his job. He will also likely need help with
    social supports as it sounds like he has few persons he can
    rely on. You become that person.

Goals: Maintain remission
        Prevent relapse
        Preserve job
        Interpersonal support

4. *Maintenance.* To prevent future episodes, Patient 3-14 will
    need to be on medication indefinitely. Any stressors that might
    precipitate an episode also need to be dealt with. A
    dexamethasone suppression test (DST) may be helpful in
    predicting relapse. (For a detailed discussion of the
    dexamethasone test, see endnote 51).[51]

Goals: Prevent future episodes
        Reduce or manage life stressors
        Continued job and social support

Quick Rounds

1. A 60-year-old man takes 300 mg of desipramine daily for maintenance treatment of a recurrent depressive illness. He complains of recent increased dysphoria (sadness and irritability) and restlessness. Because the patient is on a high dose of desipramine, fluoxetine 20 mg daily is added. A month later the patient is confused, has parathesias and myoclonic jerks. What happened?

2. A 36-year-old depressed woman was given 20 mg paroxetine. After 4 weeks her response was minimal and her dose was increased to 30 mg. Over the next 3 months her dose was raised to 50 mg, but treatment response was at best moderate. What didn't happen?

3. A 40-year-old depressed man is receiving sertraline 100 mg daily. Although his depression begins to improve he complains of dizziness when arising in the morning and after being seated or lying down for prolonged periods. His medication is reduced to 50 mg daily. What happened next, and how could it have been avoided?

4. A 49-year-old man has a nonpsychotic, first-episode major depression. He is not suicidal. He has no drug or alcohol history, and no family history of depression or alcohol or substance dependence. He is given fluoxetine 20 mg daily, which is increased to 40 mg daily. After 8 weeks, he reports about an 80% improvement, but still would like to get back to his old self. What do you do?

5. A 75-year-old man with a history of post-stroke depression repeatedly refers to his female psychiatrist as "my lovely lady doctor." What should the woman doctor do?

6. A 29-year-old man with a past nonmelancholic depression and a diagnosis of narcissistic personality disorder (self-absorbed and manipulative) often comments on his female psychiatrist's appearance and the color of her eyes. What should the woman doctor do?

7. A 50-year-old man has a chronic depression, characterized by constant fatigue, difficulty concentrating and sleeping too much. He says that most of his gloominess is from his not being able to be active. He says he has been this way for the last two years. Before his depression, he was very active. He loved the outdoors, and he misses his annual camping trips with his children. He has no past personal or family history of psychiatric illness. His internist says he is

127

in good general medical health. What has happened to this man?
(This is a hard one.)

8. A 55-year-old man with a long history of recurrent depression has
been stable on imipramine 150 mg PO qhs for the last 7 years. He
has no general medical problems (including a normal size prostate)
and has no side effects. He is assigned to a new 4th-year resident,
who tapers the imipramine, and begins sertraline because the latter
has a "better side effect profile." Six weeks later the patient is
hospitalized with a melancholic depression. How could this
depression have been avoided?

9. A 46-year-old woman, former truck driver in the 1990 Gulf War, is
anxious and agitated and has had chronic back muscle aches since
her return from the war. She has not been sleeping or eating well,
and has lost 15 pounds in the last 4 years. She has not been able to
work since her return. She feels she is living like an invalid, and
sometimes gets so frustrated that she does not wish to live. She
ruminates about the unsanitary conditions in the war and the
possibility of being exposed to chemicals. She feels her concentration
and memory are poor. She is married and has two adult children, but
has not been getting along with her family. What is the "best"
diagnosis for this patient and why?

10. A 33-year-old woman is started on nortriptyline, 100 mg daily, three
days ago. Her blood level today is 45 ng/ml (therapeutic range for
most depressed patients is 50-150). What does this level mean, and
what would you do about it?

11. A 33-year-old pregnant woman (in her tenth week of pregnancy) with
a history of recurrent depressions is again experiencing a severe
melancholic episode. She also hears voices telling her that her baby
is dead. Which antidepressant should you use?

Quick Rounds Answers

1. Fluoxetine increased desipramine levels by inhibiting CYP2D6 microsomal enzymes, and the patient became toxic (desipramine level was 400 ng/ml units). Fluoxetine interferes with many medications and is not a good choice when polypharmacy is likely.

2. Less than a third of depressed patients who show zero response to medication in one week and less than 20% of patients who show a zero response in 2-3 weeks subsequently respond to medication. Overall, only 65-70% show a marked response to remission in 4-8 weeks to medications. Limited by the general medical health of the patient and tolerance to side effects, you need to maximize your first-choice drug as soon as you can. There is no excuse for an acute depressed patient remaining essentially no better for months. If there is no response despite maximum dose of your first choice drug, think of ECT (why should your second choice drug work better than your first?!). If there is only a partial response after 2-3 weeks at maximum dose steady state of your first choice, add a new drug.

3. When a medication is working and a side effect develops, try to resolve the side effect; do not first change or lower the medication. The patient quickly relapsed. His orthostasis (did you recognize the side effect?) could have been managed by 1) instruction on how to change positions, 2) wearing support hose, and for the elderly also an abdominal binder, and 3) 1-2 cups of strong coffee in the morning. A little latte goes a long way.

4. Increase the dose further because he has shown steady improvement without substantial side effects. Although the majority of patients who respond to fluoxetine do so at 20 mg daily, some may need 60-80 mg daily. As long as the patient is improving and tolerating the medication, maximize the dose.

5. You can rarely teach old dogs new tricks, particularly after they have had strokes. What is important here is not getting the patient to be politically correct, but maintaining a therapeutic doctor-patient relationship. If his characterization of her is not overly offensive to her and if it is said in an paternal manner, the best therapeutic response might be to ignore it, or kid around with the patient (depending on his personality). Persons with brain disease get more slack when their behavior is not 100% up to code.

6. This patient's personal comments, unlike those of the man in number 5, are likely driven by personality traits not illness. More importantly, they may interfere with the doctor-patient relationship and are likely examples of the way this patient treats other people. Although unlikely to substantially change his personality, his psychiatrist is obliged to make the effort, so it would be important to not ignore the comments, but to use them to point out how the patient messes up his relationships with others.

7. Constant fatigue for two years as the primary feature of a depression in a 50-year-old without previous psychiatric disorder is atypical. Atypical means secondary until proven otherwise. For this patient, the clue is camping trips. What can you get on a camping trip that could cause a depressive-like syndrome with fatigue? Something tic-borne? You bet![52]

8. The resident violated the principle "If it ain't broke, don't fix it." Imipramine is a good antidepressant. Its substantial anticholinergic and cardiac conduction properties (only at high dosages), however, make it less suitable for elderly patients or patients whose general medical health contradicts the use of such drugs. This patient was doing great. Don't treat by ideology or theory or drug company advertising; treat by common sense and empirical data.

9. Being in a war is stressful, although to meet the diagnosis of post-traumatic stress disorder (PTSD) a person needs to have been in combat or experienced other intense stress (e.g., assigned to burial detail or working in a burn unit). Even if she also had intrusive thoughts or avoidant behavior consistent with PTSD, she also has the duck of depression. No prior behavioral problems in a 46-year-old (onset age 37) makes personality disorder unlikely. Patients who are chronically depressed often have interpersonal problems, and chronic depression may masquerade as personality disorder. Stress often precipitates major mood disorder.

10. Although this patient's blood levels appear to be less than therapeutic, we cannot increase the dose because the drug has not yet reached a steady state level. It takes about 5 half-lives to reach a steady state (i.e., the dose at which the absorption and excretion of the medication are the same) and the blood levels are constant. For nortriptyline it would be 5-7 days. So a blood level in 2-4 more days will help decide if the patient needs further increases.

11. Treatment choice is determined by efficacy (overall response and speed of response) and any specific general medical condition or

situation. All psychopharmacologic agents that are used to treat depression have a 1-2 week latency period, cross the placenta, are secreted in breast milk, and alone are ineffective in treating psychotic depression. Although the concentration of antidepressant in breast milk is lower than in maternal blood and side effects are rare, the lactation itself is inhibited by SSRI and MAO inhibitors. There are reports of irritability in infants whose mothers were on SSRIs. Systematic literature reviews do not reveal an increase in fetal abnormalities in children of mothers on psychotropics. Evidence from nonhumans and anecdotal reports warrant careful evaluation of risks versus benefits. The only antidepressant treatment that is effective in psychotic depression, works fast, and is safe in pregnancy is electroconvulsive therapy. This woman should receive ECT.

Chapter 4

Bipolar Mood Disorder

Patient 4-1: A Wolf in Sheep's Clothing

A 50-year-old man goes to his HMO generalist because of sleep problems, low energy, decreased appetite and a 10-pound weight loss over a period of several months. In the office the patient is subdued, soft-spoken, and slow in movement. The generalist quickly rules out any general medical problems, and concludes that the man is depressed. The generalist begins treatment with sertraline 50 mg HS for 3 days and 100 mg HS thereafter with an appointment in 30 days.

Ten days later the patient's wife storms into the generalist's office, shakes her finger under his nose, and informs him she will be suing him and the HMO for all their worldly goods.

What likely happened to anger Patient 4-1's wife?

This is a chapter on bipolar disorder. The generalist didn't ask about past manias (none) or hypomanias (several). A few days following the dose increase of sertraline, Patient 4-1 became energized and cheerful. He said he had never felt better and began to make several questionable business plans. He constantly spoke about these plans and became irritable if interrupted. He began to experience "waves" of euphoria and ideas that he had special powers. Several days later he was arrested by federal agents at O'Hare airport, where he was found on a runway, naked except for a red straw hat, trying to direct air traffic.

Will her suit be successful?

Antidepressants can induce mania in bipolar patients, especially if they are not receiving a mood stabilizer. Failure to inquire about mania resulted in the patient getting manic and was in a situation that resulted in his arrest. A good lawyer for the patient can make a good case for negligence.

Patient 4-1 became manic. Although the generalist had inquired about Patient 4-1's previous depressions (he had two others) and other psychiatric hospitalizations, he did not know about *bipolar II disorder* and so never discovered that Patient 4-1 had periods of hypomania.

Although the depressions in bipolar and unipolar disorder are often indistinguishable, the former is more often associated with hypersomnia (>9 hours of poor sleep), weight gain and occurrence during the winter. Look for seasonality and reversed vegetative signs.[1]

133

During these hypomanias Patient 4-1 was very productive, and so he perceived these states as his normal best. Subsequent inquiry revealed that when hypomanic he needed only 4-5 hours of sleep nightly, was hypersexual (to the annoyance of his wife), and at times inappropriately outgoing.

Not knowing is no legal excuse. Like all depressed patients with a bipolar II disorder, Patient 4-1 required coverage with a mood stabilizing drug (see Appendix 2, *Psychopharmacology at a Glance*). If mildly depressed, he might have done well with a mood stabilizer alone. If he had a more severe depression, then standard practice is to use a mood stabilizer and an antidepressant simultaneously. This is one of the rare instances where polypharmacy is appropriate early on in treatment. About 10% of bipolar patients who are depressed will spontaneously swing into a mania or hypomania. When treated with an antidepressant alone about 30% swing into a mania. Tricyclic antidepressant (TCA) drugs are more likely to do this than are SSRI agents. The assertion that bupropion is least likely to do this is not substantiated by controlled studies. We still prefer the broader spectrum antidepressants for the bipolar patient who is depressed, because we want the best results. We can minimize the potential of switching to mania or hypomania by giving the TCA with a mood stabilizer.

What mistakes, if any, did the generalist make?

Let us count the ways!

> Knowing what you do not know is okay--you can look it up or get a consultation. Not knowing your areas of ignorance is dangerous.

1. Treating patients without an adequate knowledge base
2. Not scheduling a follow-up visit within 7-10 days, a critical time in treatment for depression (see chapter 3)
3. Giving Patient 4-1 a prescription for a thirty-day supply of sertraline 100 mg, which totals 3000 mg. Although, according to the manufacturer, when used alone, sertraline in doses up to 6000 mg have not been lethal, deaths have been reported if the drug is used in combination with other drugs or alcohol.
4. Not scheduling daily phone rounds during the first several days of treatment to monitor symptoms and side effects, if any. The unfolding mania might have been caught early and treated before Patient 4-1 got into trouble.

5. Not discussing with the patient's wife the treatment plan and the possibility of a manic switch. She might have told the generalist about her husband's hypomanias.

Discussion

Bipolar patients can have extremely variable clinical presentations and illness courses. When treating any depressed patient, you must make certain they are not bipolar. Bipolar disorder should be treated by experts. *Table 4.1* displays bipolar behaviors that are often overlooked by treaters and patients until it is too late. These are referred to as the "soft bipolar spectrum."

Table 4.1. The Soft Bipolar Spectrum	
Cyclothymia	A mild life-long pattern of gradual mood swings lasting weeks or months without discrete episodes of illness. During the "ups" these people are extroverted, outgoing, cheerful, optimistic, impulsive, restless, hard working and driven, talkative, and uninhibited. They need less sleep and have increased sex drive. During the "downs" they are moody, irritable, short-tempered, lethargic, hypersomnic, taciturn, inactive, shy, unsure, pessimistic, and slow in thinking.
Hyperthymic	Over-talkative, extroverted, uninhibited, overly optimistic, restless, meddlesome, vigorous, needs less sleep, bombastic, cheerful, irritable, stubborn. As children they are misdiagnosed as having attention deficit disorder, and stimulants do not help or make them worse. Thus, some childhood history of ADHD may reflect a bipolar disorder.
Dysthymic	Hypersomnolent, brooding, anhedonic, self-blaming, passive, indecisive, irritable; no "up" period
Borderline personality disorder (50% meet DSM criteria for mood disorder)	Impulsivity, risk taking, recklessness, mood fluctuations with intense episodic dysphoria, irritability and anxiety, periods of excitement and histrionics, abuse of drugs and alcohol
Hypomania	Periods of increased energy, thoughts, activities, and speech with decreased sleep and increased appetitive behaviors that verge on dysfunction to mild dysfunction depending on tolerance of the social setting; no "down" period

Choosing an antidepressant for a bipolar patient who is presently depressed follows the same rules as choosing an antidepressant for a unipolar patient. The difference in management is that a mood stabilizing drug is also given. These include lithium, valproic acid, and carbamazepine. For a mild to moderate depression, mood stabilizers alone may be sufficient, but moderate to severe depressions need an antidepressant.

The evidence still favors lithium as the mood stabilizer of choice for the bipolar II patient. It is a better antidepressant and augmenter of antidepressants than other mood stabilizers. It is still the best antimanic agent for pure manic states, and it is the only psychotropic that has been shown to reduce suicide rates. About 50% of bipolar II patients will make a suicide attempt sometime during their lifetime, and they may have the highest completed suicide rates of all patients with mood disorder.

Lamotrigine, a newer anticonvulsant mood stabilizer, has been recently recommended for bipolar depression. However, because lamotrigine requires a dose build-up over 4-6 weeks to reach a therapeutic dose while trying to avoid its propensity to induce a serious rash and possibly Stevens-Johnson's syndrome, it is an impractical antidepressant or mood stabilizer if the patient needs rapid resolution of symptoms - - and which patient does not![2]

> Before using lithium, check to make sure the patient's renal function is adequate to excrete it and the patient does not have a cardiac conduction problem that can worsen with lithium. Also get baseline thyroid and parathyroid function studies, as 5-10% of patients on long-term lithium treatment develop hypothyroidism or hypoparathyroidism.[2]

Electroconvulsive therapy (ECT) can also be safely used to treat a bipolar depression for hospitalized patients. If a breakthrough mania does occur while the patient is safely in a hospital, ECT can be continued as the treatment of the mania. It works as well for mania as does medication (80% or more of patients have a good response).[3]

Patient 4-1's physician rushed his care and got into trouble. Blaming the "HMO" for the rush and compromise care is no excuse. Most managed care organizations will shape their monetary guidelines to fit good practice guidelines if the physician can demonstrate the reasonableness of the guidelines. We need to show how, in the long run, our practice guidelines are cost effective and necessary for patient care. Some practice guidelines for treating outpatient bipolar patients are:

1. Follow-up visits need to be about 30 minutes to ensure coverage of symptoms, the medication side effects, and life stressors. If not dealt with, they can precipitate relapse (extra outpatient time is cheaper than hospitalization).
2. Early on, follow-up visits and phone rounds need to be more frequent, perhaps 2-3 office visits the first month, two the

second and then once monthly for the next 4 months. Again, extra outpatient visits are cheaper than hospitalization.

3. Family members need to be involved. An initial meeting with the family, quarterly meetings thereafter for the first 6-12 months and your availability if needed, can help reduce relapse. Whenever possible, make the family your ally. They can be the extension of your eyes, ears and hands. Some programs for bipolar patients have family support groups. These can be very helpful in educating family members, reducing their anxieties, and giving them useful care-giver strategies others have used. These strategies will reduce family members' tendencies toward creating a too intense emotional environment (termed *expressed emotion*), a contributing factor in patient relapse.

Patient 4-2: Fast Food Chef

A 45-year-old man is hospitalized for pouring gasoline on the floor of a crowded fast food restaurant and trying to ignite it, saying he was a better cook than the restaurant's cooks are. He is brought to the hospital by the police. He has persecutory and grandiose delusions, pressured speech, is agitated and irritable and has a long history of bipolar mood disorder with poor interepisode functioning. You are called to see him. He denies illness and refuses hospitalization and treatment.

Can Patient 4-2 be admitted against his will?

Yes. Civil commitment requires the signature of a licensed physician, sometimes two physicians, on the right form. To make the commitment stick and not get into trouble, the patient should

1. Have a psychiatric illness
2. Show indications of imminent (the next few days or so) dangerousness to himself or others, *or* because of his psychiatric illness, is unable to provide his own basic health needs to guard against serious harm (e.g., too delusional to take required insulin).

Patient 4-2 was preparing to set a dangerous fire. He is psychotic and has poor judgment because of it. He can be committed.

Can Patient 4-2 be treated against his will?

Yes. You can and must begin appropriate treatment in an emergency or crisis. Not to do so is negligence.[4] To treat a patient against his will, you need to document the following:

1. He has a serious psychiatric disorder that is unlikely to resolve on its own quickly.
2. Because of his psychiatric disorder he is 1) deteriorating in function (e.g., not eating or drinking), 2) suffering (e.g., in discomfort from a dystonia), 3) threatening

> From a medical-legal perspective, the chart is everything. If you did a great job and did not record it, it never happened. Your charting should reflect what your thinking was, what you did and what happened as a result of it. If you decide you have to treat a patient involuntarily, your notes should reflect your commitment reasoning.

(e.g., verbally abusive and saying he will harm you or someone), 4) disruptive (e.g., excitement and hyperactivity that frightens other patients and staff).
3. Your proposed treatment outweighs any potential risks (e.g., he needs an antipsychotic or a mood-stabilizing drug, despite their common side effects).
4. He lacks the capacity to make a reasoned decision about the treatment (e.g., a patient had the delusion that psychotropics are poisons designed by the same persons who are putting thoughts into his head).
5. Less restrictive care does not work (e.g., he cannot be talked out of his psychosis).
6. You have made a good-faith effort to determine if the patient has executed a health care power of attorney and, if so, you have tried to contact that person.

Discussion

Manic patients are often irritable and can be violent and dangerous. Trying to talk them into voluntary admission and treatment sometimes does not work. About 25% of bipolar patients, even when recovered, do not recognize or remember the psychopathology of past manic episodes.[5] They may recall the consequences of the mania (e.g., the police came to the house), but not the mania. Nonrecognition of illness, anosognosia, can lead to refusal of admission and treatment.

We have listed the legal guidelines for you, but there is another overriding one. These legal guidelines are created to protect the patient's best interests. If by interpreting them too rigidly, we end up not doing what is in the patient's best interest, then we fail in our responsibility. Interpret the law to meet that responsibility. The concept behind this guideline is termed *beneficence*. For example, although a depressed man denies suicidal ideation, if by your evaluation you determine that if not hospitalized the man is a high risk for suicide, then you must hospitalize him with or without his consent. Beneficence is your obligation to help patients based on your medical knowledge. Interpreting the rules rather than rigidly applying them, is also supported by the concept of *therapeutic privilege*. Therapeutic privilege is your professional rationale for forgoing detailed explanations under certain circumstances. For example, you do not emphasize the details of a rare side effect when taking a medication is clearly in a patient's best interest. Another example is forgoing discussion about treatments during unsafe or critical situations so that you can treat the patient according to your medical knowledge. You must document in detail your rationale for exercising your therapeutic privilege. Therapeutic privilege is not an ironclad protection, but it gives you some legal cover to do what is medically right.

Go to court if you must to get the treatments you know to be best. Always try to include family members in your decision making. Make them allies. Document your thinking and their concurrence in the chart. More frequent and successful malpractice suits against a physician occur from a physician's not doing the right thing because of fears of legal restraints or consequences, than from the physician's "pushing the envelope" in doing the right thing.

Clinical practice is shaped by ethical, legal, and moral imperatives. If you believe you are on solid moral ground, any ethical and legal issues usually can be dealt with. If you adhere strictly to ethical and legal concerns, but you believe you are on moral quicksand, you will get into trouble despite your strict adherence to perceived rules.

Patient 4-3: You Can't Stop an Elephant with a BB Gun

A 38-year-old 6 foot 4 inch, 250 pound man is admitted in an acute excitement state. His mood is labile, rapidly shifting from euphoria to irritability. He feels he is chosen by universal forces to rule the world. He shouts angrily and points threateningly at the staff. He has shaved off the right side of his head – both hair and beard. He speaks nonstop and often is unintelligible. Speech content when understood is grandiose. He is in constant motion. He needs to be restrained in the emergency room and is placed in hospital pajamas, given 2 mg lorazepam IM, brought to the acute treatment unit, and placed in a seclusion room out of restraints and under continuous video monitoring. The lorazepam has no apparent effect, and his excitement goes unabated, although he is now restricted to the seclusion room.

What is a reasonable differential diagnosis for Patient 4-3?

Patient 4-3 is psychotic (chosen by universal forces). The differential diagnosis for a middle aged man (he is in good general medical health) in a psychotic excitement (in order of most to least likely) is

1. Mania (primary and secondary)
2. Schizoaffective disorder: manic type
3. Acute drug intoxication: stimulants, phencyclidine, prescription drugs (e.g., L-dopa)
4. Other conditions (catatonic excitement,[6] delirium)

Some clinicians would diagnose him as having schizoaffective disorder, stressing his psychotic rather than mood symptoms. Patients labeled schizoaffective by definition simultaneously have features of mood disorder and psychosis. The psychotic features are prominent, and may last longer than the mood disorder features; the long-term prognosis is not as good as nonpsychotic mood disorder. On the other hand, 30-50% of bipolar patients become chronically ill in some way, so a less than good outcome for patients with a schizoaffective disorder does not distinguish these patients from many bipolar patients. Schizoaffectives in the long run do better than schizophrenics. Although schizoaffectives have first-degree relatives at greater risk for schizophrenia, their relatives are also at greater risk for schizoaffective and mood disorder.[7]

Patient 4-3 does not use street drugs, but a drug screen would be more definitive. He is in good general medical health, and has no evidence of a specific neurologic disease. A delirium is unlikely.

Table 4.2 Acute Treatment of Manic, Mixed, and Hypomanic Episodes [8]			
Clinical Features	Therapeutic Goal	First-line Treatment	Other Alternatives
Mania with psychosis	Control psychosis, induce sleep and sedation, stabilize mood.	First, try loading with mood stabilizer while sedating with a benzodiazepine. Consider bilateral ECT early on. If needed, add an antipsychotic.	Add an antipsychotic early on rather than as a last resort. Sublingual olanzapine followed by oral dosing, or risperidone PO. Haloperidol IM and PO is always a back-up
Severe mania without psychosis	Induce sleep and sedation, stabilize mood.	Add a benzodiazepine to the mood stabilizer; consider ECT (past response or patient preference).	Add an atypical antipsychotic to the mood stabilizer, while discontinuing the benzodiazepine
Euphoric mood or "classic" mania	Induce sleep and sedation, stabilize mood.	Lithium; bilateral ECT (past response or patient's preference)	Valproate, carbamazepine, lithium plus valproate
Mixed episode or dysphoric mood	Induce sleep, stabilize mood.	Valproic acid loading Bilateral ECT	Lithium plus valproate
Rapid cycling	Break the cycle.	Bilateral ECT; valproic acid loading	Lithium plus valproate or lithium, or lithium plus carbamazepine

Table 4.2 displays some guidelines for treating acute mania. With appropriate choice and dosing, most patients will return to their pre-episode baseline within 2-4 weeks.

What should be done first? (This is a trick question.)

Diagnosis, no matter how rapid the process, is always done first. Some assessment of the etiology of Patient 4-3's excitement needs to be done. Assessment of his general medical and neurologic health needs to be done. You can restrain and fully sedate a patient such as Patient 4-3 to get this information because you must quickly rule out any life threatening or permanently disabling conditions. An unconscious patient can be examined for lung and heart disease, blood and urine can be collected, imaging studies can be obtained.

See if Patient 4-3 will agree to take larger doses (preferably IV) of lorazepam. The procedure now is to assemble a uniformed security team to present a "show of force" to the patient with the request that he submit to further sedation. Restraints may be needed, but often even the most excited patients will yield to the show of force. While the security force is present, do at least a minimally acceptable physical examination. Ask the patient for a blood and urine sample to "check" on his general medical health.

What should be done next?

If you find something critical in your assessment, you obviously need to treat it. About 15% of manic episodes are secondary.[9] Thirty to 40% of all hospitalized psychiatric patients, however, have some clinically meaningful general medical problem, so your assessment is likely to find something you need to take care of promptly. If you determine the patient has a primary manic excitement and is in good general medical health, then your next step is to stop the excitement. Manic excitement can lead to injury to the patient or others. When most severe, it looks like a delirium, and if not resolved quickly it can result in cardiovascular collapse and death. In the old days (before the Beatles), this condition was termed *Bell's mania* and prior to modern treatments 50% of such patients died.

For unknown reasons, manics often decorate their heads and wear gaudy hats, bizarre makeup, or oddly cut or shave their head and facial hair. One of the early signs of recovery is when they realize that they look odd and try to even things out.

Discussion

Trying to examine an excited manic is hard and can be dangerous. Nevertheless, it must be done. *Table 4.3* displays some suggestions on how to do this.

Table 4.3. Tactics for Examining an Acute Manic

Many patients will submit to an examination of their "general medical health," even though they deny psychiatric illness and refuse to respond to questions about that (behavioral observations, of course, can simultaneously be made).

Manic distractibility is a big problem: keep the duration of the exam short; get the patient's attention by whispering rather than raising your voice.

Manics are often angry about being hospitalized. Try to link assessment procedures to the goal of discharge as soon as possible.

Make the rules generic to the hospital, not state personal requirements, e.g., rather than "I need to get this done," "the hospital requires every patient to have this."

Link what you do to the patient's general medical complaints - - stretch the link as far as you can.

Link what you do to your concerns for the patient, e.g., "You look like you're having trouble breathing, or you're breathing too fast. I'm worried about that. Let me check that out now."

Conventional dosing strategies rarely break an acute manic excitement. A loading dose strategy is often needed, and *Table 4.4* displays that strategy for mood stabilizers and ECT.

Table 4.4 Loading Dose Strategies [10]

For Electroconvulsive Therapy

Session 1: Two bilateral treatments

Session 2 (if needed) the next day: Two bilateral treatments

Session 3 (rarely needed) the next day or 2 days later: 2 bilateral treatments

Subsequent sessions: A regular ECT schedule of Monday, Wednesday and Friday for a grand total of 12-25 treatments

---

For Mood Stabilizers

Estimate the likely daily dose needed

>For valproic acid 20-30 mg/Kg body weight initial dose

>For lithium 1200-1800 mg daily

If valproic acid is the drug of choice: On day 1 begin with the full calculated valproic acid dose. On day 2 that dose can be maintained or increased by 50%, depending on side effects and therapeutic effect. The day 2 total dose becomes the likely therapeutic dose. If the excitement is broken, you will know in a day or less, and then you give the valproic acid a full therapeutic trial, which is 2 steady state durations following that dose reaching steady state: valproic acid steady state duration is about 5 days. Thus, total duration of trial is 2 days to get to dose, 5 days to steady state, 10 days to see if it works for a total of 17 days. If excitement is not broken in 1-2 days, you need to do something else.

If lithium is the drug of choice

On day 1 begin AM dose of 600 or 900 mg with a meal.

Reevaluate in PM and determine (based on degree of reduced mania or sedation) if an equivalent PM dose can be given and if the patient is okay.

Day 1's total dose is the likely therapeutic dose and you give it a full therapeutic trial. Lithium's steady state duration varies from 4-7 days, depending on hemodynamic factors and kidney function, so the total trial is 1-2 days to get to dose, 7 days to get to steady state, 14 days to see if it works for a total of 23 days. If excitement is not broken in 1-2 days, you need to do something else.

Loading with ECT almost always works to break a mania, but because of the special technical and skill needs involved, ECT is rarely done first. From *Table 4.3* you can see that excitement will likely be broken in 1-2 days. If loading with medication is going to work, you will know it quickly. The acute manic patient will slow down, like a car running out of gas. The loading strategy is to break the excitement. It may still take a week or more to resolve the mania to the point where discharge can be considered.

We have avoided using any antipsychotics until now. This is because a patient in acute excitement might be in a state that makes antipsychotic exposure dangerous. Dehydrated, excited manics are more prone to neuroleptic malignant syndrome (NMS). Young males are prone to severe dystonias. Sometimes, however, antipsychotic use cannot be avoided. If the patient refuses all oral medication and IV valproate cannot be given, and excitement needs to be stopped, an antipsychotic IM is the only remaining choice, and haloperidol 5-10 mg or more may be needed.

If the patient will take oral medication, but not a mood stabilizer, then the oral dissolving form of olanzapine can work rapidly and is preferred over haloperidol in this situation. Once the excitement has been stopped, definitive treatment can begin.

Patient 4-4: When You Scratch a Catatonic, You Tickle a Manic

A 63-year-old woman with a 40 year history of recurrent psychoses characterized by excitement, press of speech, fluctuating intense moods, hypersexuality, and grandiose delusions is once again admitted. She is intrusive, importunate, and in a state of excitement. At other times, she stands for many minutes facing a wall and touching it with her raised palms as if the wall were about to fall. She does not spontaneously speak during these episodes, but can converse if approached. When interviewed, she sits with her legs extended above the floor for many minutes. She often walks on tiptoes as if a ballerina. She is afebrile, and her general medical health is good.

What makes Patient 4-4 catatonic?

Catatonia is a syndrome. The DSM requires 2 or more features, and we would add that their presence should be sustained for an hour or more or that they can be repeatedly elicited by clinical exam. Patient 4-4 exhibited *posturing* (standing for many minutes facing a wall, touching it with raised palms). This is also an example of *catalepsy* (prolonged posturing). She is relatively mute during these episodes. She walks on tiptoes, *stereotypic mannerism*. This is enough to say she has mania with catatonic features.

How would you treat Patient 4-4's catatonia? (This is a trick question.)

Catatonia, regardless of etiology, temporarily responds to IM lorazepam (8-20 mg daily)[11] and almost always definitively responds to bilateral ECT. If you know the specific etiology (e.g., hypothyroidism) and there is a specific treatment for it, catatonia without stupor usually resolves as the underlying condition responds to the specific treatment. In this situation, treat her catatonia by treating her mania.[12]

What are the diagnostic and treatment implications of catatonic features during a manic episode?

Manics with catatonic features are no different from manics without catatonic features in any meaningful, measurable way. Think of these features as a sign of severity, not as indicators of a different kind of mania, or as signs of schizophrenia. Treat the patient for mania. Manics with catatonic features are at greater risk for neuroleptic malignant syndrome (NMS), than are those without such features. Thus, try to avoid antipsychotics. ECT is the fastest, safest, and most parsimonious treatment for this clinical picture, because both catatonia and mania respond well to ECT.

If the catatonia is associated with stupor and immobility and the patient is not eating or drinking, neuroleptic malignant syndrome is even more likely. Do not use an antipsychotic for these patients. Give lorazepam 1-2 mg IM to disinhibit the catatonia enough for the patient to eat and drink before the drug effect wears off, and then give ECT for definitive treatment.

> Be heroic in avoiding antipsychotics. If you cannot and the patient is dehydrated, but otherwise in good general medical health, you can first rapidly run in 500-1000 cc of fluid with glucose and electrolytes and perhaps avoid NMS.

What would be the best treatment for Patient 4-4?

Patient 4-4's catatonic features present no unit or management problem. Thus, she is treated for uncomplicated mania. She is in good general medical health and had never received lithium. She is given lithium and has a full recovery.

Discussion

Among acutely ill psychotic patients, about 10% are admitted with two or more catatonic features. Among manic episodes 15% are associated with catatonic features. Among 100 patients with 2 or more catatonic features, about 50% are bipolar, 25% are unipolar, 15% have a neurologic or general medical condition that causes the catatonia, and 10% have schizophrenia.[13]

The number or combinations of catatonic features do not predict treatment response. Catatonia is a syndrome that is very responsive to lorazepam in the short-run, and ECT as a definitive treatment. If ECT is given, the catatonia often resolves with 1-2 treatments, but a full course is needed to prevent the catatonia from recurring and for treating the underlying condition, usually mania or depression.

Patient 4-5: Faux Sauerbraten and Red Cabbage

A 27-year-old woman is admitted in a moderately serve state of euphoria. Over the past several days she has gone on extravagant spending sprees and has been giving away money to strangers on the street. She has been constantly in motion, needing little sleep. On admission her speech is pressured. She speaks with a theatrical German accent and uses German phrases in her conversation. She lies in bed in odd positions (upper and lower halves of body at right angles). She has automatic obedience (see below). She is afebrile and in good general medical health. She is treated with lithium. When her illness fully resolves, she no longer speaks with a German accent, and has no recollection of doing so. She denies ever being a German speaker.

Does Patient 4-5 have one syndrome or two? (This is a semi-trick question.)

She has two syndromes: mania and catatonia, but the catatonia derives from the mania so it is one process.

How is Patient 4-5's false German accent associated with her odd posture in bed?

Speech (the utterances) is a motor behavior and catatonia is a motor dysregulation syndrome. Manneristic speech is part of the catatonia spectrum. Other catatonic speech disturbances are:

> *Verbigeration/palilalia* -- stereotypic, perseverative utterances
> *Clanging* -- stereotypic utterances associated with sound of the words
> *Prosectic speech* -- speech that slowly diminishes in volume until it becomes a mumbled whisper
> *Mutism* -- no speech or speech only when prompted *(speech-prompt catatonia)*
> *Echolalia* -- repeating the examiner's speech
> *Automatic obedience* is also a catatonic feature. To examine for it you tell the patient to hold on tightly to the arm of a chair or to a bed rail and not to let you lift his arm. Despite repeated directions not to let you do it, light pressure or stroking of the fingers and hand will compel the patient to permit you to lift his arm. Patient 4-5's twisted body is a catatonic posture.

What do you need to consider to plan the continuation and maintenance phases of Patient 4-5's treatment?

1. *For continuation:*

   a. The point in time when Patient 4-8 is in full remission of her symptoms is the end of the acute phase and the beginning of continuation, which for a mania lasts 12 months or more.
   b. The longer Patient 4-5 takes lithium, the better are her chances to remain well. Most patients who stop lithium do so because of the side effects of tremor and weight gain. If the tremor is affecting functioning, treat with beta-adrenergic receptor blockers. Weight gain is best prevented by early education of the patient about the need for diet and exercise.
   c. Patient 4-5's social and job situation cannot be too stormy. The more expressed emotion she experiences from her surroundings, the more she is likely to relapse. Expressed emotion is intense, often critical emotion expressed by significant persons in the patient's life. She will also need to practice good sleep hygiene (see *Table 4.5*), as insufficient sleep may also precipitate relapse.

Table 4.5 Good Sleep Hygiene
Going to sleep and awakening the same times each day (no sleeping in)
Sleeping about 8 hours (less than 6 and more than 9 not optimal for most adults)
No naps after 3:00 p.m. or before noon, and no nap longer than 20-30 minutes
No big meal within the 4 hours before bedtime
No bright light exposure 30 minutes before going to sleep
No work-related activity 30 minutes before going to sleep
Bedrooms for sleep (for sex only if it usually quickly leads to sleep)

2. *For maintenance:*

   a. About 70% of persons who have one mood episode will have others, but most clinicians will taper and stop medications a year after a first episode, if the patient has been asymptomatic during the continuation period. A patient with two episodes within 3 years probably requires some maintenance (2 or so years). A patient with two episodes 10 years apart may not substantially benefit from prolonged treatment because we cannot do better than that. After the third episode, maintenance is lifetime.

b. Some episodes are precipitated by stress. Others occur spontaneously. The former is a better prognostic sign than the latter because it indicates that the illness threshold is high enough that it needs a precipitant to be breached. Also, if stress is a factor in episode occurrence, you must try to reduce the stress and the patient's response to stress to perhaps prevent future episodes. Stress may be reduced through environmental changes (e.g., different job that is less demanding or does not require as long hours), stress management, and biofeedback and other meditative exercises (to reduce the patient's response to stress by training them in various relaxation techniques) and rehabilitative and cognitive psychotherapy that can help set goals and reduce false expectations.[14]

1) *Biofeedback:* signals the patient with a pleasant tone or light when muscle tension or blood pressure are in target range.
2) *Rehabilitative psychotherapy (supportive):* focuses on cognitive and personality strengths and weaknesses, and gradually uses the individual's strength to improve weakness, similar in technique and strategy one uses to rehabilitate a broken arm or leg.
3) *Cognitive psychotherapy:* assumes the perception and handling of life stress is influenced by self-attitudes and self-imposed rules and goals, and that distorted attitudes and unrealistic rules contribute to stress and can be corrected, thus reducing stress
4) *Meditation:* cultures representing over 2 billion people say it works. If it does not hurt, why not?

c. The treatment that works best during the acute phase is almost always the treatment given during the maintenance phase. The treatment given during a successful maintenance phase is almost always the treatment used during the early years of prophylaxis.

What specific things do you need to do when treating a patient with lithium?

1. Before putting a patient on lithium, you need to screen 4 organs:

   The heart. Get a good history; do a good exam. Lithium can worsen conduction defects, specifically sinus arrhythmias that can lead to multiple premature ventricular contractions, T-wave changes and further arrhythmia. Lithium EKG changes can be exacerbated by drug-drug interactions with antidepressants and thiazide.

   The kidneys. Lithium is actively excreted in the proximal tubules so adequate renal function is needed. Creatinine clearance is the best single test of renal function, but the usual urinalysis, BUN, and specific gravity are okay.

   The thyroid.: Get baseline thyroid studies, TSH, T_3, and repeat every year or so. Lithium impedes the release of T_3/T_4 from the thyroid and may also affect production. It can cause a nontoxic goiter and hypothyroidism in about 5% of lithium treated patients, and women seem to be at greater risk.

   The parathyroid. Get baseline serum calcium and parathyroid hormone levels and repeat every year or so. Lithium acts on the parathyroid the same way it acts on the thyroid. Hypoparathyroidism can lead to lethargy and depression, and about 10% of lithium treated patients experience changes in parathyroid function.

2. Watch for toxicity during the acute phase of treatment. Look for coarse tremor (fine tremor early on is a common side effect and not a sign of toxicity), lethargy, confusion, and discolored saliva (lithium is excreted in saliva).
3. Minimize and manage side effects during the early maintenance phase of treatment. Weight gain is the most common side effect and reason for stopping lithium.
4. Periodically evaluate for developing diabetes insipidus (large urinary output with low specific gravity [<10.10], normal blood glucose, low or normal serum sodium, no glucose in urine), and correct if it develops with a potassium sparing diuretic (e.g., triamterene).

> The elderly have a greater distribution of lithium into their brains than do the young, so that blood levels around .6-.8 meq/L suffice.

152

Patient 4-6: "I'm Deprived, That's Why I'm Depraved"

A 36-year-old woman is referred to you for treatment for the latest of her many manic episodes. According to the referring physician, the patient has been tried on all the usual medications and she is still symptomatic. She is now receiving valproic acid 1500 mg, lamotrigine mg, lorazepam 2 mg TID, temazepam 30 mg, olanzapine 10 mg BID, and risperidone 2 mg.

What principle of management was violated?

Patient 4-6 is receiving six psychotropics: two anticonvulsants, two benzodiazepines, and two antipsychotics. Such a regime is at best the sign of physician desperation. There is no evidence that in pharmacotherapy two of a kind beats a single ace. You may double the side effects and risks, but not the therapeutic yield.[15]

What are some of the strategies you can use to try to make sense of Patient 4-6, who is on many medications and does not seem to have responded?

1. Assume a mistake or mistakes have been made in one or more of the following: 1) the syndromal diagnosis, 2) the determination of etiology (primary or secondary), 3) the attention paid to psychiatric, specific neurologic, and general medical co-morbid conditions, 4) the use of medications regarding adequate dose and length of clinical trial, drug-drug interactions, and choice of treatments.

2. The above assumptions require a total re-evaluation. Making a life chart of the patient's episodes and treatments sometimes gives you a big picture. This can clarify what has happened. *Figure 4.1* shows Patient 4-6's life chart.

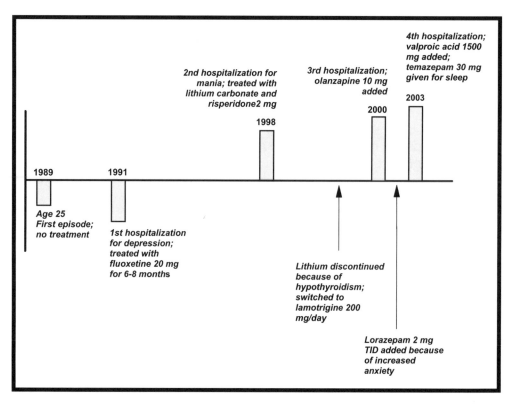

2nd hospitalization for mania; treated with lithium carbonate and risperidone2 mg

1998

4th hospitalization; valproic acid 1500 mg added; temazepam 30 mg given for sleep

3rd hospitalization; olanzapine 10 mg added

2000

2003

1989

1991

Age 25 First episode; no treatment

1st hospitalization for depression; treated with fluoxetine 20 mg for 6-8 months

Lithium discontinued because of hypothyroidism; switched to lamotrigine 200 mg/day

Lorazepam 2 mg TID added because of increased anxiety

*Lyric from West Side Story

Figure 4.1 Life Chart of Patient 4-6. Bars below the horizontal line represent depression; those above, represent mania.

What can you do to best treat Patient 4-6?

1. Whatever the etiology of Patient 4-6's condition, she is receiving too many medications, and these need to be reduced in number. After a complete re-evaluation we concluded that Patient 4-6 had primary bipolar mood disorder. Thus, the goal was to treat her for that. The choices are a mood stabilizer or a combination of mood stabilizers, or ECT. She does not need benzodiazepines, and perhaps she also does not need antipsychotics.

First step: Get rid of the medications that are unlikely to be working because of low dosing or inappropriateness. So, immediately stop the haloperidol and the temazepam.

Second step: Eliminate redundancy. So, get rid of the lamotrigine and clonazepam because the valproic acid is the best mood stabilizer in that group. But, both carbamazepine and clonazepam are anticonvulsants and must be tapered slowly. We reduced the lamotrigine by 50 mg weekly. The lorazepam was reduced more slowly to avoid withdrawal anxiety (1 mg in the first week and .5 mg weekly).

During the above taper, the patient might actually improve as the cognitive problems (almost guaranteed with such high doses of clonazepam on top of temazepam), will get better. She did improve.

Third step: Maximize the medication that is most likely to work. 1500 mg of valproic acid is a moderate dose. Unless Patient 4-6's blood levels are unusually high, she could go to 2500-3000 mg and obtain substantial benefit. Patients reach their tolerance for valproic acid around blood levels of 130, or when they develop a fine tremor or sedation, whichever comes first.

Fourth step: If Patient 4-6 substantially improves with the above strategy, wait 3 months and then consider the need to continue the modest dose of haloperidol she is on. That too may no longer be needed. All of the above was done for Patient 4-6 with good results.

2. A different strategy is to consider ECT as a better acute and continuation treatment for Patient 4-6. If so, the anticonvulsant tapers can go a bit faster (because once you can get a seizure with ECT, it then raises the seizure threshold).

Discussion

When considering treatment resistance you always check etiology and co-morbidity. *Table 4.6* and *4.7* display the more common etiologies and co-morbidities likely to lead to poor response to treatment. It is frequently a surprise to the clinician when the "second time around" suddenly reveals the condition that was "there all the time."

Patients with primary mood disorder should not be labeled treatment resistant until they have not responded to a full course of bilateral ECT. Until they receive ECT, they have only not responded to medication. Thus, they remain *treatment deprived.*

Table 4.6 Some Etiologies Explaining Treatment-Resistant Mania

Stroke (typically nondominant hemisphere, nondominant basal ganglia)

Traumatic brain injury (nondominant)

Epilepsy

Lupus (and other autoimmune diseases)

Degenerative disease (Huntington's, multiple sclerosis)

Table 4.7 Co-morbidities Likely to Lead to Poor Response

Thyroid disease

Alcoholism

Drug Abuse (particularly cocaine)

Stroke

Traumatic brain injury

Vascular dementia

Despite your best efforts, some patients will become chronically ill. The earlier the onset of illness, the more vigorous attempts to stop the chronic process. *Table 4.8* displays factors found to increase the likelihood of chronicity. Reducing environmental stressors, preventing or treating substance abuse and alcoholism, and vigorous treatment of early episodes and good maintenance offer the best hope for reduced chronicity.

Table 4.8 Factors Associated with Chronicity [16]		
Predictors of Relapse	*Predictors of Treatment Resistance*	*Predictors of Psychosocial Impairment*
Earlier age	Smaller temporal lobe	Multiple episodes
Family history of psychosis	EEG abnormalities	Treatment resistance
High expressed emotions in family	Alcohol/substance abuse	Cognitive deficits
Multiple psychosocial stressors	Presence of thought disorder	Radiologic brain abnormality
Poor socioeconomic status	Interepisodic psychosensory features	Predominant negative features, such as anhedonia, apathy

Patient 4-7: One Thing Led to Another and Yadda, Yadda, Yadda (Getting Sensitized Neurologic Style)

A 39-year-old man has experienced episodes of mania since his early twenties. Past episodes were characterized by his dressing up as Robin Hood and then going to local retailers demanding at "arrow point" money for the poor. Needless to say, the police usually got involved, and he was always hospitalized. Early episodes responded well to lithium alone, and he was usually discharged home after a few weeks.

Over the last half-dozen years, however, his episodes have become more frequent, prolonged, and no longer responsive to lithium. He has also not been able to work outside his family's farm since his late twenties. He has never married and appears to have no interest in sex. His manias are now characterized by a mixture of dysphoria and euphoria, flight of ideas with verbigeration and perseverations, pacing and sleeplessness. When well, he is pleasant and cooperative and tries to help around the farm, but he needs constant direction and can only do simple, previously learned tasks.

What happened to Patient 4-7?

Some bipolar patients appear to develop an illness pattern suggesting limbic system "sensitization" (see discussion).[17] They become chronically dysfunctional even if asymptomatic between episodes. Episodes occur with greater frequency (yearly or less) and are prolonged. Patients are no longer lithium responsive. Loss of drive, libido, ability to learn new things, and perseverativeness also suggest sensitization.

> Limbic sensitization is characterized by signs of limbic disease (what a surprise!) such as déjà vu, dysmegalopsia and dysmorphopsia, depersonalization, and derealization. These psychosensory" phenomena occur in about 30% of manias and may indicate a better response to anticonvulsants than to lithium.

What can be done now?

Limbic sensitization appears to be similar to limbic kindling, a form of laboratory-induced epilepsy (also see discussion). Antikindling drugs work better at this stage of illness than lithium. Carbamazepine and valproic acid have antikindling properties. So does ECT.

Could his chronicity have been prevented?

Thirty to 50% of bipolar patients become chronically dysfunctional after years of illness. Other neurologic disease (e.g., head trauma, stroke) and the use of street drugs (particularly cocaine) and alcoholism predispose to chronicity. Inadequate treatment also predisposes to chronicity, because it permits episodes to be prolonged, and the state of mania is physiologically sensitizing.

Repeated or chronic stress may also predispose to chronicity as stress can precipitate mood disorder episodes, particularly early on in the illness course. The more early episodes a patient has, the more later episodes he will have. *Table 4.9* displays a strategy that may help reduce the risk of chronicity. Chronic stress may also result in chronic hypercortisolemia. Prolonged high serum cortisol levels can lead to increased glutamate activity and a neurologic effect. The hippocampus is particularly sensitive to this process.[18]

Discussion

Limbic kindling is thought to underlie chronicity in epilepsy. It can be produced experimentally in lab rats by stimulating their brain with a one-second

Table 4.9 Strategy for Preventing Bipolar Chronicity
Stress management and stress reduction.
Minimize risks for head trauma.
Avoid all alcohol and street drugs.
Early episodes require vigorous management, and the shorter the illness period, the less destructive the episode to long-term function.
Treatments that prevent kindling may in the long run be the best (ECT and valproic acid can prevent it, carbamazepine and lithium cannot).

subconvulsive dose of electricity daily until the previously subconvulsive dose produces a seizure (takes about 60 days). Continued stimulations (another 30 days or so) will each produce a seizure, and when the stimulations stop, the rat will have spontaneous seizures (no electrical stimulus needed). It has become epileptic (see *Figure 4.2*).

Figure 4.2

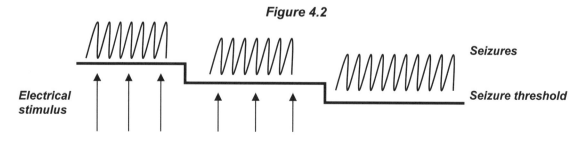

Seizures

Seizure threshold

Electrical stimulus

Sensitization works in a similar fashion, but the stimulus is chemical (e.g., cocaine) and the response behavioral change (e.g., hyperactivity and excitement). The hypothesis is that stress can trigger manias in genetically vulnerable persons, and these early manias begin the sensitization process: the episodes themselves act as a sensitizing stimuli. The more early episodes and the longer the episodes, the more sensitizing they are. After awhile, stress is no longer needed to precipitate an episode (the threshold for illness has been lowered). More episodes then lead to other limbic changes: decreased libido, perseverativeness, and problems with new learning. Chronicity occurs.

This model of illness for bipolar disorder cautions us that allowing a manic to remain even partially ill is ultimately chronicity-inducing. Loading strategies work faster than usual BID and TID dosing. If a 3 week drug trial does not resolve the mania, ECT should be offered rather than exposing the patient to many more weeks or months of trial and error drug combinations and switches.

Patient 4-8: All in the Family

A 28-year-old co-worker asks for your advice. She says her twin sister has been hospitalized for the past several days because she became extremely excited and shouted at the neighbors, who called the police. The family then discovered that the twin sister had spent all her savings on Christmas and Halloween decorations "to be ready for next year." Your co-worker says her sister has been diagnosed "schizophrenic" and has been given an antipsychotic. She says she knows schizophrenia is "genetic" and is concerned for herself as well as for her sister.

What are the odds that in a chapter on bipolar disorder, the twin sister has schizophrenia?

The same as for the snowball in you know where.

What else do you need to know about these sisters?

In the real world, mood disorder is much more common than schizophrenia. Even among acutely psychotic newly admitted patients, about 5% meet strict DSM criteria for schizophrenia, whereas 30% or more meet criteria for mood disorder, although some of these patients will be labeled schizoaffective manic. Thus, by Sutton's Law alone, the twin sister should have a mood disorder. Excitement, irritability, and a spending spree are a familiar Duck, and also suggest mood disorder.

As for the information you need, it is, are the sisters monozygotic or dizygotic twins? Monozygotic twins share 100% of their genes. Dizygotic twins share 50% of their polymorphic genes. The concordance rate for bipolar disorder (if one twin has it, so does the other) is about 65% for monozygotic and about 25% for dizygotic twins. Also in about 20% of twin pairs where both twins are ill, one will be bipolar and the other unipolar.

Assuming either schizophrenia or bipolar mood disorder, what would you tell your co-worker about her risks of each?

Table 4.10 shows the risk figures for schizophrenia and bipolar mood disorder. MR stands for morbid risk. Morbid risk is the prevalence of the disorder (old plus new cases) corrected for the age distribution of the sample being counted.

Table 4.10 Morbid Risk in Family Members [19]			
Population	**The first-degree relative's risk of developing**		
	Bipolar Disorder	**Schizophrenic**	**Schizoaffective**
Bipolar disorder	5-10%	0.3%	0.1 % acute 1.6% chronic
Schizophrenia	1.3%	3.1%	5.0 % acute
Schizoaffective – acute	11.7%	4.9%	5.8% acute 1.6% chronic
Schizoaffective – chronic	8.8%	1.7%	0 acute 2.5% chronic
General population	1.2%	0.6%	0.6% acute 0 chronic

Note: The risk of schizophrenia and bipolar mood disorder is higher a) in monozygotic twins, b) if both parents are ill.

You can determine a rough measure of heritability (how much of why someone will get the disorder is due to genes) by doubling the difference between monozygotic and dizygotic concordance rates. Thus, for bipolar disorder, the heritability is about 2 (65-25)=2(40)=80%. That's a lot, but it also means 20% comes from something else. Gestational, labor and delivery, and neonatal problems have been implicated in that 20%.

So, you could tell your co-worker that her risk is substantially higher than the general population, but depending on how much she shares genes and early problems with her sister, an illness is not inevitable.

In what ways does knowing the family history help in diagnosis and treatment?

This information is overrated. The most important information you have is the patient in front of you. The patient's family history is secondary. It becomes helpful for diagnosis only when you cannot figure out the patient's illness from your direct evaluation of the patient. Then you hope another family member was also ill and that some other clinician was able to make the diagnosis. Then, if you know the illness to be familial you can with some assurance say, "Well if the relative has X, maybe my patient also has X." But, in the case of Patient 4-8, the sister was probably misdiagnosed. So, family history even when available, can be misleading.

For treatment, family history can tell you about relationships, who you can count on, the degree of stress in the family, and thus what you may need to do to minimize these stressors in your patient's life. The idea that families also respond to the same treatments (if the twin sister gets better with eye of newt, so will your patient) is fallacious. There are too many confounding variables that can influence response for you to bet on the patient responding to the same medication as the family, so stick to the patient and ask yourself, based on the patient's condition, what is your first choice treatment.

Patient 4-9: Famous Fathers, Troubled Sons

A 33-year-old man is hospitalized for excitement, irritability, and grandiose delusions. He says he has 29 fathers including John F. Kennedy, Martin Luther King, and Elton John. His mother, he says, is Marilyn Monroe, and he has been left several fortunes. He says he became invisible and was somehow transported to his present location. He is verbally abusive, has pressured speech with flight of ideas. He also has strings of jargon, and paraphasic speech with neologisms. He is highly distractible and moves somewhat "stiffly" for his age.

What are the most striking elements of Patient 4-9's patterns of psychopathology?

1. Fantastic delusions (becoming invisible and being transported)
2. Flight of ideas with formal thought disorder (the aphasic-like speech)[20]
3. His stiffness

Note the exact content of Patient 4-9's psychopathology (who his fathers are and what is the nature of his fantastic delusion) are not diagnostically important. The form of this psychopathology is what diagnostically counts.

What do the Duck Principle and Sutton's Law suggest about Patient 4-9?

Patient 4-9's mood, grandiosity and flight of ideas suggest the Duck is mania. But, the patterns above are not typical. It is an odd looking Duck. Whenever a patient is somewhat atypical, the likelihood substantially increases that the syndrome will be secondary.

Sutton's Law suggests the most likely cause of a secondary mania in a young man will be what?

How should Patient 4-9 be treated?

Patient 4-9 likely has a drug-induced psychosis. Urine screening, blood for medication levels, and a careful history looking for drug use need to be done. In fact, Patient 4-9

> Drug-induced psychosis can result from intoxication, but also from the neurotoxic effects of the drug producing brain damage. In addition, cocaine intoxication can cause seizures and small strokes from vascular spasms, and these events can also result in brain damage and psychosis. [21]

abused almost everything ever bottled or packaged by humans, and in large quantities. His drugs of choice were marijuana and phencyclidine.

Antipsychotics are often needed for such patients, but they can make motor features of the condition worse,[22] and, as in patients with traumatic brain injuries, they can slow recovery. Sometimes they cause a confusional dementia-like state. Try to avoid antipsychotics in patients with drug-induced psychoses.

If the patient is in an acute intoxication, a structured calm setting, good nursing, and mild sedation may be all that is needed for the process to resolve. If there is no resolution within 48 hours or it becomes clear the patient is not in an acute intoxication, but has a recurrence from the brain-damaging effects of past drug use (late-occurring psychotic disorder), then he will need more intrusive treatment. Try anticonvulsants first; add lithium if the patient is very manic. If these medications do not work quickly, give ECT. Once the acute phase of treatment is over, these patients need to be evaluated and treated as if they had a traumatic brain injury (which they do, it's just molecular).

If you cannot avoid an antipsychotic, select one that has the least motor side effects to avoid exacerbating any motor problems associated with chronic drug abuse. Atypical antipsychotics, such as quetiapine, is one option. If the patient refuses oral medication, the oral-dissolving form of olanzapine might still be accepted. If not, then a typical antipsychotic is your last resort. Chlorpromazine is the typical antipsychotic pharmacodynamically most like the atypicals, so IM 50 mg several times daily might be a good choice. Haloperidol IM is always available.

Discussion

Secondary manias respond to general treatments for mood disorder as well as to any specific treatment of the etiologic process. Prognosis is based on the cause, as continuation and maintenance. For a *late-occurring drug induced psychotic* disorder (which is what Patient 4-9 has), the patient has suffered a biochemical traumatic brain injury that may have produced secondary structural and intraneuronal genetic changes. Assessment, prognosis, rehabilitation, medication usage are similar to those for patients with more gross traumatic brain injury.[23] Unfortunately, if the drug abusing patient continues to use drugs, the trauma is repeated, increasing the likelihood of chronicity.

Assessment of prognosis of patients who have chronically used drugs should minimally include:

1. *Level of self-sufficiency in activities of daily living.* Can the patient live independently? Does he have adequate hygiene? Will he be able to prepare his meals, keep his home reasonably clean and organized, shop, and deal with the agencies and people needed to maintain a home? If he cannot do these things, how bad are the deficits? Good frontal lobe function is required to live independently. These skills can all be systematically assessed. Match his placement with his strengths in these areas.
2. *Level of social skills.* How well does the patient interact with others? Does he stand too close when he speaks to others? Does he speak too loudly, have adequate emotional expression, speech and language function? Does he express odd ideas that will put people off? Does he look clean and neat? Good self-monitoring is needed to govern oneself in social situations.
3. *Level of motor behavior.* Is he motorically normal? If he has motor problems, what are their nature and severity?
4. *Level of cognition.* Test attention, abstract thinking, new learning, and visuospatial function. Based on this assessment decide if more elaborate neuropsychological testing is needed.

Patient 4-9 has adequate emotional expression, and some volition, although he has not worked in years. His formal thought disorder and "stiffness" during the acute episode are poor prognostic features. When he recovered from his acute psychosis, he still had substantial executive, visuospatial, and abstract thinking problems. He could live independently if he stopped using drugs.

165

Patient 4-10: Once Crazy, Always Crazy

A 60-year-old woman with a long history of bipolar mood disorder, hypertension, and coronary artery disease is transferred from a nursing home for sudden worsening of her condition. On examination, she is hyperactive, irritable, disoriented to day, and labile in her mood. Her speech is often paraphasic, and her understanding of your questions and comments is variable.

What is the first step in managing Patient 4-10? (This is a trick question.)

The first step in management is always assessment, a definitive diagnosis being the best result. A sudden change in behavior in a psychiatric patient with general medical problems should always alert you the present illness may be related to those general medical problems. Do not be like Patient 4-10's nursing home caregivers and her admitting doctor. Do not automatically assume the behavioral change must be her psychiatric illness. Psychiatric illness does not protect a person from other illness.

So what is the diagnosis? A sudden behavioral change, paraphasic speech, a history of hypertension and coronary artery disease, a 60-year-old woman: This Duck is a stroke.

In the US, women are now slightly more at risk for stroke than are males. See what smoking and over-weight can do for you!

Although the *location* of the stroke will not change Patient 4-10's treatments or management, being able to locate it will help you become sensitive to behavior-brain relationships and better at identifying strokes in other patients. So, how do you figure it out for Patient 4-10?

Your best bet for locating Patient 4-10's stroke is her language problems. She is fluent (talks a ton) and spontaneous in her speech, and she has no problems with articulation or emotional expression (prosody). Her anterior language systems are okay! The fact that she has no motor deficits is consistent with this. She does have paraphasic speech and variable understanding of your questions and comments. These features suggest posterior language systems are involved. Further elaboration would require you to figure out if this variable understanding was related to the complexity of what you are saying. Difficulties like that suggest some auditory comprehension problems. You would test her repetition: Poor repetition suggests cortical involvement in or near Wernicke's area;

adequate repetition suggests subcortical or transcortical involvement. Testing her reading and writing and naming would help. We will discuss stroke in more detail in chapter 7, but Patient 4-10 had a stroke in the watershed area[24] involving the temporoparietal cortex.

What should be your overall plan for helping her?

Patients with bipolar disorder often do not do well under stress. Older persons with cognitive problems also often do not do well under stress. Persons who have strokes that give them cognitive difficulties can become upset about not understanding others or not being understood. Persons being hospitalized on a psychiatric unit when their illness is a stroke can be upset (we would, wouldn't you?). So, the best overall management plan for Patient 4-10 is to manage her stroke and be empathic. Then, her other behaviors are likely to lessen, if not resolve. If all the above stressors precipitated a mania then the mania gets treated. But, in Patient 4-10's situation her "mania" disappeared as she was treated for stroke. Her baseline was mild hypomania, and she returned to it within one week.

Patient 4-11: Three's a Crowd

A 43-year-old man is being followed in a primary care clinic for recurrent tension headaches and hypertension. During one visit, Patient 4-11 complains of tiredness and increased thirst. Further questioning reveals he also has increased micturition. Suspecting diabetes mellitus, the primary care physician orders blood chemistry and a urinalysis. Before leaving the office Patient 4-11 tells his primary physician that he has recently also been diagnosed as having bipolar mood disorder, and that his psychiatrist is planning to put him on medication. The primary care physician calls you for advice.

> May patients with migraine also have tension headache and *vice versa,* so look for other migraine features in these patients and their families (it's familial). Migraine also is co-morbid with epilepsy, so look for seizure disorder in these patients, particularly if the patient's behavioral syndrome

There are two big diagnostic concerns you need to resolve before you can advise Patient 4-11's physician. What are they?

Always make a diagnosis first. For Patient 4-11, you need to know if he really has headaches and hypertension that meet the threshold for illness, and if he is bipolar. Then apply the Rule of Parsimony, because three different illness processes are too many.

Let us assume his signs and symptoms all reach the threshold of illness and that you are satisfied that Patient 4-11 is indeed hypertensive, bipolar, and has a headache disorder. Headache is often a manifestation of hypertension, so you first need to see if Patient 4-11's hypertension can explain his headaches. Then treating the hypertension should take care of the headaches. Bipolar disorder can sometimes result in hypertension (much higher systolic rise than diastolic, although both are elevated). So, if his bipolar disorder is the cause of the hypertension and the hypertension is the cause of his headache, treating the bipolar disorder could take care of everything, except the diabetes. The Rule of Parsimony might also lead to the conclusion that his diabetes has caused vascular changes that have led to small strokes and that his bipolar disorder is secondary to the diabetes, as are his hypertension and headaches.

But, in Patient 4-11's situation it turns out that his diabetes does account for his hypertension and headache, but not for his bipolar disorder. So the treatment problem becomes how to treat a bipolar patient who also has diabetes and will need antihypertensive medication.

Also, because he is prone to headache (this should markedly improve with control of his hypertension), he may occasionally take analgesics and so drug-drug interactions may become a problem.

What factors will help you decide if Patient 4-11, in fact, needs a mood stabilizer?

The importance of this question should now be clearer after the discussion above: If Patient 4-11 does not need a mood stabilizer it would make therapeutic life a lot easier. How do you decide? *First,* does his bipolar disorder reach the threshold of dysfunction that indicates that treatment is needed? *Second,* if previously treated, what stage of treatment is he in: acute, continuation, maintenance? *Third,* if he is in one of the first 2 stages, will he need the third, i.e., treatment for years or a lifetime?

Patient 4-11 is cyclothymic. Cyclothymia was at first recognized as a low-grade, chronic disorder with gradual swings from weeks of highs or irritability to weeks of downs. It then got mistakenly placed among the personality disorders and only recently has it been switched back into what is now Axis I mood disorders. If the dips and crests of cyclothymia are great enough, problems ensue, and Patient 4-11 has had interpersonal and employment difficulties because of it. He needs treatment. Because cyclothymia is continuous rather than episodic and because Patient 4-11 has been that way since a teen, he will need treatment indefinitely. Because he has never been treated for his cyclothymia, he is in the acute phase of treatment.

> There is no evidence that bipolar prophylaxis with a mood stabilizer can do better than an episode every 5 years. However, most of the time patients with two or more episodes - regardless of interepisode duration - get indefinite maintenance treatment.

If Patient 4-11 had an episodic form of bipolar disorder, then your questions would be, is he in an episode now? If not, how many previous episodes has he had? If more than two, he is likely to get ill again and so needs treatment. If he has had only one previous episode, although he is still likely to have another, you might opt to wait on treatment, particularly if that episode was more than 5 years ago.

Which mood stabilizer will be best for Patient 4-11, and what factors will influence your decision?

Lithium and then valproic acid are still the first-line medications for bipolar mood disorder. For acute manic episodes, ECT also is a first-line treatment and works as well as medication.

The most important factor determining your choice of medication for Patient 4-11, who is not in an episode, is his general medical condition, specifically his diabetes. Lithium has an insulin-like effect on carbohydrate metabolism and will interfere with treatments for diabetes. The renal effects of lithium also cause initial polyuria/polydipsia, and diabetes insipidus is an adverse renal consequence of lithium use for some patients. It is, therefore, likely that lithium's effects could mask his diabetes mellitus features and the diagnosis of diabetes mellitus is missed. However, lithium may also exacerbate diabetes mellitus due to its hyperglycemic effects. Further, if lithium is used, then diuretics for his hypertension should be avoided. Nonsteroidal antiinflammatory analgesics interfere with lithium levels, and can lead to toxicity, and because of his hypertension and headaches, he might be prescribed thiazide and nonsteroidals. Thus, lithium, although a first choice drug in uncomplicated mania, may not be practical for Patient 4-11. In all treatment, what you do has a risk and a benefit. If the patient's diabetes is mild and easily controlled; if he is smart enough to avoid potentially problematic drug-drug interactions, then lithium can be used, with perhaps more frequent check-ups to ensure all is going well. If you decide his diabetes is more brittle or he is unlikely to watch the medications he is given, then valproic acid will be a better choice, especially if his headaches were migraine variants, as valproic acid works for mania and migraine.[25]

Tables *4.11* and *4.12* display the side effects of lithium and its common drug-drug interactions.

Table 4.11 Side Effects of Lithium	
Nausea Vomiting Diarrhea Increased thirst Polyuria	Occur at the beginning Often transient
Fine tremor Polyuria (60%) Nephrogenic diabetes insipidus (5-10%) Hypoparathyroidism (10%) Hypothyroidism (5%) Insulin-like effect on carbohydrate metabolism	Long-term effects seen in patients on prophylactic treatment
Coarse tremors Confusion Seizure Renal failure Coma	Occur during toxicity

Table 4.12 Drug/Drug Interactions	
NSAIDS	Increased lithium level due to effect of NSAIDS on renal prostaglandin level
Thiazide diuretic	Increased lithium level due to decreased clearance
Theophylline	Decreased lithium level due to increased excretion
Acetazolamide	Decreased lithium level due to increased excretion
Fluoxetine	Increased lithium level and toxicity, mechanism unknown

Quick Rounds

1. You give a hospitalized excited, 44-year-old manic woman lithium, 1200 mg daily. The next day she tells you she is tired, feels slow, and would prefer to sleep than talk with you. What do you do?

2. You give a 27-year-old manic man lithium, 1500 mg daily. After 10 days of treatment he seems almost fully recovered. Two days later he tells you he feels a bit down and unsure of the future. Sleep and appetite are okay. What do you tell him?

3. A bipolar patient, now melancholic, is given ECT. After 4 treatments she becomes hypomanic. What do you do?

4. You have a bipolar patient on 2500 mg of valproic acid for three weeks. He is doing well. However, over the next week he becomes motorically and cognitively slow, and he sleeps during the day. What do you do?

5. You put a 36-year-old manic man on valproic acid. At 1500 mg daily his blood level is 50. He is only somewhat improved. You go to 2000 mg daily. The blood level goes to 65. You go to 2500 mg daily. The blood level goes to 55 and he remains only modestly better. What happened?

6. A very wealthy manic patient recovers and tells you he wants to give you a gift of $50,000. What do you do?

7. The emergency room physician calls you because one of your patients is in the ER complaining of a rash. The patient has a history of bipolar mood disorder and is taking sodium valproate 1500/day and lamotrigine 100 mg/day. Lamotrigine 50 mg BID was added a week ago to treat depressive symptoms. What do you do?

8. A manic woman slaps a nurse's aide, who in a reasonable manner was trying to help the patient get dressed. The nurse's aide wants to call the police and press charges against the patient. What do you do?

9. A 60-year-old man with bipolar mood disorder who is being followed by the same psychiatrist for 15 years notices the psychiatrist's weight loss and comments on how young and attractive she looks. How should the psychiatrist respond?

10. A 28-year-old man is being admitted from the ER for irritability, hyperactivity, and lack of sleep. He is loud, speaks fast, and is constantly cursing. When asked to change into his pajamas, he strikes an ER nurse. What should the ER staff do now?

11. A 47-year-old man was diagnosed 15 years ago as having bipolar mood disorder, mixed type, his mood rapidly alternating between euphoria and dysphoria. He achieved a full remission with lithium treatment, stopped taking it after 5 years, and remained asymptomatic until now. His current episode is identical to his previous ones. What should you do for him now, and what do you have to check first before doing it?

12. A 65-year-old man was diagnosed five years ago as having mania secondary to a stroke in the right temporal lobe. He was treated successfully with valproic acid, and he has not had another episode. He now requests that you stop the medication. He has no past personal or family history of psychiatric illness. What should you do?

13. A 28-year-old man was diagnosed six years ago as having bipolar mood disorder. He was given lithium carbonate and has not had any manic episodes since then. He now wants to stop the lithium. He had his first manic episode at the age of 16, and two more episodes before he was finally diagnosed and put on lithium. He also has a family history of bipolar illness. What do you do?

14. A 48-year-old man with bipolar mood disorder is given lithium as an outpatient. He responds, but also develops a bilateral fine tremor. Following an increase in the dose, the tremor becomes severe so that he cannot hold a full glass of water without spilling it. What should you do now?

15. A 30-year-old man with bipolar mood disorder is taking lithium carbonate 900 mg po BID for several weeks, and experiences severe tremors about two hours after taking a dose. Lithium blood levels are about .8 meq/L. Why does this man have tremors, and what can you do about it?

16. An acutely manic woman is agitated, verbally abusive and threatening to blow up the inpatient unit and hurt others. She needs immediate treatment. What drug would you give, how would you give it, and why?

17. A 40-year-old man is taking valproic acid for his mania. His valproic acid levels are at the upper limit, yet he is not responding, although in the past, he responded well. What is the reason for nonresponse, and what will you do about it?

18. A 45-year-old man with a history of several episodes of mania and depression returns to the hospital in an acute manic state. About 5 years ago he was taken off lithium because he had been psychiatrically asymptomatic for more than 10 years. He has been diagnosed as having degenerative arthritis and diabetic nephropathy. Should you put him back on lithium? If "no," why not, and what would you do instead?

Quick Rounds Answers

1. You check her saliva. If it is clear (most likely) then her complaints mean she is getting better. You smile and tell her so. Her experiences are the first signs of improvement with lithium.

2. About 30-50% of manics responding to lithium have a mild transient rebound depression that usually requires no further treatment other than patient education.

3. Give more ECT until she is better. ECT works as well for mania as any medication.

4. Get liver functions and ammonia level. Valproic acid-related liver dysfunction mostly occurs in epileptic children receiving two or more anticonvulsants. Lethargy after steady state is rarely from liver disease, but can be from valproic's interference with the urea cycle, leading to increased ammonia levels with otherwise normal liver function. You can correct the interference with a food supplement, carnitine 1 gm, without having to stop the valproic acid.

5. Sometimes valproic acid autoinduces its protein binding so less free valproic acid is available. The more you give the faster this happens. For these patients, valproic is maxed out. You need to enhance or do something else.

6. A minor gift from a patient is acceptable after the patient has recovered. Expensive gifts or money is not acceptable. Respectfully decline, and tell the patient you got paid: he got better. The patient can also donate large monetary gifts to your medical school or to a worthy mood disorder program.

7. One of the side effects of lamotrigine is rash, which could also be Steven Johnson's syndrome (a potentially lethal reaction). To avoid this reaction, lamotrigine should be started slowly. The manufacturer recommends that due to drug interaction, when prescribing in patients already on valproic acid, the starting dose should be 50% of the routine starting dose (50 mg).

8. Patient behavior due to disease needs to be treated not criminalized. This patient will not be prosecuted, and the aide needs empathic education. Anyone working on an inpatient psychiatric unit must be prepared for occasional aggressive or violent behavior. You cannot work in this setting if you are not capable of dealing with violence, just

as no one can work on an ICU who cannot do CPR. If you don't like the sight of blood, don't become a surgeon. If you are uncomfortable around patients who act oddly and who are occasionally aggressive or assaultive, don't work in psychiatry.

9. The psychiatrist should smile and thank the patient: It wasn't easy losing all that weight! Socially acceptable comments by a patient or anyone else deserve responses that fit social norms. The patient was in remission, and appropriately complimented someone he knew for 15 years.

10. This patient is violent and needs to be controlled so that he does not hurt anyone else: other staff, other ER patients, himself. If he can verbally and with a show of force be calmed and gotten into pajamas, fine. If not, he needs to be restrained, sedated, and placed into hospital clothes. Having the patient change into hospital clothes in the ER is a safety precaution to check for weapons, without making it seem like a strip search.

11. If nothing else has changed, what worked in the past will likely work now, so go for the lithium. If lithium does not work now, or the man's general medical health has changed making lithium treatment too risky, then valproic acid is the next best choice. So, checking his heart, kidney, thyroid, and parathyroid functioning should tell you about the risks with lithium. Checking his liver function should tell you about his risks with valproic acid.

12. If this man had primary mood disorder, we would have no hesitation agreeing to his request. However, because he has a mania secondary to a lesion in a mood regulating area (i.e., temporal lobe), the risk of relapse is very high, and we would not recommend discontinuing medication.

13. The decision is clear-cut here: medication for life. However, education about bipolar illness, its course, recurrence, genetic risk factor is essential to the patient's cooperation. Remember that if not convinced, patients can always stop the medication on their own. It is absolutely necessary that the patient understands the reasons behind your recommendation.

14. When a patient does well on a medication but a mild side effect occurs, try to treat the side effect rather than lowering the medication dose or stopping it. When side effects are severe, we, of course, switch the drug. It is working, after all! In this man's situation, try to manage the tremor by 1) switching the dosing to one dose in the

evening so peak effect occurs while he is sleeping, and 2) if he is a coffee drinker (they are more likely to have lithium tremors), get him to cut down or stop (do the latter gradually as caffeine addiction and its withdrawal are unpleasant). If these steps are not enough, give propranolol (20-120 mg daily). Other beta blockers may induce depression. Do not use beta blockers if a patient is asthmatic, diabetic, has hyperthyroidism, or is pregnant. If the last contraindication pertained in this patient's case, report it in a medical journal --you will become famous.

15. Rates of absorption and peak plasma levels differ for each medication. Sometimes side effects are most prominent at peak plasma levels. After a drug is absorbed, it reaches a peak concentration and then the concentration drops due to redistribution. Sometimes that peak concentration is above a tolerable pharmacodynamic range, and then the patient experiences side effects, in this situation severe tremors. To avoid this side effect, lithium could be given in TID doses instead of BID, or most of the drug given at night (with a snack please) so peak concentration occurs when the patient is asleep. If tremors persist, they can be treated with beta adrenergic receptor blockers (metoprolol 50 mg qid or propranolol 10-15 mg/day). If the total daily lithium dose is 1200 mg or less, giving lithium once daily at bedtime can avoid other side effects and may offer some protection from long-term lithium-induced renal problems.

16. Efficacy of the drug is related to its minimal effective concentration (MEC), and MEC is related to route of administration. To exert a therapeutic effect, each drug must reach its minimum effective concentration in the blood. Route of administration becomes important in situations like this. Giving intravenous or intramuscular medication will reduce the time required for the drug to achieve minimum effective concentration. Because the situation calls for rapid sedation, a sedative is the drug of choice. Most often it will be lorazepam. For an acute manic, 2-4 mg may be needed, although 2 is often enough. Of course, do not attempt to give the drug until the patient has been restrained or is otherwise subdued.

17. Therapeutic effect is often correlated with free drug levels, i.e., *bioavailability*. Valproic acid is 90% or more protein bound. However, its therapeutic effect is achieved with the drug that is protein free in plasma. Less than 10% is not much "bang for the buck" but the idea of dosing is to saturate the system so the active stuff remains at a reasonable concentration. This patient may have adequate total blood valproic acid blood levels, but insufficient free drug levels. To

confirm your suspicions, you must order free valproic acid levels. If the free valproic acid levels are low, then you need to increase the total dose.

18. Drug choice is always decided in part on the patient's general medical condition, and any medications that the patient is already receiving. ("Discretion is the better part of valor.") Lithium is a good medication, but probably not for this patient. Treatment for arthritis relies on nonsteroidal anti-inflammatory drugs. Many of these agents (aspirin is an exception) can substantially affect lithium blood levels. Nonsteroidals increase lithium levels by inhibiting the proximal tubule secretion of lithium. Chronic use of these agents may also affect renal function and lithium elimination by the kidney. This patient is also diabetic with evidence of vascular changes due to diabetes affecting his kidneys, again making lithium a problem choice. Thus, this patient is at risk of developing lithium toxicity. Alternatives would be valproic acid or ECT for his acute mania, and valproic acid for continuation and maintenance.

Chapter 5

Anxiety Disorders

Patient 5-1: Am I Scared to Death?

A 30-year-old woman comes to a primary care clinic because she has been experiencing episodes of extreme anxiety over the last 10 years. Lately, these episodes occur almost weekly and last about 20-30 minutes. During these attacks she becomes overwhelmed with fear and thinks she is going to die. Her heart beats rapidly, She feels dizzy and numb, and has difficulty breathing. She is constantly worried about having another attack and sometimes drinks alcohol to relieve her worries.

What is the first step in treating this woman? (This is a trick question)

The "trick" of course is to diagnose first, then treat. Patient 5-1's episodes appear to be anxiety or panic attacks. Normal persons (e.g., medical students) under severe threat, persons with anxiety disorders, and persons with any one of many general medical and neurologic conditions can have *panic attacks*. *Table 5.1* lists features of basic anxiety or panic syndromes.

Tables 5.2 and 5.3 list some of the causes of secondary anxiety disorder.

Table 5.1   Basic Anxiety Syndrome
Mood: apprehension, fear
Cognition: notion of impending doom, inability to concentrate, depersonalization
Fight/flight phenomena: dilated pupils, exophthalmus, piloerection, increased muscle tone, tachycardia, sweating, vascular shunting
Nonadaptive features: tremors, dry mouth, blurred vision, chest pain/discomfort, palpitations, air hunger, dyspnea, hyperventilation, paresthesias, weakness, fatigue, easy fatigability, inner shakiness, lump in throat, vascular throbbing, increased bowel motility, urinary urgency/incontinence

Secondary anxiety disorders often begin later in life rather than in the teens or early 20s. *Table 5.4* compares the common primary anxiety disorders. Persons with a specific phobia also have anxiety attacks, but these attacks occur in proximity to or anticipation of the phobic object (e.g., a horse) or situation (e.g., air travel). The anxiety attacks of panic disorder are unrelated to anything specific. They are spontaneous and sudden. The patient goes from calm to panic within a few minutes.

Table 5.2   General Medical Conditions Causing Secondary Anxiety Disorder

Cardiovascular disease: angina pectoris, arrhythmias, congestive heart failure, hypertension, hypovolemia, myocardial infarction, syncope (multiple causes), valvular disease, vascular collapse (shock); hypertension; mimics generalized anxiety disorder (GAD)

Endocrine disorders: hyperthyroidism, Cushing's disease, diabetes with hypoglycemia; mimics panic, GAD

Mitral valve prolapse: fatigue, easy fatigability, palpitations; mimics panic disorder, GAD

Pulmonary embolus: mimics panic disorder

Asthma: mimics panic disorder

Chronic obstructive pulmonary disease: mimics panic and GAD

Hypoglycemia: mimics panic disorder, GAD

Irritable bowel syndrome: mimics panic disorder, GAD

Secreting tumors (pheochromocytoma, carcinoid, insulinoma): always mentioned, rarely found; mimics panic disorder

Anemia: mimics GAD

> In the ER, a panic attack can be confused with an acute cardiovascular event, particularly an MI. In a primary panic attack, however, pulse is strong and rapid, systolic blood pressure is up, chest discomfort is tightness but not crushing nor radiating, and the patient is usually younger than the typical cardiac patient.

Table 5.3   Some Traditional Neurologic Conditions Causing Secondary Anxiety Disorder

Temporal lobe epilepsy: mimics panic disorder

Parkinson's disease: mimics GAD

Postconcussion syndrome: mimics GAD

Multiple sclerosis: mimics GAD

Withdrawal states: mimics panic disorder, GAD

Caffeinism: mimics panic disorder, GAD

Drug abuse (stimulants, dopaminergics, sympathomimetics, and anticholinergics): mimics panic disorder

Table 5.4	Comparison of Anxiety Disorders				
	Panic Disorder With and Without Agoraphobia	**Specific Phobia**	**Generalized Anxiety Disorder (GAD)**	**Post-Traumatic Stress Disorder**	**Social Phobia**
Prevalence in general population	3.5%	Specific 11.3%	5.1%	1-14%	13.3%
Gender differences	Female:Male 3:1	Female:Male 2:1	Female:Male 2:1	Female:Male 1:1	Female:Male 2:1
Age of onset	Teens through mid-30s	Childhood to early adulthood	Childhood	Variable	Childhood to early adulthood

What would you tell Patient 5-1 about her illness and long-term prognosis?

Assuming Patient 5-1 has no evidence for a secondary panic disorder, you would then tell her that she has panic disorder, that her condition is very common, and that women are at greater risk than men. She should know that panic disorder occurs early in life, runs in families and is a brain disease. Although she will always have the risk of having other attacks, the prognosis is good with proper treatment. The only "fly" in this ointment is her drinking. If she is self-medicating, then controlling her anxiety disorder will control her drinking. If she is also prone to alcohol dependence, then, "We got a problem, Houston!" Family history and personality assessment can help here. Women alcoholics often have alcoholic first-degree relatives, so ask about this. Patient 5-1 has none. Women alcoholics often have impulsive, thrill-seeking temperaments. Patient 5-1 does not. So, a good prognosis is, indeed, more likely.

> Morbid risks in first-degree relatives is about 20% within the broad anxiety disorder category versus 4-6% in the general population; MZ twin concordance is 50-60%, DZ twin concordance is 20-30% for anxiety disorders in general, indicating that about 40-50% of the cause is genetic. No genes have been identified yet, however.

What are the comorbidities of her condition?

About 60% of anxiety disorder patients have a premorbid (anxious-fearful) personality disorder. Most patients experience occasional depressions (nonmelancholic) and may become home-bound, fearful of having an attack in public (agoraphobia). Some patients (particularly men) may abuse alcohol to relieve anxiety, and as a result develop alcohol dependency.

How would you care for her?

1. *Anxiety disorders reflect brain disease. Medications are often needed.* Persons with anxiety disorders often are sensitive to drug side-effects. Thus, start low and go slow with dose increases. Educating the patient and family is essential for good compliance. Phone rounds and other strategies to treat mood disorder patients apply equally to patients with anxiety disorders. Full response may take weeks or several months, so don't give up prematurely. Once maximum improvement has been obtained, continuation and then maintenance treatment may be needed. SSRIs, tricyclic antidepressants and MAOIs have all been shown to be effective in treating panic disorder, due to their favorable cardiac profile and relative ease in use. SSRIs have become first-line treatments.[1] Often panic disorder patients experience worsening of symptoms after initiation of the antidepressant treatment and may stop taking medication. It may help to add a benzodiazepine, such as clonazepam .25 - .5 mg TID, for a few weeks to cover this period.

2. *Phobic-like responses to physiologic signs of anxiety exacerbate anxiety disorders. Behavioral interventions help.* Compliance and perhaps quality of improvement is maximized by counseling, encouragement, and support. Combined medication plus behavioral techniques are best for severely ill patients. Behavioral techniques used in the treatment of anxiety disorder:

   a. *Relaxation training.* Patients are taught to relax their muscles and minds through a series of commands from the therapist.
   b. *Rebreathing training.* The therapist teaches the patient to use abdominal breathing as anxiety management.
   c. *Systematic desensitization.* Patients are asked to visualize anxiety-provoking situations first in the therapist's office and then in actual settings. For example, this patient would be asked to imagine she is having a panic attack and would then practice relaxation.

d. *Education.* Patients are educated about the biological nature of their attacks and reassured that they will not die.

Discussion

Acute anxiety is an adaptive physiologic state that is part of flight/fight behavior to avoid or defend against danger. In humans, at least, it occurs with subjective experience of fear. The flight/fight system is activated by strong, typically sudden and often unexpected stimuli, or stimuli that evoke memories.

Flight/fight mechanisms are integrated with the brain's arousal system. Sleep to full wakefulness occurs with the activation of the reticular activating system (RAS) and locus ceruleus interacting with the thalamus. The thalamus projects this arousal tone to the cortex and helps focus cortical attention to stimuli for further processing and action. Too much or too little arousal can lead to attention problems. Intoxications and delirium are examples of disrupted arousal causing problems with attention.

Cortical processing in flight/fight involves *attribution*, e.g., this pattern of stimuli is good, that pattern is bad or sad or potentially dangerous. For example, if you are called into the Dean's office and you think you are being called because someone complained about you, you will be anxious, but if you think you will receive an award, you will experience elation. If the stimuli are sudden, unexpected, intense, or novel, however, the thalamus initially bypasses the cortex and sends this information directly to the amygdala, hippocampus, and parahippocampus, like express mail, for very rapid processing. Getting to the cortex and having it process this information before initial action takes too long, and our ancestors would have been lunch had they depended on the cortex to make the initial decision about flight/fight. The hippocampus/parahippocampus try to match the stimulus pattern with past patterns (memories) of danger. Even an approximate match (e.g., a dark alley) will trigger the hippocampus to alert the basal ganglia, leading to flight/fight behavior. Simultaneously, the thalamus sends the new potentially dangerous information to the nucleus accumbens, septal nuclei, and cerebral cortex. Through a feedback loop, the hippocampus/parahippocampus gets further information from the amygdala about the emotion that is being attached to the stimulus pattern. This information is also sent to the nucleus accumbens, septal nuclei, and striatum. The thalamus also simultaneously sends the stimulus information to the hypothalamus. This input plus feedback from the amygdala/hippocampus/parahippocampus stimulates the hypothalamus to arouse the sympathetic nervous system to produce the physiologic state necessary for rapid, intense activity. The system is fueled by dopamine in the RAS arousal system and mediated by norepinephrine from the locus ceruleus. Serotonin projections from the median raphe nucleus modify the system.

The intensity of the stimulus pattern, the degree of danger and fear that the hippocampus/parahippocampus/amygdala attach to the stimulus pattern. The greater the intensity, the greater the flight/fight reaction. This process relates to what is termed somatic anxiety.

Flight/fight behavior, therefore, involves several steps:

1. Arousal
2. Thalamic channeling of the stimulus pattern
3. Hippocampus/parahippocampus/amygdala processing
4. Basal ganglia and septal nuclei motor programming and attention
5. Cortical processing and attribution
6. Action brain integrated responses

The steps in the flight/fight process also are a framework for reorganizing the DSM anxiety disorders into more clinically meaningful groupings and for developing more specific treatment strategies for primary and secondary anxiety-related conditions.

Several neurotransmitter systems are involved in flight/fight, which is one reason why different drugs can alleviate anxiety (e.g., antidepressants, benzodiazepines, alcohol, buspirone). Norepinephrine (NE) appears to be the initiating factor in flight/fight, and its activity underlies many of the central and peripheral features of anxiety. Serotonergic (5-HT) activity underlies many homeostatic processes and appears to modulate NE activity with dorsal and medial raphe nuclei projections to the locus ceruleus and again to the thalamus/parahippocampus/hippocampus/septal system. Too much NE activity can produce central and peripheral anxiety. Too much serotonergic activity reduces the inhibition of the NE system and leads to central features of anxiety. GABA (gamma amino butyric acid) distribution in the brain is more widespread than that of NE or 5-HT. Its involvement in anxiety disorder is probably indirect and as a modulating factor (i.e., high or low activity will influence the effects of NE/5-HT on flight/fight systems). It is also a chronicity factor: The longer-lasting or more severe the anxiety disorder, the more likely GABAergic function is disrupted, the more likely excitatory amino acids are released and limbic sensitization with its behavior (psychosensory features) and cognitive

185

(memory problems) consequences is likely to occur. *Table 5.5* lists the evidence supporting this notion.

Table 5.5   Biology of Anxiety Disorders
Autonomic arousal: baseline and during habituation
At rest: increased BP, elevated pulse, increased respiration, increased galvanic skin response, fast activity on EEG.
Repeated stimuli do not lead to habituation.
Panic response to changes in blood pH
IV infusions of sodium lactate, CO_2 or yohimbine will produce a typical anxiety response.
Some patients become anxious after exercise.
Premorbid personality: 60% have premorbid personality disorder, most commonly from cluster C (anxious-fearful).
Genetics: familial (15-20% MRs in relatives versus 4-6% in general population); MZ twin concordance 50-60%, DZ twin concordance 20-30%.
Neurochemical abnormalities: increased noradrenergic activity (increased CSF and plasma methyl hydroxy phenylglycol (MHPG) in anxiety disorder patients, stimulation of locus ceruleus leads to fear response in monkeys); increased serotonergic turnover.

Anxiety disorder probably arises from the flight/fight system's hypersensitivity to stimuli. The more ambiguous, novel, or potentially dangerous the stimulus pattern, the more intense the response. Thus, the flight/fight system in anxious patients responds to stimuli that do not produce a flight/fight response in nonanxious persons (the threshold is lower). It also over-responds to stimuli that produce a modest response in nonanxious persons (once over the threshold, the response is more intense and of greater duration). *Table 5.6* lists the proposed theories of etiology.

Table 5.6 Theories of Etiology
Carbon dioxide supersensitivity: Panic attacks can be reproduced by infusion of sodium lactate or respiration of 5% carbon dioxide in panic disorder patients, but not control subjects. These findings have led to the hypothesis that panic disorder occurs because of brainstem hypersensitivity to CO_2.
Locus ceruleus theory: Locus ceruleus has 50% of all noradrenergic neurons. Stimulation of locus ceruleus causes fear and anxiety in nonhumans. Abnormal firing of locus ceruleus is thought to be involved in causing anxiety disorders, and resultant hyperadrenergic state and catecholamine sensitivity.
GABA receptor theory: GABA receptors are distributed throughout the brain. Benzodiazepine, which relieves anxiety, blocks these receptors. GABA receptors are thought to be malfunctioning in anxiety disorders.

Patient 5-2: Home Sweet Home. That's Where I Prefer to Stay.

A 35-year-old woman comes to her appointment driven by her husband. After being involved in a "fender bender" three years ago, she developed panic attacks and was given alprazolam 2 mg TID, which she still takes. Although she no longer has panic attacks, she is afraid to leave her house alone. She wants you to increase her alprazolam so she can go out on her own.

Should you increase her medication? (Another trick? You bet!)

First, diagnose! Just because Patient 5-2 was diagnosed as having panic attacks does not necessarily mean she has panic disorder. It is important to define the syndrome and then decide if it is primary or secondary to a general medical or neurologic condition.

Patient 5-2 had "panic attacks" after a stress event. That sounds like a phobia. However, a *specific phobia* is unrealistic anxiety only in the phobic situation. Patient 5-2 had subsequent panic attacks without getting into a car, and she is afraid to even walk outside by herself. Her problem is more pervasive than a specific phobia. Patient 5-2's fender bender experience likely triggered something associated with panic attacks, that is more continuous and restricting. She fears going outside.

> Specific phobias often come with Greek prefixes to make students' lives more difficult. So we get *acrophobia* (fear of heights), *claustrophobia* (fear of closed-in space), etc. All you need to know and ask about are the big subtypes: animal, situational, ecological (storms, water), blood-injection-injury, and a miscellaneous category (fear of vomiting, getting ill, etc.)

Avoiding going outside one's house is the essential feature of agoraphobia. These patients fear being in public places or situations where escape may be difficult or where help may not be available. Fearing future panic attacks can sometimes lead to agoraphobia.[2] Patients usually avoid panic-inducing situations or only go out if accompanied. Agoraphobia is not diagnosed if the patient's symptoms are due to other disorders, such as social phobia[3] or specific phobia (fear of a circumscribed situation or object, e.g., fear of flying or fear of spiders). Assuming Patient 5-2 has primary panic disorder, her diagnosis would be panic disorder with agoraphobia. Although she no longer has panic attacks, she is agoraphobic and needs treatment.

Patient 5-2 requests an increase in her alprazolam, and high doses (4-6 mg) of alprazolam may be more effective than lower doses. However, her dose is 8 mg. That's high enough. Although alprazolam is one of the medications used to treat panic disorder, we prefer not to use it for the following reasons: a) Patients become addicted to alprazolam and develop benzodiazepine tolerance and need escalating doses, and b) alprazolam is an intermediate acting benzodiazepine and requires multiple dosing daily. In our experience it is extremely difficult to wean a patient off alprazolam. We prefer to use antidepressants as the main drug treatment for anxiety disorder. Good results have been achieved with tricyclics, such as imipramine or nortriptyline, in doses lower than those used to treat depression. Pure SSRIs, such as venlafaxine, may also be used. However, pure SSRIs may worsen the anxiety in the beginning of treatment and may need adjunctive benzodiazepine therapy. As with tricyclics, patients with panic disorder need doses of SSRIs lower than what is needed to treat depression. *Table 5.7* has the starting doses of all the SSRIs. If Patient 5-2 were still experiencing panic attacks, it would be advisable to add an antidepressant. However, since at this time she only has agoraphobia, nonpsychopharmacologic intervention will be the next best step.

Table 5.7 SSRI Doses in Panic Disorder		
	Starting Dose	*Therapeutic Dose*
Citalopram	10 mg	20-40 mg
Escitalopram	10 mg	20-40 mg
Fluvoxamine	50 mg	100-200 mg
Paroxetine	10 mg	20-50 mg
Sertraline	25 mg	50-200 mg

Is there anything else you need to do?

Cognitive behavioral therapy (CBT) for panic disorder is a symptom-oriented approach and includes:

1. *Psychoeducation.* This is usually the first phase. Patient is asked to identify each symptom, and the biological nature of the symptom is explained.
2. *Monitoring of symptoms.* Patient is asked to keep a diary for panic attacks.
3. *Breathing retraining.* Patient is asked to learn to breath abdominally which reduces panic.
4. *Cognitive restructuring* is focused on correcting the bodily sensation. Anxiety disorder patients often overestimate their body sensations. For example, increased heart rate may be interpreted as having a heart attack or GI sensations may accompany fear of losing sphincter control.

5. *Exposure to fear cues.* Final stage is actual exposure to the phobic situation.

Exposure to fear cues is used to treat agoraphobia. In order to do that we would refer the patient to a psychologist.[4] The anxiety for each situation is rated from 1-10. The patient is asked to enter in each situation at low level of anxiety on a daily basis until the fear is attenuated and then proceed further. A more intense exposure (sink or swim), also called *flooding* is rarely used and borders on patient abuse.

Group therapy is also helpful for patients with agoraphobia. Exposure to fear cures is often conducted in group. Sometimes, the patient's spouse is an inadvertent accomplice, who accompanies the patient or does chores with him/her. Studies that include spouses in treatment demonstrate increased efficacy.[5]

What is her long-term prognosis?

Panic disorder responds well to a combination of medication and therapy. The course of agoraphobia is variable. Although agoraphobia theoretically can occur without panic attacks, in almost all clinical situations, agoraphobia is accompanied by panic attacks. In some patients, decrease in panic attack correlates with decrease in phobic avoidance. In others, agoraphobia may become chronic regardless of panic attacks. About 20-30% of these patients remain the same or become worse. We do not know the predictors of chronicity.

Patient 5-3: The Hair Collector

A 26-year-old man comes to your office complaining of being continuously anxious since a teenager. He says that he is afraid that his hair is contaminating others, and that they might develop an illness from his hair. He collects his hair and has been storing it in bags for many years. The bags now fill his house. He spends 8-10 hours daily collecting his hair, and a similar amount of time worrying about his hair contaminating others.

What syndrome best defines Patient 5-3's problem?

Patient 3 is overwhelmed by his clearly false ideas about his hair. Do these represent a delusion or an obsession? A *delusion* is a false, fixed belief that develops from faulty thinking or from misperceptions (e.g., hallucinations). *Obsessions* are intrusive unwanted thoughts or images that cause marked anxiety. Obsessions are often exaggerations of common concerns. For example, food workers and hospital workers often wear caps to minimize the risk of their hair contaminating their fields of work. Their lives, however, are not consumed by this concern. Obsessive thoughts are different, not in content, but by being unstoppably intrusive. Patients try to ignore or suppress them, but can't.   They often recognize their thoughts as their own imagination and as unreasonable. However, resisting these thoughts causes significant anxiety. Most patients develop ritualistic, repetitive behaviors in response to these obsessions. These behaviors are called compulsions. Compulsions are aimed at reducing anxiety. Compulsions can be mental list making, or mental counting, or specific rituals. For example, many normal persons have rituals that they do to relieve mild anxiety. Some will "knock on wood" after making a positive statement to avoid bad luck. A person with obsessions about bad luck might knock on wood a certain number of times and then incorporate other repetitive actions to help. Compulsions are repetitive and almost stereotypic. They are often procedural memories gone haywire.[6] When obsessions and compulsions occur independently of general medical or neurologic disorder, the patient is diagnosed as having obsessive compulsive disorder (OCD).

> Subtypes of OCD: a) Hand washers (75%) to avoid contamination, b) checkers (40%) to avoid disaster, c) orderers (9%) need for symmetry and order, d) repeaters (8%) to feel comfortable and avoid something bad, and e) pure obsessionals (7%) only obsessions are experienced (no rituals present).

What other information would be helpful to make a definitive diagnosis?

The first goal in diagnosis is defining the syndrome. So, do we have enough information to say with reasonable certainty that patient 3 suffers from primary OCD? *Table 5.8* describes demographic features of OCD. Patients with primary OCD typically experience signs of obsessive thinking for years before the OCD becomes paramount in their lives. They often have a premorbid anxious-fearful personality disorder, and anxiety traits appear in their relatives. Their OCD symptoms emerge gradually and then fluctuate in severity, but rarely fully resolve. Patient 5-3 has all these features.

Table 5.8	*Demographics of OCD*
Prevalence in general population	4-6% with recent increase
Age of onset	Early to late teens
Gender difference	Men = women
Course and prognosis	One-third episodic with complete remission, one-third episodic with partial remission, and one-third chronic

How would you treat Patient 5-3?

OCD can be treated with a combination of behavioral therapy and serotonin reuptake inhibitors.

1. *Behavioral therapy* works best[1] for OCD patients like Patient 5-3 with well-defined rituals. Treatment will focus on exposing him to his hair, but preventing him from collecting it. In the beginning, he may be asked to visualize that his hair is all over his house, but that he is not collecting it. Once he is more comfortable in imagining these circumstances, exposure may be attempted in fact (in vivo). This type of exposure and response prevention is often facilitated by concomitant relaxation training. Other techniques include thought stopping by the therapist or the patient himself (interrupting obsessions by shouting "stop") or paradoxical intention and mass practice (asking the patient to think continuously of the obsession to the point of fatigue). Thus, behavioral interventions for OCD are relaxation training, thought therapy, in vitro and then in vivo exposure with response prevention.

2. *Pharmacotherapy:* Clomipramine (200-300 mg for at least 12 weeks) is still the first choice, and about 70% of OCD patients respond. Other SSRIs, such as fluvoxamine (300 mg), fluoxetine (60-80 mg), sertraline (100-200 mg) and paroxetine (40-60 mg), also work. Because OCD patients often obsess

about side effects, begin with low doses and go slowly. As always, when choosing a drug, consider the side effects that may be most bothersome to the patient, resulting in noncompliance (e.g., sexual side effects of fluoxetine in this young man must be considered and if they occur, they may be either treated by dose reduction or bupropion 75-100 mg). many patients who respond will need to be on medication indefinitely.

In what other psychiatric disorders do patient 3's symptoms occur?

Several seemingly different syndromes share common features of intrusive thoughts or actions. These include Gilles de la Tourette's (GTS) syndrome, impulse control disorders, such as kleptomania, trichotillomania, pathologic gambling, eating disorders, hypochondriasis, self-mutilation, obsessive hoarding, some paraphilias, and some PTSD.[2] Patients with mania or schizophrenia may experience classic obsessive compulsive behaviors secondary, but some of these patients are actually experiencing the stereotypies and ritual-like behavior have catatonia not OCD. Obsessive-like ruminations and perseverative motor behavior are common in melancholia. This can be a diagnostic challenge because nonmelancholic depression is comorbid in 60% of OCD patients. Lack of vegetative signs and a reactive mood distinguish depression superimposed on OCD from melancholia.

The relationship between obsessive compulsive personality and OCD is unclear. Although one-third of OCD patients have an obsessive compulsive personality, only a small percentage of persons with obsessive compulsive personality develop OCD. The majority of OCD patients have other cluster C (anxious, fearful) personality traits.

Discussion

Although in the DSM, OCD is listed as an anxiety disorder, OCD differs from other anxiety disorders. The risk for developing OCD in men and women is equal, whereas for most anxiety disorders the risk is higher for women. There is also increased risk of tic disorder in the families of OCD patients. OCD patients (particularly males)

PANDAS (Pediatric Autoimmune Neuropsychiatric Disorder Associated with Strep Infection). Childhood mood disorder with OCD is difficult to treat and has a guarded prognosis. PANDAS children have high DNA antibodies for strep, swollen basal ganglia on MRI, and present with OCD and tics. Plasma exchange, steroids, immunoglobulins, vitamin E, and antibiotics acutely treat and may prevent chronicity. [9]

also have a history of tic disorder. The converse is also true, and about two-thirds of Tourette's patients have OCD.

Table 5.9 compares the phenomenology of OCD with other anxiety disorders. OCD patients have an increased prevalence of labor/delivery and gestational problems. They have increased rates of non-specific EEG abnormalities. Neuroimaging studies show reduced caudate volume on CT and MRI. Functional imaging studies show hypermetabolism in the orbitomesial frontal cortex and caudate nucleus. In addition, OCD patients also have deficits in frontal lobe and right hemispheric function, e.g., visual memory problems, problems matching patterns with verbal cues.

Table 5.9 OCD and Other Anxiety Disorders					
Disorder	Obsession	Compulsion	Avoidance	Anticipation/ Worry	Panic Attack
OCD	Yes	Yes	Maybe	Maybe	Maybe
Panic disorder	No	No	Yes	Yes	Yes
Phobia	No	No	Yes	Yes	Maybe
Generalized	No	No	No/maybe	Yes	No

These findings suggest the involvement of basal ganglia, especially the caudate and globus pallidus. Basal ganglia lesions or dysfunction produce OCD-like symptoms in patients. When OCD-like symptoms occur for the first time after age 35, these secondary causes become more likely. Table 5.10 lists the secondary causes of OCD.

Table 5.10   Some Causes of Secondary OCD
Basal ganglia disease
Epilepsy
Stimulant drug abuse
Benzodiazepine withdrawal
Right frontal lobe infarct
Multiple sclerosis

193

Patient 5-4: I Wash My Hands Because I Must

A 39-year-old man frequently fantasizes butchering small animals and seeing blood splattered over the room. Whenever he thinks this, he feels he must thoroughly wash his hands and face. He is unable to stop these thoughts and actions. His symptoms began in his early teens. Now they are worse, and he thinks he is "going crazy." He has been treated with fluoxetine and behavioral therapy without much success. He is taking Clomipramine.

What should you do next?

Any patient who has not responded to the treatment needs to be re-evaluated. Is the syndromal diagnosis correct? Has an underlying etiology been missed? Are there co-occurring conditions that interfered with treatments? Are there pharmacokinetic or compliance problems? Let us assume that you have checked and that none of these explain patient 4's nonresponse.

Next check treatments. How long has he been taking clomipramine and at what dose? OCD is often initially treatment-resistant, so it is often necessary to give a maximum dose (300 mg or more) for 12 weeks or more. Also, determine the dose and duration of other drug trials.

What alternative treatments are available for this patient?

Over 50% of treatment resistant patients respond to IV clomipramine.[10] For these patients, IV clomipramine over a two to three week period (doses given over one hour starting at 25 to 50 mg and increasing to 200 to 250 mg) can substantially relieve symptoms for weeks or months in some patients or can make a previously unresponsive patient much more responsive to oral clomipramine. However, do not use IV clomipramine if you are concerned about a seizure disorder (tricyclics lower seizure threshold) or if the patient has heart disease (may cause arrhythmia or heart attack). Repeated intravenous dosing over a 1-2 year period may be needed before trying to discontinue the drug.

MAOIs (phenelzine 90 mg daily) should be tried for those patients not responding to reuptake inhibitors, and a small proportion of treatment resistant OCD patients will respond. However, do not combine with an SSRI, as the combination may precipitate a serotonin syndrome.

Dopamine agonists (e.g., amphetamine 10-20 mg or bromocriptine 12.5-30 mg daily) may also work for a small proportion of patients with mostly pure obsessions due to coarse basal ganglia disease. Do not use these agents, however, if the patient or family has tic disorder, as they may worsen or induce that condition.

Clonidine (0.25-1 mg daily), a presynaptic alpha$_2$-agonist that decreases norepinephrine release, may help in tic disorder and can be combined with clomipramine for OCD. Some OCD patients may get worse with clonidine, but some substantially improve (20%). Sedation and orthostasis are the major side effects of clonidine. Clonidine is also used for Tourette's disorder, and 40-60% of patients respond over an 8-12 week course of treatment. Associated attention deficit and OCD symptoms will also improve.

Benzodiazepines are helpful for short-term relief of anxiety until other drugs work or as a temporary sleep aid. Clonazepam 4-10 mg daily also has some serotonergic properties and may more specifically benefit some patients (20%). Lithium carbonate may help if the OCD is associated with a mood disorder. Carbamazepine and valproate may help if you suspect epilepsy spectrum disorder.[11]

Antipsychotics have also been used to treat OCD patients who also have tics. Because of the risk for tardive dyskinesia, these are drugs of last resort, and pimozide the agent of choice followed by haloperidol. Doses are the same as when used for GTS. Pimozide (2-12 mg) and haloperidol (6-16 mg) help 70% of GTS patients. Risperidone (2-6 mg) may be used, but is not as effective. For most patients, pimozide is preferred because of fewer extrapyramidal side effects. Because pimozide can cause prolonged Q-T cardiac conduction problems, it is not used in patients with heart block arrhythmias.

Table 5.11 Drugs for Treatment Resistant OCD	
Drug	Dose
IV clomipramine	200-250 mg
Monoamine oxidase inhibitor phenelzine	90 mg
Dopamine agonist amphetamines	10-20 mg
Bromocriptine	12.5-30 mg
Clonidine added to clomipramine	0.25-1 mg
Clonazepam	4-10 mg
Lithium carbonate added to clomipramine	900-1200 mg

If nothing else works, then the patient may benefit from psychosurgery. Stereotactic capsulotomy, anterior cingulotomy, or subcaudate tractotomy have been used for over 25 years to treat OCD patients who have failed to respond to all other treatments (including modern pharmacotherapy). As patients who undergo this procedure for OCD are typically in good general health and have no other neurologic disease, side effects from neurosurgery (bleeding, infection, seizures) are infrequent and, when they occur, remediable. An additional side effect is a 2-3 month postoperative period of fatigue, decreased initiative, and mild bradyphrenia that correlate with the degree of the transient edema from surgery. Long-term cognitive problems have not been demonstrated, but if present are far outweighed by the therapeutic response. Patients whose personalities and family support structure remain intact are the best candidates, and about 40-50% will experience substantial improvement.

Patient 5-5: Fear Has No Reason

After failing his final exam three months ago, a 22-year-old man has had ten episodes of sudden apprehension, associated with a sense of doom, hypervigilance, irritability, and fatigue. He also notes dizziness, shortness of breath, and palpitations with these episodes. The episodes are not associated with exertion, life threatening situations or frightening stimuli. He reports no problems between episodes. Physical and laboratory examinations reveal no evidence of any general medical or traditional neurologic illness.

Does this man have PTSD?

The term PTSD (post-traumatic stress disorder) was introduced in 1980 as a "recognition" of psychiatric symptoms of war veterans, especially Vietnam combat veterans. In addition to victims who experience combat, burial detail, and working in a burn unit, current criteria include victims of any life threatening, or maiming event, i.e., rape, kidnapping. PTSD is a syndrome that occurs after an individual has been exposed to one of these extremely stressful events. Thus, by definition, Patient 5-5 does not meet the criterion for the stress.

PTSD is characterized by recurrent re-experiences of the original traumatic event in the form of flashbacks or intrusive thoughts. PTSD patients often complain of psychological numbness, depression, hypervigilance, and irritability.   They have sleep disturbances and associated nightmares. *Table 5.12* lists DSM criteria for PTSD.

From the description above and from DSM criteria, Patient 5-5 does not have PTSD.

Eighty percent of PTSD patients have at least one additional diagnosis. Psychiatric disorders that commonly occur with PTSD are major depression, dysthymia, panic disorder, generalized anxiety disorder, substance abuse, obsessive compulsive disorder, phobia, somatization disorder, dissociative disorder, sleep disorder, personality disorder, and traumatic brain injury.

Table 5.12 Diagnostic Criteria for Post-traumatic Stress Disorder
The person has been exposed to a life-threatening traumatic event.
The traumatic event is persistently re-experienced as: (1) recurrent and intrusive distressing recollections of the event. (2) recurrent distressing dreams of the event (3) acting or feeling as if the traumatic event were recurring. (4) intense psychological distress or physiologic reactivity at exposure to internal or external cues of the traumatic event
Persistent avoidance of stimuli associated with the trauma and numbing of general responsiveness (not present before the trauma).
Persistent symptoms of increased arousal (not present before the trauma).
Duration of the disturbance (symptoms in Criteria B, C, and D) is more than 1 month.
The disturbance causes clinically significant distress or impairment in social, occupational, or other important areas of functioning

What other disorders could Patient 5-5 have?

Table 5.13 lists the different causes of acute anxiety in a 25-year-old man. Based on what we now know, it is likely that Patient 5-5 has an anxiety disorder. He is experiencing recurrent episodes of acute anxiety. Although one panic attack does not constitute a disorder, recurrent episodes of panic without a physical etiology suggest panic disorder.

What is wrong with Patient 5-5?

Anxiety disorders have a significant biological component. Genetic biochemical and CNS factors contribute to development of anxiety disorders. In 30% of monozygotic twin pairs, both have panic disorder, whereas in dizygotic twins, rates are similar to unrelated individuals.

Normal anxiety occurs as an adaptive response to fight/flight situations. The fight/flight system is activated by strong and typically sudden and unexpected stimuli or stimuli that evoke memories of previous dangers. The brain structures involved in fight/flight include the reticular activating system (arousal), locus ceruleus (norepinephrine release), and thalamus regulating arousal and cortical structure involving attribution, i.e., deciding if the stimulus is dangerous or not. The thalamus also simultaneously sends stimuli to the amygdala/hippocampus and parahippocampus, which, in turn, stimulates the hypothalamus to produce

Table 5.13   Differential Diagnosis of Acute Anxiety in Young Men

Caffeine intoxication: history of caffeine intake, occupation that requires long hours or night duties (e.g., truck driver, physician, nurse)

Cocaine dependence or abuse: history of cocaine abuse, other high novelty seeking behaviors, such as involvement in high risk activity (e.g., race car driving, mountain climbing)

Seizure disorder: history of head injury with either loss of consciousness or strong acceleration-deceleration impact, episodes of anxiety followed by some confusion. History of generalized or febrile seizures.

Anxiety disorders: onset in childhood or late teen anxiety (paroxysmal or generalized; specific or nonspecific), family history of anxiety disorder, no medical or neurologic problem

Alcohol withdrawal: long history of alcohol use, family history of alcoholism, abnormal liver function test, primary anxiety disorders, pattern since childhood or teenage years, high harm avoidant personality traits, family history of some anxiety disorder

Depression: anxiety with sadness, presence of vegetative symptoms, depressive thought content, family history of depression

needed sympathetic responses. In extreme situations, cortical processing is bypassed and stimuli are processed through the amygdala/hippocampus and parahippocampus.

The anxiety produced by cortical attribution is called *cognitive anxiety*, whereas the anxiety produced hypothalamic stimulation is called *somatic anxiety*. Anxiety disorder probably arises from the flight/fight system's hypersensitivity to stimuli. The more ambiguous, novel, or potentially dangerous the stimulus pattern, the more intense the response. Thus, the flight/fight system in anxious patients responds to stimuli that do not produce a flight/fight response in nonanxious persons (the threshold is lower). It also over-responds to stimuli that produce a modest response in nonanxious persons (once over the threshold, the response is more intense and of greater duration).[12]

Many panic disorder patients experience panic attacks due to sodium lactate infusion or hyperventilation, suggesting that these patients exhibit hypersensitivity to carbon dioxide. A variety of neurotransmitters are capable of inducing panic by stimulating noradrenergic and dopaminergic systems. Stimulation of the locus ceruleus, which contains 90% noradrenergic neurons, causes fear and anxiety. Serotonin and GABA are also involved in producing anxiety by modulating noradrenergic activity. Medications that relieve anxiety work on these neurotransmitters.

Patient 5-6: Nightmare on School Street

One week after she was an observer in a school shooting in which many children were hurt, a 30-year-old teacher complains of episodes of apprehension associated with fearful and constant visual scanning for new danger. She experiences a sense of doom, numbness and tingling in her arms and legs. During these episodes she is dizzy, has a dry mouth and palpitations. Between episodes, she feels "numb." She prefers to be in large, open spaces, rather than in regular rooms. Frequently, she daydreams and has nightmares about the shooting. She has no history of a sustained sad mood. Other than the nightmares that awaken her for a few minutes, she has no other sleep problems. She denies any suicidal ideation and is not psychotic.

Does Patient 5-6 have PTSD?

Patient 5-6 was in the middle of a shooting during which she saw children hurt. This level of trauma definitely qualifies for PTSD. She re-experiences the event in her nightmares and daydreams. She is hypervigilant and has anxiety attacks. She also experiences numbness between episodes. All these features could be explained by depression, but Patient 5-6 has no sustained sad mood. She has no general medical or traditional neurologic illness that can explain her condition (*Table 5.14* lists the differential diagnosis for PTSD). So Patient 5-6 meets most DSM criteria for PTSD. However, the DSM also requires symptoms persisting for at least one month. Thus, Patient 5-6 has all the features consistent with an acute stress response, but not necessarily a disorder. Most persons would respond as she has, but most persons would also get over it. Those that don't get the PTSD diagnosis.

Table 5.14   Differential Diagnosis of PTSD
Depression
Obsessive compulsive disorder (when intrusive thoughts are present)
Epilepsy (especially when flashbacks are present)
Adjustment disorder with anxiety
Other anxiety disorders, such as phobia or generalized anxiety disorder
Psychotic disorder, primary or secondary (if flashbacks present)
Delirium (if hypervigilance and flashback present)

How would you treat her?

Most persons with an acute stress response get better within a month. Counseling and occasional use of benzodiazepine is sufficient for many and should be tried first. Factors that may cause a person to have persistent PTSD features requiring further and different treatments are a past history of anxiety disorder. Women also have a higher risk of PTSD than do men, particularly when the stressor occurs when young. Women with PTSD also have more symptoms and a longer illness duration.

Patient 5-7: A Caterpillar Who Wants to Be a Butterfly

A 48-year-old professional woman comes to you because of her concern about her recent increase in alcohol consumption. This coincides with a recent promotion to a position which requires her to frequently attend dinner meetings and speak in front of large gatherings. She often takes a few drinks before she goes out. Although she does not get drunk and does not have any general medical disease, she often experiences a headache in the morning. She denies any other symptoms. Her sleep and appetite are unchanged. She has always been a quiet, socially inhibited person.

What should you tell Patient 5-7?

As always, start with diagnosis. Is Patient 5-7 anxious or depressed before she drinks? Is she drinking because it relaxes her? The increase in drinking occurred after she was promoted to a job that requires a lot of socializing. Has she had past difficulty interacting with people? *Social anxiety disorder* (SAD) or social phobia, as it was previously known is a fear of several or most social or performance situations. The nongeneralized form is characterized by fear of a single situation, usually public speaking.

You need to tell patient 7 that SAD is the most common form of anxiety disorder with a lifetime prevalence of 13-14%. It develops early, usually appearing in adolescence.[13] Persons with SAD experience anticipatory anxiety before the feared situation, and exposure to these feared events precipitate intense anxiety symptoms. The anxiety is usually worsened by negative cognitions around their performances.

What is her prognosis?

About 70-80% of individuals with SAD experience depression, generalized anxiety, panic disorder, substance abuse, and personality disorder.[14]

Without treatment, SAD is a chronic illness that can last several years. Less than 40% recover without treatment. Individuals with SAD experience considerable impairment and disability. Patients who have comorbid depression or alcohol and substance abuse have a worse prognosis. Other factors that predict poor outcome include earlier onset, severe symptoms, and positive family history of SAD.[15]

How would you treat her problem?

Cognitive behavior therapy as described for Patient 5-2 helps to reduce anxiety. SSRIs (such as sertraline, fluvoxamine and paroxetine) have all been shown to be helpful as has venlafaxine. Medication choice depends on tolerability of side effects and comorbid conditions. If reuptake inhibitors do not help, an MAOI, like phenelzine, may help. Benzodiazepines can reduce anxiety rather quickly and may be used initially. However, they are not effective in treating comorbid depression or OCD and can cause tolerance. They should not be used on a long-term basis.[16]

What should we do about drinking? Isn't that what she came to us for? Well, treating her social anxiety effectively will automatically reduce her drinking. For once, we are lucky.

Quick Rounds

1. A 35-year-old woman is taking sertraline 200 mg PO qhs and lorazepam 1 mg PO BID. During an office visit, she complains of increased anxiety in the afternoon. What should you do?

2. A 40-year-old woman is taking alprazolam 1 mg TID for the last 10 years for panic attack along with nortriptyline 100 mg PO qhs. You would like her to get off the alprazolam, but she tells you that this was attempted three times in the past and she couldn't do it. What should you do?

3. A 25-year-old college student is taking sertraline 50 mg for generalized anxiety disorder. She reports doing well except that 2-3 days before her menstrual period, she experiences worsening of symptoms that resolves 1-2 days after her period. What is the cause of her anxiety, and what should you do?

4. A 60-year-old man is taking citalopram 20 mg daily for post-stroke depression. He has been under more stress recently due to increased financial problems, and he complains of increased depression. You increase his citalopram to 30 mg daily, but instead he takes 40 mg. Three to four days later he calls you because of worsening symptoms. He also is experiencing anxiety, sleeplessness, and agitation. What is your next step?

5. A 35-year-old college professor complains of anxiety when giving lectures. She often finds herself sweating, her face gets flushed, and she experiences palpitations and dry mouth, leading to obvious difficulty presenting. What medication should you give her?

6. Twenty-four hours after an elective surgery, a 46-year-old woman with panic disorder develops anxiety, tremulousness, and restlessness. She has a temperature off 99^0 F, and her pulse is 120/minute. The patient is alert, oriented, and has not received any medications except Tylenol. What happened?

Quick Rounds Answers

1. The patient is experiencing withdrawal anxiety because lorazepam is a relatively short-acting benzodiazepine. Replacing lorazepam with an equivalent dose of a long-acting benzodiazepine, such as clonazepam will also relieve the anxiety.

2. Alprazolam is one of the most difficult benzodiazepines to stop taking. The best way to discontinue alprazolam is to replace it with an equal dose of clonazepam and then slowly taper clonazepam. Because of clonazepam's long half-life, it is easier to taper.

3. The reason she is experiencing anxiety premenstrually is twofold. First, progesterone and its metabolite tetrahydroprogesterone are GABA A agonists, and premenstrually their levels go down. Some patients experience this as anxiety, akin to benzodiazepine withdrawal. Second, sertraline levels may go down premenstrually because of increased renal clearance. Increasing sertraline to 75 mg for one week starting 4-5 days premenstrually should relieve her problem.

4. This patient's worsening symptoms are due to the serotonergic effects of citalopram, especially since the dose has doubled. You should tell him to stop the citalopram for the day and come right in for an evaluation so you can assess him for the presence of serotonin syndrome. If his symptoms are mild and he has normal blood pressure, pulse and temperature, then he should resume citalopram at 30 mg daily, wait for a couple of weeks, re-evaluate and increase, if needed.

5. She is experiencing performance anxiety. However, anxiety can be categorized into somatic anxiety marked with more autonomic features and cognitive anxiety associated with cognitions, such as worry, fear, etc. Benzodiazepines work better if cognitive anxiety is associated with somatic anxiety. If somatic anxiety is the only predominant feature then a beta blocker, such as propranolol 10-20 mg, can be used. Word of caution: Ask the patient to take a trial dose before the lecture, just to ensure it will be tolerated.

6. You first need to ask the woman what medication she takes for her panic disorder. Most likely, she is experiencing withdrawal from her anxiolytic medication since she has not taken her medication for more than 24 hours. The next step is to restart her on her medication.

Chapter 6

The Differential Diagnosis of Psychosis

Patient 6-1: Take the Road Less Traveled

A 28-year-old man is hospitalized involuntarily after being brought to the ER by the police for trying to stab his mother. He destroyed some of her furniture and then threatened persons in the street. He has a long history of this behavior with exacerbations associated with persecutory ideas, perceptual distortions (faces look misshaped and odd in color), and auditory hallucinations (voices). He has been diagnosed schizophrenic.

> Schizophrenia is an uncommon disorder when specific diagnostic criteria are used "as directed." Population base rates from modern studies are around 0.5%. Only about 5% of acutely psychotic hospitalized patients meet criteria. Schizophrenia there is never your first consideration, and best used as the last resort diagnosis after you have ruled out treatable medical and more common mood disorders.

If not schizophrenia, what?

It is always easy to rely on past diagnoses. Patient 6-1 has for years been diagnosed schizophrenic, so stick with the plan, put him on the latest antipsychotic, fasten your seat belt, and hope for the best. Most likely, the best will be a rehash of the past: "Past is prologue" with chronic illness.

BUT, Patient 6-1 is only 28 years old. He potentially has another 50 years of life. You could go down the well traveled schizophrenia path or try the road less traveled and see what happens. Your only road signs are: Do no harm, and make the diagnosis for which you have good treatments, because even if you are wrong the patient got a trial of medications that could have helped him.

So, what else might Patient 6-1 have to explain his condition? *Table 6.1* also answers the question: **How do you figure out "the what?"**

What is schizophrenia?

Schizophrenia is a psychiatric illness that is characterized by the presence of hallucinations, delusions, disorganized thinking, negative symptoms, such as decreased motivation or pleasure in the absence of mood disorder and lasting more than 6 months. Hallucinations are perceptions without real stimuli and occur in all sensory modalities (e.g., auditory, visual, etc.). Auditory hallucinations are most common. Some hallucinations are elaborate or well formed: hearing a specific voice and what it says, seeing a specific person in full detail. Some hallucinations are vague: dim, flimsy, unformed like a sound or light but not a voice or figure. These are termed elementary hallucinations.

Table 6.1 What You Might Find on a Road Less Traveled	
Condition	**What to Consider**
Mood disorder	Assess for the presence of mood symptoms lasting a week or longer. Does he have an episode illness? If more continuous than episodic, a bipolar disorder is likely to begin in childhood so look for a history of hyperactivity, oppositional personality disorder, or an atypical attention deficit disorder that did not respond to stimulants. Family history will likely also be positive for mood disorder. Substance abuse, unfortunately, is also likely in such patients.
Substance abuse	Substances to first consider when violence is a concern are: inhalant abuse, phencyclidine (PCP), LSD, and chronic stimulant use. History with collateral confirmation is always important for this choice. Inhalant abuse can be the most dangerous. Recent abuse can produce a perioral or facial rash. PCP abuse may be associated with periods of catatonia and cerebellar dysfunction. LSD may be associated with distorted visual hallucinations, fantastic delusional content (e.g., spaceships, previous lives), synesthesias and the combination of flight of ideas with formal thought disorder. Chronic stimulant use may be associated with movement disorders.
Epilepsy	Usually with a mesial frontotemporal focus and associated features discussed in chapter 7.
Head trauma	Typically involving frontal regions or the nondominant hemisphere.

What are the treatments for "the whats" in a patient like Patient 6-1?

If *mood disorder*, carbamazepine or valproic acid, or ECT may offer the best outcomes rather than an antipsychotic. An antipsychotic with ECT may also work, if the antipsychotic or ECT is only partially effective.[1]

If *substance abuse,* treatment choices are the same as for mood disorder. Patients with drug related psychoses, particularly late recurring psychotic disorders (psychotic episodes from drug use cause brain damage) have cognitive impairment that can substantially reduce interepisode functioning. Antipsychotics can delay cognitive recovery, so they should be used briefly or as last resorts in such patients.

If *epilepsy,* decide if the psychosis is post-ictal or interictal and treat as discussed in Chapter 7.

If *head trauma,* anticonvulsants can be used to control both psychosis and aggressive behavior. Although we have frequently used carbamazepine because of reports its effectiveness in intermittent explosive disorder,[2] there is no clear evidence that carbamazepine is superior to valproic acid.

> Schizophrenics have reduced libido and thus fertility (10% of norm for males, 20% for females). The age of onset of the first psychosis is typically 15-25 for males and 5 years later for females. Males have a more chronic form, but females a greater family history for schizophrenia.

Discussion

By now you've noticed that we are not quick to label a psychotic patient schizophrenic, especially in the absence of symptoms, such as loss of emotional expression, anhedonia (lack of pleasure), apathy (lack of interest), also known as *negative symptoms*. We think that once a patient is labeled schizophrenic, he will likely be given antipsychotics and will not receive any other medication, nor further evaluation. We prefer to call these patients "Positive Symptoms, Nonaffective Psychosis." In our experience this label, though not a DSM diagnosis, accurately portrays the clinical presentation. There is schizophrenia and there is schizophrenia. The DSM schizophrenia is a group of psychoses with varying symptoms and outcomes (DSM-IV-R). However, the schizophrenia defined by stricter criteria appears to be a neurodevelopmental disorder. The neurodevelopmental hypothesis suggests that genetic vulnerabilities are impacted by events occurring during critical periods of neuronal growth (during the second trimester) that adversely affect brain development. Schizophrenia has demonstrated genetic liability. Chronic schizophrenia is typically associated with problems in childhood. These include emotional aloofness and irritability; deficits in attention; working memory and cognitive flexibility; neuromotor awkwardness; delayed motor landmarks; poor school performance and learning difficulties. Many of these patients do not have a chronic deteriorating course. *Table 6.2* lists other causes of chronic positive symptom psychosis.

Table 6.2 *Other Causes of Positive Symptoms*
Space occupying lesions
Wilson's disease
Herpes encephalitis
Normal pressure hydrocephalus
Chronic alcoholic hallucinosis

Patient 6-2: Love by Remote Control

Patient 6-2 is a well-dressed and well-groomed 52-year-old housewife. She is pleasant and looks younger than her age. She complains that someone has put a video camera in her bathroom so that "Harrison Ford" can watch her in the shower. She believes that Mr. Ford is in love with her. Although she can not see the camera, she knows it is there. She has moved three times, but Mr. Ford has had every apartment bugged. Patient 6-2 has never been depressed nor manic. Her general medical health is good. Although she never worked outside the house, she is a meticulous housewife and has raised three daughters.

What psychopathology does Patient 6-2 have?

The only psychopathology mentioned in this vignette is the primary delusional ideas about the video camera and Harrison Ford. *Table 6.3* defines different delusional phenomena and their diagnostic implications.

Table 6.3 Delusional Phenomena and Their Diagnostic Implications

Phenomena	Implications
Delusional mood: a feeling of ill-ease and suspicion as if some as yet undefinable thing is wrong and potentially dangerous	An early sign of psychosis; the experience (but more intense) of a "bad trip" on a street drug
Ideas of reference: a delusional mood with more definition, where the actions of others appear directed at the patient: "People are looking at me, talking about me."	An early sign of psychosis; diagnostically nonspecific
Primary delusion: a fixed, false idea from arbitrary or illogical thinking that becomes central to the person's life	Patient 6-2 had a primary delusion as do many psychotic patients. It is nonspecific unless it occurs alone in an elaborated form with mundane content. Then it is diagnostic of delusional disorder.
Secondary delusion: a delusion that is based on other psychopathology that is accepted as true: the hallucinating patient believes the hallucinated content and develops a delusion based on that. Intense moods, depression, euphoria can lead to delusions of great guilt or grandiosity.	Also diagnostically nonspecific.
Delusions of "first rank": based on a subjective experience. If the experience is of being controlled by external forces (e.g., electromagnetic) it is termed *experience of control.* If the experience is of thinking someone else's thoughts or having a body part that belongs to someone else or having a demon or foreign body inside oneself, it is termed *experience of alienation.* If the experience is of understanding hidden significance and meaning in everyday events or objects, it is termed *delusional perception.*	These were incorrectly thought pathognomonic of schizophrenia. They occur in many primary and secondary psychoses, but are particularly common in schizophrenics, 60-75% of whom have had such an experience.

What diagnostically important psychopathology does Patient 6-2 *not* have?

What a patient does not have is also diagnostically important. We already know Patient 6-2 is neither depressed nor manic. Although in a real world evaluation you would have to specifically ask or make observations about these phenomena, from the vignette we may assume that the following are *not* present:

1. Emotional blunting
2. Speech and language problems
3. Motor abnormalities
4. Other delusions (see *Table 6.3*)
5. Hallucinations or other perceptual problems

Assuming all the information we have is correct, what disorder is Patient 6-2 not likely to have? What does she have?

Because Patient 6-2 does not have emotional blunting, i.e., patient has normal emotional expression and is volitional, and has functioned reasonably well as a mother and housewife, schizophrenia is highly unlikely. On the other hand, *delusional disorder* is the most likely syndromal diagnosis. The essence of delusional disorder is the presence of nonbizarre delusions (involving situations that can occur in real life, e.g., being followed, being cheated on).

Delusional disorder is a psychosis occurring later on in life (>age 30) than most schizophrenic psychoses. It usually occurs in a previously reasonably high functioning person who then develops a delusional story about themselves: a person loves them or hates them, there is some corporate or government plot to defraud them or others, they are a member of a well-known family. Other psychopathology is usually absent.[3]

Delusional disorder appears distinct from other psychoses. It is not a variant of schizophrenia or mood disorders. Family members are not at greater risk for other psychoses, but may be more likely to have *paranoid personality disorder*.

What might be the etiologies of Patient 6-2's condition?

Many conditions can cause delusional disorder.[4] What could affect the brain to such an extent? The patient's age, gender, the rate of development of the psychosis, general medical problems that affect brain function, and intrinsic neurologic disease that can cause psychosis. If the vignette is correct (why should we lie now) her general medical health is good. Thus, if she is not a substance abuser or an alcoholic (she is not) any likely condition will be neurologic. For neurologic disease, search first for "neighborhood" signs. Does she have any motor dysfunction and, if so, is it localizable? (She does not.) Does she have other psychopathology that suggests a region and, therefore, an illness? (She does not.) Does she have speech or language dysfunction? (She does not.) Does she have dyspraxias (difficulty performing an action despite normal motor strength and sensory system) or agnosias (difficulty using a sensory modality despite normal sensory system, i.e., a patient cannot identify an object by looking at it) suggestive of cortical disease? (She does not.)

> If a patient's general medical health "below the neck" is good, the likelihood of cardiovascular, endocrine, or metabolic disorders affecting the health "above the neck" is slim.

Traumatic brain injury or a significant infection involving the brain (e.g., herpes, mononucleosis) can cause psychosis and needs to be ruled out. (She has had none.) Finally, does the patient have risks for stroke, as small basal ganglia strokes and nondominant hemisphere strokes can go clinically undetected, but can cause psychosis. (She did not, and her MRI was normal.) Thus, her delusional disorder is primary.

How would you treat Patient 6-2?

Without mood disturbance or an episodic pattern to patient's 2's delusional disorder, ECT, or mood stabilizers are unlikely to be of benefit, although ECT should be tried if antipsychotics do not work. Low doses of an atypical antipsychotic would be a reasonable choice, i.e., risperidone 1-4 mg daily, or olanzapine 10-20 mg daily. The prognosis for delusional disorder is generally no deterioration, but only modest improvement.

Educating the family about the patient's illness may reduce their anxieties and family conflict over the delusion. Trying to convince Patient 6-2 of the false nature of her ideas or trying to cognitively restructure her ideas will not work. Be a good listener. Be honest and matter of fact in your disagreement. Help Patient 6-2 with other concerns she may have. Perhaps she will feel somewhat comforted in seeing you and, thus, more likely comply with her medication.

Patient 6-3: Caught in the Revolving Door

A 32-year-old man with a history of many hospitalizations despite being on adequate doses of antipsychotics, once again is admitted because he became agitated, angry and threatened his mother. He has the delusion that his mother is poisoning him. She, in turn, constantly nags him to eat more, and gets very angry because he refuses to eat anything she cooks. He has also experienced people talking to him (when no one is there), off and on for several years. When not threatening, he is avolitional and shows little emotional expression. As soon as he is on the inpatient unit, he usually is much better. He has been taking olanzapine 30 mg daily and has minimal side effects.

> Delusions of being poisoned -- more so than other content -- are associated with attacks on the presumed poisoner. If a patient thinks you are involved in the poisoning delusion, hospitalize that patient and take precautions because these are the patients that kill their doctor.[5]

What, if anything, can be done to get Patient 6-3 out of the revolving door? (This is a semi-trick question, followed by new stuff.)

The semi-trick, of course, is let's make a diagnosis first and then see what the appropriate treatments should be. All we know about Patient 6-3 is that he is psychotic. *Table 6.4* lists the differential diagnosis of psychosis the list and the common things to look for. They are listed in the order of likely occurrence (Sutton's Law) on an acute community hospital adult psychiatric service. In some private hospitals depression is the most commonly seen condition, and mania much less than expected. (Manics are hard on the decor and require longer hospitalizations than many insurance carriers tolerate.)

Patient 6-3 meets criteria for schizophrenia. He has experienced auditory hallucinations on and off for years, has a chronic condition with poor emotional expression, and avolition. No specific etiology could be determined, although like so many schizophrenics his mother had a difficulty pregnancy and delivery with him.

> Always ask about the patient's gestation, labor, and delivery, as problems here can cause brain damage which is a risk factor for later illness. Say, "I know it was a long time ago and you may not have been told, but did your mother (family) every say she had medical problems during her pregnancy with you, or that she had a difficult labor or delivery?" If possible, ask the patient's mother, or if he has one, a sister or aunt. In our experience, male relatives are less likely to know these details. Perhaps the next generation will be different.

Table 6.4   The Differential Diagnosis of Psychosis

Choice	What Else to Look For
Drug related mood disorder	Drug abuse history Episodic course Spared emotional expression, although avolitional other than drug-seeking Manias with flight of ideas *and* formal thought disorder Motor problems with chronic stimulant abuse and PCP use Often have a family history of mood disorder
Mania with psychosis	Mood symptoms take precedent over all psychotic features. Chronic course does not rule this out; 30-50% of bipolar patients are chronic. Always apply the Duck principle and then Sutton's Law. Catatonia will be present in 15-20% of bipolar episodes.
Psychotic depression	Vegetative signs do not lie. Apprehension and anxiety is more likely than sadness. Anhedonia rules. Mood symptoms take precedent over all psychotic features.
Nonmood disorders, drug related psychoses	This will be a nonaffective positive symptom psychosis. Emotional expression is spared but the patient often is avolitional. Drug history prominent: hallucinogens, inhalants (patient can be violent). Young male patients are more likely to be dangerous to staff.
Delirium	Most common in elderly patients with general medical problems who are receiving several medications. Fluctuating course during the day. Apprehension and agitation with "confusion": disorientation, memory lapses.
Dementia	Most likely in patients with vascular or alcohol related dementias. Elderly demented psychotic patient can be dangerous to staff members.
Epilepsy	Epilepsy takes many forms – it is the great mimic of psychiatry. Psychosensory features or auras can be present. Panoramic hallucinations and multiple hallucinations in multiple sensory modalities can be present. Onset is usually rapid with intense moods.
Traumatic brain injury	Frontal and nondominant injuries most likely to cause psychosis. Injuries are usually substantial unless in the elderly where "bumps" on the head can cause subdural hematoma.

Table 6.4 The Differential Diagnosis of Psychosis (con't)	
Choice	*What Else to Look For*
Stroke	Small strokes in tertiary cortices or related subcortical structures are likely. Motor and speech and language signs of stroke are often absent. Cognitive testing can help localization. Psychopathology is often isolated, rare in type, or atypical in some way.
Psychotic disorders from the DSM: schizophrenia, delusional disorder, brief psychosis, atypical psychosis	The patient meets specific criteria. Everything else is ruled out.
Space occupying lesions	Look for fronto-temporal vascular malformations, hematomas, and intrinsic brain tumors in the central core of the brain.

What should be your major concerns for each of the three stages of treatment for Patient 6-3?

1. *Acute phase*

   a. Minimize dangerousness and control irritability.
   b. Provide as much socialization and activities as he can tolerate (at first not a lot).
   c. Olanzapine 30 mg daily has not worked. He needs a total re-evaluation of his medications toward starting him on one that may stop his delusion.
   d. If the patient has not been on a typical antipsychotic, then an adequate trial of a high potency antipsychotic is warranted (e.g., haloperidol).
   e. If the patient has received an adequate trial of a typical antipsychotic, then a trial of clozapine at a maximum tolerable dose (300-600) should be given. (Note: Monitor CBC regularly to assess development of agranulocytosis.)[6]
   f. If the patient does not respond to clozapine, then we have two options: a) try another atypical antipsychotic (e.g.,

quetiapine), or b) ECT. There is evidence that in agitated psychotic patients, ECT may help. ECT and clozapine have also been reported to help some patients resistant to clozapine alone.[7]

2. *Continuation phase*

   a. Assuming Patient 6-3 leaves the hospital delusion free, and is not irritable, he is then continued on the treatments that worked.
   b. Early in hospitalization his mother needs to be educated toward her behaviors and emotionality as likely precipitants of relapse and a factor in her son's hospitalization. Her behavior, intense negative emotion is termed *expressed emotion*. She will need to markedly reduce this behavior to stop the revolving door. When expressed emotion is controlled, relapse rates *drop* 50%, even when medications are kept stable.[8]

3. *Maintenance phase*

   a. Constant reinforcement of good compliance with medication or ECT plus medication, and expressed emotion control for Patient 6-3 *and* his mother.
   b. Assessment of Patient 6-3's vocational, social, and cognitive strengths and weaknesses toward trying to rehabilitate some of his deficits.

Acute psychoses are analogous to broken bones. The acute treatment phase is equivalent to being in the cast. Continuation is like acute rehab. Maintenance is like better safety precautions (e.g., not riding the Harley-Davidson at 100 mph) and continued strength and flexibility training.

Patient 6-4: You've Got Mail

A 22-year-old man is diagnosed as schizophrenic and is hospitalized for the first time because he feels he is receiving messages from his computer even when the computer is off. He also believes that there are persons literally in his computer who take his thoughts away, and make him into a robot that functions at their command. These experiences are not just ideas he has but are "felt."[9] He has no history of any head injury or seizure disorder. His general medical and traditional neurologic examinations are within normal limits.

Patient 6-4 is treated with an antipsychotic and his delusions and hallucinations resolve, leaving him with mild loss of emotional expression and modest avolition. Although he is ready for discharge, his parents are very anxious about his homecoming. His mother is also worried about her other children getting the same illness.

> Unlike mania or psychoses with great emotionality or uproar, the psychosis associated with schizophrenia can respond to lower doses of antipsychotics. The big concern is to avoid tardive dyskinesia and its debilitating and socially disruptive motor features and its moderate cognitive impairment. First-choice antipsychotics might be olanzapine, or risperidone. In an otherwise healthy young male, chlorpromazine might be a backup. Clozapine would be the last choice, if Patient 6-4 still did not respond.

What can you do to help Patient 6-4's parents and maximize Patient 6-4's response to medication?

Patient 6-4 has completed acute treatment. Getting a schizophrenic to have no positive symptoms and only modest negative symptoms is the most you can expect, for most patients. Continuation of the good response to prevent relapse of this episode is the next challenge. Steps to do are:

> Without medication 75% of schizophrenics will relapse during the 6-12 months following an episode.

1. Educate the family about his illness, treatments over the next year, what they can expect over the long run, and risks of their other children getting schizophrenia.
2. Evaluate their other children to see if they have any of the *risk factors* predictive of psychosis, and take preventative steps if they do.

3. Assess the family for *expressed emotion* and minimize this influence on relapse rates. Provide family counseling, if needed.
4. Provide reinforcement for *compliance* with treatment, and continue Patient 6-4 on the medication that worked for the acute episode, and at the same dose that worked.
5. Assess Patient 6-4 for the appropriateness of cognitive, vocational, and social rehabilitation programs.

Discussion

Schizophrenia is a lifelong condition that in most patients likely begins from some interaction between a genetic vulnerability and gestational factors. The adverse uterine and gestational events are followed by prepsychotic neuromotor childhood abnormalities and then psychosis.[10] *Table 6.5* summarizes the genetics of schizophrenia.

Table 6.5 Morbid Risk for Schizophrenia	
In first-degree relatives	4-15%
Monozygotic concordance	50%
Dizygotic	5-15%
If one parent has it	10-15%
If two parents have it	30-40%
General population rate	.5-1%

Table 6.6 summarizes the factors that have been found in persons who later in life develop a schizophrenic psychosis. The severity of these factors predicts the likelihood and severity of the psychosis of schizophrenia. They also predict early childhood problems that in turn also predict the psychosis. Thus, Patient 6-4's siblings need to be evaluated for the factors in *Table 6.6,* and for the prepsychotic features predicting psychosis. These are displayed in *Table 6.7*.

The developmental model of schizophrenia is important because it suggests preventative strategies. Because there seems to be no specific single gene for schizophrenia and there may be a genetic overlap between schizophrenia and psychotic mood disorder, which families are at risk and then what to do about

Table 6.6   Factors Increasing the Risk for Schizophrenia
Maternal starvation or severe malnourishment
Second trimester exposure to influenza
Fetal distress or signs of anoxic problems
Prolonged and difficult labor and delivery
Use of marijuana in early teens

it is knowable. *Table 6.8* summarizes these strategies. Persons at high risk typically develop their first psychosis during the decade after puberty. Once the psychosis develops, further cognitive and social decline is likely, but this decline seems to plateau after 3-5 years. Preventing this decline is the focus for Patient 6-4, who has had his first psychosis. *Table 6.8* also shows steps in tertiary prevention.

Table 6.7 Childhood Prepsychotic Features of Schizophrenia

Delayed motor landmarks

Neuromotor problems and soft neurologic signs[11]

Problems with sustained attention and cognitive flexibility

Emotional aloofness and reduced animation and responsiveness to interpersonal cues

Minor physical anomalies

Table 6.8 Preventative Strategies for Schizophrenia

	Target	What to do
Primary prevention	Pregnant woman with personal, family, or spousal history of mood disorder or schizophrenia	Treat as high risk pregnancy. Provide flu shots before conception if planned pregnancy. Avoid viral infection during second trimester as if immune compromised. Maximize diet. Avoid all toxins to neural development.
Secondary prevention	Child of high risk woman	Assess for features shown in *Table 6.7*, getting baseline cognitive, motor and behavioral ratings. If no factors present, follow. If factors present begin rehabilitation program similar to those for children with better understood developmental disorders.
Tertiary prevention	First episode psychosis	Resolve quickly with treatment least likely to cause tardive dyskinesia. Begin rehabilitation during the later stages of hospitalization and continue these for at least a year after discharge. Maintain medication to prevent relapse and further decline. Reduce environmental stressors to prevent relapse and further decline.

Patient 6-5: Psychosis Lite

A 27-year-old man comes to the emergency room because he keeps seeing fireflies from the corners of his eyes. When he is driving, he sometimes mistakes shadows for water on the road when there is none. He has no hallucinations or delusions. His speech is vague and elliptical, and he converses in a slow, deliberate manner. He speaks with minimal gesturing or facial expression. He has never been treated for any psychiatric illness, but his visual experiences have become more frequent and annoying. He thinks what he sees are examples of magic.

Elliptical speech is speech that never really gets to the point, but which is always around the topic. *Flight of ideas* keeps on going away from the topic. *Circumstantial speech* gives too much detail and parenthetic information before reaching the point. An example of elliptical speech is, in answering why he does not work, Patient 6-5 talks about work in general, but not what he has done and not why he does not work.

What is Patient 6-5's syndromal (DSM) diagnosis? To answer question 1, you will need some additional information. What are the "big ticket" items in the information supermarket you want to get?

1. Always get the Duck. This Duck is a young man with frequent chronic illusions or vague (elementary) hallucinations,[12] vague speech, and loss of emotional expression, and, at least, odd ideas.
2. Your big ticket purchases to complete this picture are

    a. Does he have any delusions or other hallucinations?
    b. Does he have past or present manic or depressive symptoms?

In Patient 6-5's case the answers are all "no." He has been this way since childhood. He has never been depressed or manic and has never had other perceptual disturbances. He says he believes in magic and ghosts and sprits, but he has no other ideas that might be delusional. He says he knows some people do not believe in these things, but if they were not real, why would the Harry Potter books be so popular?

As it stands, Patient 6-5 does not meet criteria for any Axis I condition. However, he does meet criteria for schizotypal personality disorder, an Axis II condition. See *Table 6.9* for a summary of schizotypal behaviors.

What should you do after you have solved question 1? (This should be "old hat" by now.)

Once you have established the likely syndrome, you *always* search for etiology. What is the differential diagnosis of schizotypal personality disorder? *Table 6.10* displays the more common causes. When *drug abuse* is the cause, abuse will have typically begin around puberty, hallucinogens will be the culprits, and some genetic vulnerability will be likely, so look for a family history of psychiatric illness, particularly mood disorder. When *head injury* is the cause, look for falls or auto accidents with coup/counter-coup injuries most likely. If due to a *seizure disorder* look for the fits (see Chapter 7). If a *vascular malformation* is the cause, vascular malformations elsewhere may be present, and again look for seizures and get an MRI. A previous *viral infection* need not appear severe, but meningitic-like signs would usually have been present. *Psychotic spectrum disorder* means that schizotypal (indeed all of Axis II, odd-eccentric personality disorders) is really not a personality disorder at all, but a low-grade, chronic variant of psychosis, usually schizophrenia, but occasionally mood disorder. Schizotypal patients in this category rarely develop psychosis because they are not in a premorbid or early phase. They are in their part of the spectrum from a lesser "dose" of whatever causes psychosis.

Table 6.9 Schizotypal Behaviors
Reduced volition
Reduced emotional expression
Vague, empty or elliptical speech
Illusions and other perceptual distortions
Odd beliefs or magical thinking, e.g., belief in sixth sense
Thinking that focuses on details and misses the point or big picture
Excessive social anxiety
Odd, eccentric behavior
Suspiciousness

Table 6.10 The Differential Diagnosis of Schizotypal Personality Disorder
Chronic drug abuse (particularly hallucinogens)
Head injury (closed head injury, usually to frontotemporal poles as in coup/counter-coup)
Seizure disorder (complex partial with frontal or temporal focus)
Vascular malformation (also frontotemporal, often causing complex partial seizures)
Viral infection (herpes, Epstein-Barr)
Psychotic spectrum disorder

Discussion

DSM Axis II is divided into three personality disorder clusters. They are poetically referred to as A, B, and C. Cluster A is likely a mistake.[13] Cluster A includes schizotypal, schizoid, and paranoid "personality disorders." But, these are not conditions that are variations of normal traits. *Paranoid personality disorder* (irritable, suspicious, litigious, begrudging) is low grade delusional disorder and is observed in families of delusional disorder patients. *Schizoid personality disorder* (low energy, reduced emotional expression, social and motor awkwardness) is typical of children and teens who later develop a schizophrenic psychosis. *Schizotypal personality disorder* is more common in the relatives of patients with schizophrenia and perhaps in the relatives of persons with psychotic mood disorder. Schizotypal persons also have laboratory abnormalities similar to those seen in schizophrenia. *Table 6.11* summarizes these.

Schizotypal symptoms can also occur in other disorders. Treatment of schizotypal disorder is based on the etiology, and *Table 6.12* summarizes these.

Table 6.11 **Laboratory Findings in Schizotypal Personality Disorder**
Abnormal smooth pursuit eye tracking
Nonspecific EEG and evoked potential abnormalities
Decreased platelet monoamine oxidase
MRI abnormalities
Cognitive impairment
Information processing deficits

Table 6.12 Treatments for Schizotypal Personality Disorder	
Etiology	*Suggestions*
Drug abuse	Abstinence programs Anticonvulsant medications (valproic acid often first choice) Control expressed emotion in the family Rehabilitation
Head injury	Anticonvulsants or medications to modulate aggression, if present Control expressed emotion Rehabilitation
Vascular malformation	Surgery if operable Same as for head injury
Seizure disorder	Anticonvulsants Comprehensive treatments for epilepsy (see Chapter 7)
Viral infection	Same as for head injury
Psychotic spectrum disorder	Anticonvulsant mood stabilizers if family history of mood disorder Low dose atypical antipsychotics if family history of schizophrenia Control expressed emotion in the family Rehabilitation

Patient 6-6: Déjà Vu All Over Again

A 40-year-old man with chronic schizophrenia lives in a community group home. In the last 5 years he has been hospitalized many times for worsening of his psychosis. Once in the hospital, he is quickly stabilized on haloperidol 20 mg po, and his auditory hallucinations and irritability resolve. However, as soon as he is discharged, he stops taking his medications, and is readmitted within 4-6 weeks.

What are the possible reasons for Patient 6-6's noncompliance with treatment?

1. *Bad diagnosis.* Noncompliance can result from incorrect diagnosis, and the real illness rears its ugly head as soon as the patient is discharged. Then the patient stops treatment because of his symptoms.

2. *Bad treatment.* Sometimes treatments are inadequate, and patients who are still ill are discharged too soon or on too low a dose of medication. No one would discharge a patient getting IV antibiotics for a systemic infection before the patient is afebrile and the infection seems to be resolved or resolving. But we in essence do this all the time with psychiatric patients. A longer hospitalization in some circumstances can maximize response, stopping the revolving door. Bad treatment also means not paying attention to treatment side effects and cost. If a patient does not accept treatment side effects or cannot afford treatment, noncompliance is guaranteed.[14]

3. *Bad assessment.* Many acutely hospitalized psychiatric patients and most chronically ill psychiatric patients have *general medical problems* such as CHF, kidney disease, that can cause fatigue, and decreased motivation which can interfere with treatment, by making compliance difficult. Many psychiatric patients have *cognitive impairment,* particularly frontal lobe executive deficits, that make it difficult for them to follow instructions. They do not recall information well, and forget to remember. If cognition is a problem, the patient should be discharged to a situation where someone will administer the medication following your written and oral instructions.

4. *Bad vibes.* If I do not like you, if you or others around you have been mean or curt or disrespectful, why should I listen to you? If you have not been direct and truthful with me, if you have not

seemed skillful in your examinations, if you have not been caring and empathic, why should I listen to you? The quality of the doctor-patient relationship directly influences compliance.

5. *Bad temperament.* Whatever axis I condition a patient has, he also has a personality. *Normal* personality variations do not correlate with psychotic illness. Psychotic patients, however, may have some variant of cluster A personality disorder. Persons, particularly those with mood disorder, may have normal variations of personality that make them less cooperative or more self-directed than the average person. These patients, even if fully better from their axis I illness, will tend to be contrary.

6. *Bad placement.* Placements that have too much expressed emotion and not enough empathy and caring can lead to relapse. Placements that demand higher functioning than the patient has will lead to frustration, noncompliance, and relapse. Placement that is below the patient's abilities will lead to boredom, noncompliance, and relapse. Social skills and cognitive assessment at the end of hospitalization or the acute phase of treatment can guide placement.

What can be done to maximize compliance in chronic psychiatric patients like Patient 6-6?

1. Correct all the problems listed above.
2. All patients can, to some degree, be conditioned to reinforcers. Severely mentally retarded children can modify their disruptive behaviors when reinforced with such things as M&Ms, so most psychiatric patients can also respond to rewarding reinforcers. Medication blood levels indicate compliance. The trick is finding the reinforcers for a specific patient and getting the funds to give these at each clinic visit.
3. When all else fails, long-lasting depot haloperidol or fluphenazine can be helpful. Their use requires:

   a. The patient has a condition likely to respond to antipsychotics.
   b. Recurrent hospitalization due to noncompliance with oral medication is the problem.
   c. The patient cannot be trusted to take medication as directed.

   To use a depot preparation, first establish a daily effective dose with the corresponding oral agent.

d. Calculate the depot dose according to the manufacturer's instruction. In our and some of our colleagues' experience, patients require haldol decanoate every 2-3 weeks. For haloperidol the decanoate dose is 10 times the oral dose, whereas for fluphenazine the decanoate dose is 1.25 times the oral dose. However, some authors recommend using this as a guideline and not an absolute rule (Perry et al, 1997). Intramuscular forms of olanzapine and ziprasidone will also be available. However, we as of yet do not have any personal experience with these forms (Jones et al, 2001).

e. Adjust the frequency and the depot dose according to the individual patient's response.

f. The simultaneous use of antiparkinsonian medication, such as benztropine, is a matter of controversy. Some clinicians recommend routine use of antiparkinsonian medication to enhance compliance. However, general consensus is to use antiparkinsonian medication prophylactically only in patients who are at high risk for developing extrapyramidal side effects (EPS). These include younger age, male, high dose intramuscular use, and past history of EPS.[15]

Patient 6-7: Schizophrenia It Ain't!

A 22-year-old man is admitted from the emergency room where he was brought by friends for being "confused" and acting "strangely." The ER physician determines Patient 6-7 is physiologically stable, and the psychiatric consultant diagnoses "acute schizophrenia" and gives Patient 6-7 haloperidol 10 mg IM.

On the unit, you find Patient 6-7 lying supine, staring in ecstasy at the air above his head, and slowly reaching for things in the air that you do not see. His face is flushed, his eyes unfocused, and he speaks continuously but mostly incoherently about "heavenly hosts." He does not respond to verbal interactions, and resists being physically moved, although with effort you can do this, and put him into odd postures that he maintains for many minutes before returning to his "reaching" behavior. Muscle tone is increased bilaterally. You cannot find obvious neurologic problems that explain his behavior, and his general medical health seems good.

What grade would you give to the actions of the psychiatric consultant in the ER, and why?

We give him an "F." True, he did not kill Patient 6-7, or throw Patient 6-7 into a neuroleptic malignant syndrome, but not from want of trying. What specifically was poorly done?[16]

Did you recognize that Patient 6-7's resisting being moved and posturing with catalepsy were catatonic features? Lying supine but not sleeping or reading is an odd behavior. Most patients move about. Whenever a patient does something motorically odd, always assess for catatonia. Table 6.13 displays some odd behaviors that should trigger an assessment for catatonia.

1. *Treating without an adequate diagnosis.* Psychosis is not synonymous with schizophrenia. Many things can cause an acute psychosis (we assume psychosis because of Patient 6-7's incoherence and reaching for things we cannot see, i.e., hallucinations, and his catatonic features). Some suspects are drug intoxications, complex partial or nonconvulsive status, bipolar mood disorder, and delirium from vasculitis. These are most likely in Patient 6-7's age group, satisfying Sutton's Law.

Table 6.13 Odd Behaviors Warranting an Assessment for Catatonia
Speech, facial or hand mannerisms (repetitive, stilted and premorbidly absent, e.g., speaking in a foreign accent or with unusual enunciation, grimacing, holding hands or fingers in a unique way)
Odd, fluctuating, "nonneurologic" gaits (hopping, skipping, tip-toe walking)
Intermittent compulsive-like behaviors (checking, straightening, ritualistic sequences)
Socially odd repetitive behavior (standing at attention, saluting, marching in place)

2. *Giving an antipsychotic.* Antipsychotic medication is definitive treatment after you have decided the patient has a condition that a) is likely to respond to an antipsychotic, and b) is not likely to get worse from the antipsychotic. Most psychoses will respond to some degree to antipsychotic medication, but sometimes antipsychotics make a psychotic episode worse (some epileptic psychoses and psychosis secondary to stroke or head injury) or put a patient at too much risk for adverse effects (like NMS). Also, Patient 6-7 has catatonic features on the inpatient unit, but did he have these features in the ER? Have they been tested? So, is his catatonia due to his illness, or was it triggered by the haloperidol? Giving an antipsychotic often confuses symptoms, making diagnosis more difficult. If the consultant thought Patient 6-7 would be unmanageable on the inpatient unit, then sedation would have been warranted, and a benzodiazepine or diphenhydramine the choices. But Patient 6-7 is not bothering anyone, and so he may not have needed any sedation.

What additional information, if any, would you now like to know?

Lots! But, diagnostically most helpful would be:

1. Drug screen results and any blood levels of psychotropic medication
2. Patient 6-7's substance abuse history
3. Patient 6-7's past psychiatric history
4. An EEG to see if he is in some form of "status" or has an encephalopathy (if we can get one that is not full of movement artifacts, making reading impossible)

5. EKG, chest X-ray, and any other test that will clear Patient 6-7 for general anesthesia

Patient 6-7 was not taking any psychotropic medications. A drug screen was not done, but a friend called the hospital telling us he used mescaline at a party. Patient 6-7 previously was a regular marijuana smoker. Patient 6-7 has no psychiatric history. His mother, however, was treated for recurrent depression.

> 3,4-methylenedioxymethamphetamine, MDMA, a synthetic amphetamine derivative, whose street name is "ecstasy," has a similar effect to mescaline and has a specific neurotoxic effect on serotonergic neurons in the dorsal raphe nucleus. Fiber tracts from the dorsal raphe nucleus parallel dopaminergic systems and modify them. In addition to the acute intoxication, long-term damage and dysfunction occurs.

At this point the most likely diagnosis is drug-induced psychosis, and the patient's striking features of altered responsivity, catatonia, and reverie are typical of mescaline intoxication. An EEG would be important to rule out partial complex status or nonconvulsive status, but to get an adequate tracing, Patient 6-7 would need to stop moving. Otherwise muscle artifacts would make a reading impossible. An EEG tracing was attempted, however, and no obvious epileptic pattern was seen.

What would be your management plan for him?

Based on what you now know about Patient 6-7, you can reasonably conclude that he is a young, generally healthy man, with an acute drug-induced psychosis, the result of intoxication with mescaline. Drug intoxications sometimes result in signature features and *Table 6.14* summarizes these patterns.

Table 6.14 Signature Features of Drug Intoxications	
Alcohol	Ataxia, nystagmus, slurred speech, altered consciousness
Marijuana	Reduced arousal, injected conjunctiva, altered time sense
Stimulants	Hyperarousal (motor, emotion, sympathetic nervous system), tactile hallucinations of insects on or under the skin, geometric or herringbone visual hallucinations, suspiciousness and persecutory hallucinations
LSD	Anxiety, synesthesias,[17] irritability with euphoria, flight of ideas with formal thought disorder, and visual hallucinations and distortions
Mescaline/ peyote	Ecstasy, catatonia, grandiose delusions, panoramic hallucinations
Phencyclidine	Violence, excitement, psychosis, catatonia, generalized analgesia, cerebellar signs, sympathetic hyperarousal

For Patient 6-7 there are three options for acute treatment:

1. Wait another 24 hours to see if the intoxication resolves on its own while maintaining adequate nutrition and fluid intake. This would be the most conservative approach.
2. Treat the catatonic features with lorazepam, and maintain nutrition and fluid intake and, if needed, begin an anticonvulsant. Because Patient 6-7 has catatonia, an antipsychotic is relatively contraindicated. If one eventually would be used, an atypical might prove safest and in low doses (e.g., olanzapine 15 mg or risperidone 1-2 mg).
3. Assuming it is safe to use a general anesthetic, give bilateral ECT, which works as well if not better than, drugs for many prolonged drug induced psychoses.[19]

For many acute drug induced hallucinatory states, deep limbic excitation is hypothesized and anticonvulsants can sometimes work as well as antipsychotics.[18]

231

Discussion

Whatever your choice, remember that treatment is a three-legged stool. So you also need to plan what to do when the acute intoxication resolves. Continuation treatment may not require medication or continuation ECT if the acute intoxication fully resolves and the drug is completely excreted. Marijuana and phencyclidine will remain in the body the longest, intoxication from the latter almost always requires 8-12 months of continuation of treatment. If ECT is used, continuation ECT may follow to prevent relapse: 3 months of once weekly, shifting to every other week treatments.

Even if no continuation drug treatment is needed, rehabilitation is. Patient 6-7 will need to be assessed for cognitive problems, personality disorder or traits that might increase drug abuse risks, and strengths and weaknesses in his social and job situation.

Patients who chronically abuse drugs (such as cocaine, amphetamines, ecstasy), have abnormal brain perfusion, cognitive deficits, and cerebral atrophy.[20] Metabolism is decreased in the medial orbitofrontal cortex and basal ganglia. They have persistent deficits in short-term recall, deficits in memory (new learning) and concentration, plus deficits in nonverbal abstraction and problem solving.

Cognitive functioning affects treatment outcome in substance abusers.[21] The more deficits, the worse overall functioning and inability to understand and comply with treatment.

Quick Rounds

1. A 37-year-old man with a long history of recurrent psychoses has been stable for the last seven years on haloperidol 10 mg twice daily. During a routine follow-up you notice the patient frequently rolls his tongue in his mouth. When you ask him to stop, he is able to do so for a few minutes. What does this patient have and what do you do now?

2. A 50-year-old unemployed executive comes to you for evaluation of treatment resistant depression. The patient reports a major depression 7 years ago. At that time the patient was given imipramine 300 mg and trifluoperazine 10 mg (which he is still taking). The patient now denies any sadness but reports anhedonia and not wanting to do anything. He denies any sleep or appetite disturbances but reports staying in bed most of the day. The patient has been tried on various antidepressants and ECT. The patient admits to not wanting to live like this and is feeling like a burden on his family. Examination reveals a well nourished, slightly disheveled man, who is dressed casually. He has an expressionless face and talks in a monotone. What does this patient have?

3. A 40-year-old man with a diagnosis of bipolar complains of a rash on both his arms and his face. Upon examination you notice a macular rash on both of his arms with a clear end line just above the elbow. He also has a similar rash on his face extending to his neck. The patient has been taking lithium carbonate 600 mg BID for the last 10 years and his present blood level is 0.8 meq/L (n .6-1.2). However, he was recently started on chlorpromazine 100 mg for mild insomnia and increased suspiciousness. What caused this rash?

4. A 32-year-old woman with mood disorder and mild mental retardation is acutely psychotic, with persecutory delusions, and agitation. She has not been eating for several days and appears dehydrated. She refuses all oral medication. Your colleague attempts to treat her with intramuscular haloperidol. Shortly after administering 10 mg, she develops muscular rigidity, fever to 104° F, diaphoresis, and becomes obtunded. She is tachycardic with rapidly fluctuating blood pressures. A thorough medical evaluation cannot find a source of infection. What do you advise your colleague?

5. A 32-year-old man with bipolar mood disorder had been treated for years with haloperidol 20 mg/day. He had developed abnormal movements involving the neck and head. He is unable to keep his

head straight because his posterior neck muscles are in contraction and his head keeps tilting back. These movements have worsened since haloperidol was discontinued. What is your next step?

6. A 29-year-old man complains of hearing voices just before going to bed. He does not hear the voices at any other time. There is no evidence of any other psychopathology. What does this man have?

Quick Rounds Answers

1. This patient has tardive dyskinesia, which often begins with tongue movements or choreoathetotic movements in the fingers of the preferred hand. Cholinergic dopamine imbalance and cell loss in the substantia nigra is the pathology caused by exposure to antipsychotics and sometimes strong serotonergic drugs. The goal is to stop the antipsychotic, minimize the dose of the antipsychotic, or switch to an antipsychotic with less risk of tardive dyskinesia. Each of these choices has risks and benefits. There is no free lunch in therapeutics. We prefer to switch treatments if possible to an atypical drug to prevent any further damage.

2. Although this patient has some depressive symptoms, he does not seem to have a full depressive syndrome. The fact that he has an expressionless face and monotone voice, is 50 years old, and was once a high-functioning executive suggests neurologic disease, specifically Parkinsonism. When looking for the etiology of this syndrome, we need not go any further than the usual suspect, i.e., antipsychotic. His trifluoperazine is a potent typical agent. Typical antipsychotics can cause avolition, anhedonia, emotional blunting and can, thus, mimic depressive symptoms. Gradually discontinuing his antipsychotic relieved most of this patient's symptoms.

3. This patient has erythematosus, a macular rash that is confined to exposed areas. Considering the recent addition of chlorpromazine, this rash is most likely a result of photosensitivity due to chlorpromazine. Two things done differently could have avoided this. First, when starting an antipsychotic, patients must be warned about photosensitivity and those with lighter skin must be instructed to use sunscreens. Second, rather than starting a new medication for re-emergence of manic symptoms, the dose of lithium could have been increased to control the mania.

4. Autonomic instability, fever, rigidity and altered consciousness in absence of infection suggest neuroleptic malignant syndrome (NMS) due to haloperidol. Depot or IM neuroleptics are more likely to cause NMS. The other factors that increase the risk of NMS include manic excitement, dehydration, starvation and other motor system disease. Although, conventionally, dopamine agonists such as bromocriptine or dantrolene sodium are still used to treat NMS, many NMS experts now accept the idea that NMS is another form of malignant catatonia and should be treated the same way: lorazepam 1-2 mg TID IM increasing every day or so, if needed, to 12-15 mg or higher and, if

that does not work, bilateral ECT. ECT can also be used as the first-line treatment of the NMS and also for the associated psychosis. The death rate for NMS is 10-15%. If ECT is given within 5 days of onset, the death rate is zero, after 5 days the rate is also 10-15%.

5. This patient has tardive dystonia secondary to antipsychotics. Although the exact mechanisms of tardive syndromes are unknown, it is thought to be caused by a functional hyperactivity of CNS dopaminergic and noradrenergic systems with reduced activity of GABA and anticholinergic system. This effect is thought to be the result of prolonged dopamine blockage by the antipsychotic. No specific treatment has proved satisfactory for TD. Treatments such as vitamin E have been tried, but they do not work. For dystonic conditions like this patient's, anticholinergic drugs or botulinum toxin injections are helpful. This particular patient received botulinum toxin injections (under EMG monitoring) once every three months subcutaneously. He had a remarkable improvement. Botulinum toxin blocks the release of acetylcholine at neuromuscular junction. This denervates the muscle and leads to paralysis of the local muscle spindles. Clinical use of the toxin aims to reduce the muscle activity without producing significant weakness.

6. Hearing voices just before going to bed are called hypnagogic hallucinations. Recurrent hypnogogic hallucinations occur in patients who have either narcolepsy or epilepsy. He sleeps well at night, but still reports the need for frequent daytime naps. In this man, sleep studies showed shortened REM latency, confirming the diagnosis of narcolepsy. He was treated with protriptyline 15 mg po qd.

Chapter 7

Neuropsychiatric Syndromes

Patient 7-1: Not Everybody Is Named "Murray"

A 72-year-old man is brought to the hospital because over the past several weeks he has become psychotic. He believes family members have been leaving their trash in his house. The trash "comes and goes," he says. He also thinks a stranger has moved into his next door neighbor's house, and the stranger has been calling him on the phone only to hang up when he answers. His daughter and son deny all this and say he also has "other memory problems."

Elderly patients almost always need smaller doses of antipsychotics, but not necessarily smaller doses of antidepressants or mood stabilizers. Although risperidone is a better choice than a typical antipsychotic, because of lower risks for extrapyramidal side effects, it is not without side effects. Clozapine is often too sedating and is a powerful anticholinergic, so we do not use it in elderly patients, certainly not those who are demented. They have enough troubles without adding an anticholinergic delirium, arrhythmia, paralytic ileus, urinary retention – well, you get the picture.

Patient 7-1 is seen in the clinic, and is prescribed risperidone 1 mg BID. Within an hour of the first dose, he becomes rigid and develops a shuffling gait. His memory deteriorates over the next two days to the point that he is unable to care for himself. After several weeks, he is placed in a nursing home with a diagnosis of Alzheimer's disease.

Why does Patient 7-1 *not* have Alzheimer's?

1. Although persons with Alzheimer's disease often have difficulties recognizing people, it usually unfolds over many months or years, rather than over weeks.
2. Although Alzheimer's disease represents 50% of all diagnosed patients with dementia, psychosis is more likely in dementias that affect the action brain or that result in more focal lesions, as does dementia secondary to cerebrovascular disease (vascular dementia).
3. Persons with Alzheimer's disease who are psychotic usually respond well to low doses of antipsychotics. They can be delusional, but Patient 7-1's psychotic features are different. He thinks his old neighbor is someone else. Misidentification delusions are not typical early-on in Alzheimer's disease. He is also apparently "seeing" garbage in his house that "comes and goes." He confirms he sees these objects. Visual hallucinations are also rare in Alzheimer's disease.
4. Finally, just because a patient is demented, it does not automatically follow that he will have Alzheimer's disease. A

diagnostic evaluation is needed, and several etiologies could explain Patient 7-1's dementia (assuming he is demented!). Not all dementia is named Alzheimer's disease, just as not everybody is named "Murray."

Given the information you have, what is a leading possibility explaining Patient 7-1's behavior, assuming he is demented?[1]

Most demented patients who become psychotic respond to antipsychotic medication or ECT. Patient 7-1 not only did not respond, he got worse. The dementing process most likely to do this is diffuse Lewy body dementia. Why this occurs is unclear, but persons with this condition typically rapidly deteriorate cognitively and motorically after receiving even low doses of antipsychotic medication. They have a hypersensitivity to antipsychotics.

What other possibilities should you consider in a person with such a history?

Table 7.1   Medications That Commonly Cause Dementia
Anticholinergics (antidepressants, antiparkinsonians, neuroleptics)
Antihistamines (cold and sleep preparations)
Antiarrhythmics (quinidine)
Sedative-hypnotics
Lithium carbonate
Narcotic analgesics
H_2 receptor blockers (cimetidine)
Digitalis
Anticonvulsants
Beta-blockers
Antihypertensives
Corticosteroids
Antibiotics
Metoclopramide
Benzodiazepines

Medication effect is the single largest category of reversible dementia. If caught early and the medication stopped, full recovery usually occurs. If a patient is taking a medication that crosses the blood-brain barrier and adverse behavioral change has occurred, proximate to the introduction of that medication or its dose increase, that is the cause of the adverse behavioral change until proven otherwise. Table 7.1 displays some of the most common offending agents.

Depression is the single most common disease causing reversible dementia. In persons aged 50-70, it is 4 times as common as Alzheimer's disease.

239

Vascular dementia represents 15% of diagnosed dementias. Men are at greater risk for it than are women. Psychosis is more common in vascular dementias than in Alzheimer's disease. If the cardiovascular problem causing the dementia can be controlled or stopped, the progression of the dementia can be slowed or stopped.

> If a patient has substantial cardiovascular problems below the neck, this may be a clue to look for similar problems above the neck.

Primary psychiatric disorders occur at all ages. Psychiatric disorder often produces cognitive impairment, and in older persons the combination of normal aging changes plus illness can result in cognitive function dipping into the demented range. Pseudodementia is the best known syndrome like this, but any major psychiatric disorder can result in a dementing-like picture in an elderly patient.

Discussion

Lewy body dementia[2] is a group of syndromes in which the common denominator is the presence of small rounded cytoplasmic eosinophilic inclusions near the neuronal nucleus or in dendrites. About 10% of dementias are associated with Lewy body inclusions. *Table 7.2* summarizes the classic "big picture" features of Lewy body dementia. Four overlapping subtypes are described. The most common, involving the brain stem and basal ganglia, is identical to Parkinson's disease, and patients are treated for Parkinson's. A second variation has primarily a neocortical distribution, and clinically has an anterior, frontotemporal pattern or idiopathic frontal lobe degeneration. Ten to 15% have both patterns and are clinically diagnosed as having Alzheimer's disease. These patients have the "sporadic" or nonfamilial form of Alzheimer's. A diffuse pattern with cortical and subcortical involvement and a fluctuating course is also observed. Early on, these patients may develop a positive symptom, nonaffective psychosis that resembles a late onset schizophreniform disorder.[3]

Table 7.2 Lewy Body Dementia
Fluctuating episodes of confusion and lucidity and cognitive impairment, delirium
Classical Parkinsonism with early dementia
Behavioral changes early in the illness
Antipsychotic sensitivity syndrome
Repeated unexplained falls

Unlike Alzheimer's patients, patients with diffuse Lewy body dementia early on have memory difficulties that can be helped by giving cues. They also have problems with working memory and with executive functions. They perseverate responses and have trouble shifting from one set of rules to another to solve new problems. Early on, they may have a tremor, rigidity and myoclonus, and can be mistaken as having Parkinson's disease. Unlike Parkinsonian patients, however, patients with Lewy body dementia may have frontotemporal bursts of slow waves on EEG and frontal atrophy on MRI. Fifty to 80% are hypersensitive to antipsychotics, as was Patient 7-1, and when exposed they can develop severe Parkinsonian features and NMS. The pattern is:

Frontal lobe dementia pattern
Parkinsonian features with myoclonus
Late-life psychosis with sparing of emotional expression
Frontal atrophy on MRI
Abnormal EEG frontotemporally

Patients with Lewy body dementia can be mistaken for having Alzheimer's disease, although the latter is initially a temporoparietal, not a frontal or diffuse pattern. Muscle rigidity can occur in the early onset form of Alzheimer's disease. These patients also have a significant family history of Alzheimer's disease. *Table 7.3* summarizes other differences (in percentage of patients) between Alzheimer's and Lewy body dementia.

The psychosis in patients with Lewy body dementia is best treated with ECT to avoid antipsychotics and anticholinergics. If an antipsychotic is the only option, quetiapine is the least offensive because of its minimal extrapyramidal and anticholinergic side effects.

Table 7.3 Lewy Body Dementia		
	LBD	AD
Visual hallucinations	50	13
Auditory hallucinations	20	1-2
Major depression	20-25	8
Anxiety	36	33
Delusions	50	25
Misidentification delusions	45	15
Apathy	40	Rare
Irritability/violence	25-33	<10 (?)

Unlike patients with vascular dementia, patients with cortical involvement with Lewy body dementia have loss of cholinergic neurons and can modestly benefit from cholinergic enhancing strategies similar to those described for Alzheimer's disease.

Patient 7-2: Sometimes a Cigar Is Just a Cigar

A 72-year-old woman is referred to you for depression. She has been having memory problems for the past six months. She has been complaining of difficulty remembering the names of objects and finding objects such as keys and her purse. She says she worries about her children, but does not report sleep or appetite disturbances. Both of her parents were diagnosed as having Alzheimer's disease. Patient 7-2 has no history of any psychiatric problems.

Is Patient 7-2 depressed?

Persons who are depressed *must* have an abnormal mood. The notion of "masked" depression is invalidated. In our experience "the limbic system never lies."[4] If it is upset it will tell you. So, if no sadness, gloominess, apprehension or anxiety, no depression. Patient 7-2 also has no vegetative signs.

How can you help Patient 7-2?

> Episodic memory is memory for events in one's life: your graduation ceremony, a great date, where you put your keys when you came into the house carrying all those groceries. Episodic memory is visual.[5]

1. *Make a diagnosis*. Sometimes a cigar is just a cigar: the obvious diagnosis is what the patient has. So, Alzheimer's disease is probable, but you need to know more. Alzheimer's typically begins in the mid-seventies. Early complaints focus on memory problems. Patient 7-2 has some naming problems and perhaps problems with episodic memory. For you to determine if Patient 7-2 has Alzheimer's disease, you need to know what to look for. What are the important features that should be present and what things should not be present for the diagnosis? *Table 7.4* displays these features.

Table 7.4   Early Clinical Features to Assess in the Diagnosis of Alzheimer's Disease [6]

Feature	Description
Bilateral temporo-parietal function	Gradual difficulties with new learning, episodic memory, forgetting to remember, recognizing faces, topographic orientation, visual-spatial processing. Look for: fender-benders, losing things, forgetting names, not immediately recognizing familiar people.
Motor function	No abnormalities until late in the course. Patients with a strong family history and earlier onsets may develop moderate rigidity without tremor. If several basal ganglia or cerebellar motor signs present, look for other causes of dementia.
Cranial and peripheral nerves	Intact. If abnormal findings, look for other causes of dementia. The one exception is olfaction which is dysfunctional (poor discrimination of odor) early on in patients with Alzheimer's disease as some basal forebrain structures and enterorhinal cortex develop plaques and neuronal loss early on.
Mood	Normal. Substantial features of depression or mania suggest action brain disease, not Alzheimer's. Alzheimer's patients often minimize problems; depressed patients maximize their difficulties.
Speech and language	Some word finding and naming problems may be present, but no clear pattern of aphasia. Exception is early onset form with a strong family history when transcortical sensory aphasia (involving medial aspects of parietal lobe) can occur. This aphasia may also occur late in the illness course of patients whose dementia develops at a more typical age.
Cardiovascular function	Should be normal for age or, if dysfunctional, clearly not contributory to the brain dysfunction you are concerned about.
General medical health	Should be acceptable for age, or if dysfunctional, clearly not contributory to the brain dysfunction you are concerned about.

Laboratory findings in Alzheimer's patients early on are generally negative, with the following exceptions:

The *EEG* may show some nonspecific, lower amplitude slowing, and is rarely of use. The *MRI* typically reveals mild to moderate sulcal widening, ventricular enlargement and reduced hippocampal volumes (most helpful when patient is under 70. Over 70, normal age changes can confuse the picture). It is also useful in assessing co-occurring vascular disease. *SPECT* reveals bilateral temporoparietal hypoperfusion, and this can be present several years before the dementia unfolds.

Patients with Alzheimer's disease have perceptual-integrating brain problems early on (see Chapter 2). Patients with Alzheimer's disease will often have a positive family history for it, although a sporadic (nonfamilial) type occurs. In persons with the rare onset in their 50s, the family history is usually particularly strong and may also include persons with Down's syndrome (50% of persons with Down's syndrome die in their 40s or 50s with Alzheimer's disease) or myeloproliferative disease. *Table 7.5* summarizes the present understanding of the genetics of Alzheimer's disease. As we write, new insights about the genetic influences in Alzheimer's disease are occurring rapidly.[7]

Table 7.5 The Genetics of Alzheimer's Disease		
Chromosome 21	Beta amyloid precursor protein (APP)	5-20% of early onset (ages 30-60) familial Alzheimer's
		APP induces cholinergic hypofunction, particularly in hippocampus and cortex
		APP disrupts neuronal calcium homeostasis (overload) leading to neurotoxicity
Chromosome 14	Presenilin 1	70% of early onset familial Alzheimer's
		Gamma-secretase enhances APP build-up
Chromosome 1	Presenilin 2	Rare cases between ages 50-70
		Gamma-secretase enhances APP build-up
Chromosome 19	Apoprotein-0-epsilon (APOE)	APOE is a lipoprotein involved in neuronal growth and response to injury. Several alleles are present in humans.
		Presence of 3/4 and 4/4 allele seen in 40% of late onset familial Alzheimer's
		50% risk factor in sporadic cases

2. Patient 7-2 met all the indicators for Alzheimer's disease. Once Alzheimer's disease is diagnosed, the initial goals of treatment are 1) prepare the patient and family for the worst, and 2) treat to delay the worst. In subsequent vignettes we will discuss treatment.

Patient 7-3: Early Bad News, Late Good News

You are treating a 46-year-old woman for recurrent major depression. She is doing well, maintained for several years on sertraline 100 mg daily. On a routine visit she tells you her mother was recently diagnosed as having Alzheimer's disease. She is fearful she too will get it, and wants to know more about the illness and its effect.

What should you tell the daughter about her mother's future?

This is an example of how your knowledge can help patients and families just by discussing their concerns with expertise.

Alzheimer's disease is progressive. Once diagnosed, if early on in the course, the treatment goals are 1) to lessen the degree of decline, and 2) prepare the patient and family for the more severe times ahead. The decline may be lessened by enhancing the cholinergic system which decays in Alzheimer's disease. For this strategy to work, the system still has to be functional.[8]

1. Then the patient is given Lecithin and choline dietary supplements as acetylcholine precursors plus donepezil (a long-acting acetylcholinesterase inhibitor) 5-10 mg once daily.[9]
2. The patient's response is monitored with cognitive testing and general level of functioning. When a plateau seems to be reached, "enhancers" may then be added. These include *naltrexone,* which stimulates acetylcholine release by inhibiting endorphins.

> Donepezil side effects include syncope, nausea, diarrhea, vomiting. These can be minimized by taking the medication with food. Donepezil also produces REM sleep disturbances.

3. Regular cognitive and physical exercise helps. The former is based on the principle of "use it or lose it." Because synaptogenesis and neuronal pruning continue throughout life, the more you use your brain, the less the decline (so read on). Aerobic exercise and strength training in the normal elderly improves general health and ability to do things, and cognition.[10]
4. Once Alzheimer's has been diagnosed, the usefulness of nonsteroidal anti-inflammatory agents, vitamin E, and estrogen to moderate the illness progression is unclear, but many clinicians continue to use these. If there are no contraindications, we do it. The combination of the above

interventions may reduce the scope of the decline, adding 2 or more years of better functioning for the patient.

5. The patient and caregivers are educated about the illness, and the patient's living quarters and daily habits are structured to make everyone's life easier.

6. The family and specific caregivers are strongly advised to join a local Alzheimer's support group.

7. The patient is cognitively monitored. The diagnostic process should have included SPECT or equivalent, EEG, and MRI. SPECT and MRI may be repeated after a year to see if any substantial change has occurred. Once the diagnosis is firmly established, cognitive testing at regular intervals is sufficient follow-up.

What is the likelihood that that the daughter will get the illness?

Persons with a first-degree relative with Alzheimer's disease are at substantial risk for it.[11] The daughter needs to know this. There are also other factors that for good or ill alter this risk. *Table 7.6* displays these, and you and the daughter need to assess where she stands on these.

Table 7.6 Some Factors Affecting One's Risk for Alzheimer's Disease	
Increasing the Risk	**Decreasing the Risk**
Family history of Alzheimer's, Down's syndrome, myeloproliferative disease	Several years of education beyond college or other evidence of baseline good brain reserve
First depression after age 50	Regular use of nonsteroidal anti-inflammatory agents, and perhaps vitamin E
Thyroid disease after age 50	

However, before doing any genetic testing for Alzheimer APOE risk, you need to assess the daughter for her ability to cope with bad news. What will her response be? Will she give up on life? Will she ignore whatever responsibilities she has and prematurely ruin her life? If she is at risk will she comply with strategies to reduce it?

You review with her the risk factors we discussed with Patient 7-2 and the possibility of testing for APOE. Depending on your conclusions of her risk, she might do nothing more or she might do the following:

1. Get base-line SPECT, MRI, and cognitive testing. Early cognitive testing, even years before any cognitive decline, can predict fairly well the likelihood of an Alzheimer's dementia.[12]
2. Begin use of a nonsteroidal anti-inflammatory agent, if not contraindicated. The evidence is fairly robust that regular use reduces risk, even with aspirin. The use of vitamin E (doses 1000-1500 mg daily) remains unproven, but higher risk patients often use it.
3. Begin a cognitive and physical exercise program.

> Several nonviolent video games can help overall speed and accuracy of cognitive processing, particularly visuospatial function and perceptual motor coordination. Word games and memory games also help.

Discussion

Persons who get Alzheimer's disease typically have some subtle signs several years to a decade or more before the dementia. Mild, but reduced temporal volume and mild temporoparietal hypoperfusion on SPECT can be detected at least 5 years before the dementia.[13] Thus, efforts to delay the onset of the dementia can be planned. Because most patients with Alzheimer's disease become demented after age 75, a delay of only several years can be *preventative* because some patients will die from something else. Others will die from something else before the worst of Alzheimer's hits. *Table 7.7* displays the overall treatment strategy for a patient with Alzheimer's disease.

Table 7.7 Strategy for Treating a Patient with Alzheimer's Disease

Phase 1

High risk patient in the "preclinical" stage (The guiding principle is prevention or delay of onset.)

1. Base-line SPECT, EEG, and MRI.
2. Monitor preventative efforts with baseline and repeated cognitive testing.
3. Begin nonsteroidal anti-inflammatory agents, and perhaps vitamin E.
4. Aerobic and cognitive exercises.
5. Patient and family education and counseling; link family with a support group or organization.

Phase 2

Clinical Alzheimer's stage 1 (The guiding principle is to moderate the decline.)

1. Monitor treatment efforts with cognitive testing.
2. Maintain nonsteroidal anti-inflammatory agents, vitamin E.
3. Treat with a cholinergic enhancing drug, acetylcholine precursors.
4. Continue aerobic and cognitive exercises.
5. Continue patient and family counseling.
6. Begin to structure patient's living situation.

Phase 3

Clinical Alzheimer's stages 2 and 3 (The guiding principle is to maximize the patient's quality of life.)

1. Monitor treatment efforts with cognitive testing.
2. Value of continuing nonsteroidal agents and vitamin E is unclear.
3. As decline has continued, cholinergic enhancement less likely to be of benefit; switch to selegiline (10 mg daily) and postsynaptic receptor stimulators (arecoline, succinimide, velnacrine).[14]
4. Treat behavioral problems.
5. Continue aerobic and cognitive exercises.
6. Provide interesting sensory excursions and activities to punctuate needed structure and routine.
7. Continue family counseling and support group.

Patient 7-4: All in the Family

Patient 7-4 is a 45-year-old man who lives in a nursing home. He has been hospitalized several times for depression. He complains of progressive memory problems, and you are told that cognitive testing done in the past 6 months showed him to have mild impairment for his age. He reports sudden jerky movements in his arms that wake him at night. He makes intermittent grunting noises associated with a facial tic. His father and grandfather had similar symptoms. His father died of a heart attack when he was 50, and his grandfather died in an institution.

What big-category syndrome might this man have, and how can you prove it?

A patient with a history of recurrent depressions who now has memory and other cognitive problems might likely have another episode of depression. So depression would be the first thing to look for. Unfortunately, Patient 7-4 is subdued and clearly avolitional, but not typically depressed. You need to hunt for another Duck. There are two other clues: grunting noises and a facial tic, and "progressive memory problems." The grunting noises and facial tic and a family history of similar problems suggests Giles de la Tourette's disorder. This, however, almost always develops in childhood (Patient 7-4 was okay then), and most of the difficulties faced by Tourette's patients relate to obsessive compulsive disorder. Patient 7-4 has no obsessive or compulsive features. So again, no Duck here. That leaves progressing memory problems, and that suggests dementia. What, then, are the criteria for the syndrome of dementia, and does Patient 7-4 meet those criteria? Before you look at *Table 7.8* for the answer, see if you can come up with these criteria.

Five percent of the US population over 65 has dementia and 20% of the US population over 80 has dementia. Twelve percent of the US population is now over 65, and by 2020 that percent will increase to 20%.

Table 7.8   Criteria for Dementia
Arousal is not reduced (i.e., the patient is not delirious).
Cognitive impairment is present and substantial.
The pattern of cognitive impairment is diffuse or if within a brain system (action versus perceptual-integrating), it nevertheless involves memory.

Your behavioral examination of Patient 7-4 should determine if he is in a state of reduced arousal (he is not). A screening cognitive examination such as the Mini-Mental State Examination (MMSE),[15] will help you decide if Patient 7-4 is cognitively in a dementia range. Top score is 30, but scores of 27-30 are normal in persons over 75. The norm for Patient 7-4 is 30. A score of 22 or less suggests substantial cognitive impairment consistent with dementia, but not positive for dementia. You must do further cognitive testing. The score of 22 was picked because patients with that score or lower are more likely also to show structural brain changes consistent with dementia. Patient 7-4 scores a 22. Now what?

What logic tree can you use to help you determine the etiology of Patient 7-4's syndrome?

When a physician faces a patient who is likely demented, we have observed the following physician responses:

1. Oh boy, that's terrible. There's no hope. Off to the nursing home.
2. Ah, Alzheimer's disease! Here's some donepezil.
3. Which dementia could it be? I'll order $2 million worth of lab tests and maybe one of them will indicate the etiology.

None of these responses is helpful. Response 1 is clearly the worst. You must be a therapeutic optimist and at least consider possible reversible dementias. Response 2 is not a good bet because only half of persons with dementia are said to have Alzheimer's disease. Response 3 is the most common, but if you order 20 tests 1 or 2 will be positive by chance alone and you will not be able to interpret the finding. So, instead – *use your head to help the patient's head!*

There are two overlapping ways of trying to *figure out* the etiology of dementia. One is the age of onset of the cognitive decline and the other is whether the dementing process begins by affecting the action brain or perceptual-integrating brain, or both. *Table 7.9* displays the more common dementing processes organized by age and brain systems initially involved. Within the table, conditions are listed in decreasing prevalence.

Table 7.9 Dementias by Age and Brain Systems Typically Initially Involved

Under 50 Years	50-70 Years	Over 70 Years
Action brain	*Action brain*	*Action brain*
Alcohol dementia	Depression	Vascular
Head trauma	Vascular	Hypoxemia
Basal ganglia diseases (Huntington's, Wilson's)	Basal ganglia (Parkinson's)	*Perceptual-integrating*
Normal pressure hydrocephalus	Non-Alzheimer neurodegenerative disease (olivopontocerebellar degeneration, primary frontal lobe degeneration, Pick's disease)	Alzheimer's disease
Multiple sclerosis		*Diffuse*
Prion disease		Medication
Diffuse		Metabolic imbalance
Infection	Alcohol-related (alcohol dementia or Korsakoff's)	Head trauma
Nutritional	Hypoxemia	
Collagen-vascular disease	Space-occupying lesions and systemic effects of neoplasms (paraneoplastic)	
Endocrinopathies	*Diffuse*	
	Medication	
	Cancer and cancer therapy	
	Nutritional	
	Lewy body disease	
	Head trauma	

Patient 7-4 has some depressive features, memory problems, motor abnormalities, and dementia at age 45, and a family history of dementia.

There are four choices in the *Under 50* column of *Table 7.9* that have striking motor features. Can you name them before looking at *Table 7.10*?

Table 7.10 Motor Symptoms in Dementia	
Likely Choices	**Motor Signs**
1. Basal ganglia disease, Huntington's disease, Wilson's disease	Choreiform tic-like movement, choreoathetosis, arm beating, tremors, rigidity
2. Normal pressure hydrocephalus	Rapid development of ataxia
3. Multiple sclerosis (MS)	Dysarthria, cerebellar signs, bradykinesia
4. Prion disease	Rapid development of ataxia, myoclonus, tics, cerebellar signs

Patient 7-4's history seems to indicate a gradual decline, so choices 2 and 4 are less likely. MS is possible, and you would carefully examine Patient 7-4 for scanning speech, nystagmus and other cerebellar-like signs, plus slowing of movement. He has none. That leaves basal ganglia dementias. Persons with Wilson's disease have onsets typically in the late teens and early twenties, and liver and basal ganglia copper deposition from insufficient ceruloplasmin. Liver degeneration can be identified with liver function tests, and among patients with central nervous involvement, 98% will have Kayser-Fleischer rings along the edge of their corneas. Twenty-four hour urine copper level (elevated) is the best single test for Wilson's disease. Serum ceruloplasmin levels are low. Patient 7-4 has none of this. So, with a family history of movement disorder (and everything else ruled out), Huntington's disease is the most likely diagnosis.

> When classic neurologic and behavioral features are both present, the neurologic features usually represent the brain process that also accounts for the behavioral features. Do not assume the behavior is "a reaction" to the other "medical or neurologic" symptoms. Remember the motor system's left/right, back/front/ top/bottom organization helps circumscribe and identify brain disease. Always turn to it first for help.

What can you do to confirm your etiologic choice?

To confirm Huntington's specifically (a CT scan will show atrophy of the basal ganglia, but that is not specific to Huntington's), genetic testing is done, looking for the number of CAG trinucleotide repeats. Thirty-six or more repeats result in varying degrees of illness, and repeats

can go as high as 150. The more repeats, the more severe the form.
Patient 7-4 had 40.

Discussion

Besides your learning a little bit about Huntington's disease, the important lesson Patient 7-4 has to teach you is that the differential diagnosis of dementia changes dramatically with age of onset. Most dementias beginning before age 70 most commonly initially or exclusively

> A third of Huntington's patients have major depressions, typically preceding the movement problems. Five to 10% will have a bipolar picture.[16]

affect the action brain or are diffuse in pattern from their onset. Alzheimer's typically begins with a perceptual-integrating brain pattern. It is not a diagnosis of exclusion. If Patient 7-4 were to become depressed again, choice of drug is as always a challenge. These patients are cognitively sensitive to anticholinergic drugs, and pure SSRIs can make their motor features worse. Venlafaxine may be the best choice. Quetiapine and ziprasidone might be least problematic if the patient becomes psychotic.[17]

Patient 7-5: Sad, Stiff and Senile?

Patient 7-5 is a 72-year-old man diagnosed with nonmelancholic depression and cognitive difficulties. He has complained of progressive memory problems. He is unable to do daily chores, such as cooking, playing the piano, and writing letters, because he has difficulty with the sequence of steps for these activities. He also is not able to concentrate and do tasks as fast as in the past. He can learn new information, although it takes him longer to commit it to memory.

Patient 7-5 is a tall man with stooped posture, expressionless face and a short-stepped gait. Both his arms are modestly rigid, more so on the right. He has been treated for over a year with fluoxetine 20 mg daily with only modest improvement in his depression, but with worsening of his motor problems. He describes the depression as a feeling of no energy or interest, mild moodiness with a tendency toward tearfulness and anhedonia. He has lost 10 pounds over the past year (normal weight 185). He says he sleeps well at night, and occasionally naps during the day. He assumes his life is almost over.

Can all of Patient 7-5's symptoms be explained by one disease process? If so, which one?

Parsimony rules until overthrown by data. Patient 7-5's big picture is:

1. Depression
2. Progressive memory problems for procedural steps
3. Bradyphrenia (takes longer to learn)
4. Concentration difficulties
5. Muscle rigidity

When in doubt, ask yourself if the pattern fits action brain or perceptual-integrating brain disease. In Patient 7-5's situation the answer is what?

You guessed it!

Action brain it is! And once you have decided that, your next step is to determine if the dysfunction is in the frontal circuits or anterior limbic system, or in the cerebellar-pons. Those are the components of the action brain. As in most such situations, the motor exam helps. In Patient 7-5's situation, he has no cerebellar features, but he does have rigidity, which suggesting frontal circuitry, specifically the basal ganglia.

Patient 7-5 has all the classic features of basal ganglia disease. Given his age, Parkinson's disease or stroke are most likely. Because he has bilateral rigidity, depression, and concentration problems, a bilateral basal ganglia problem is most likely. You need to check his blood pressure and other cardiovascular function, but Parkinson's is a good bet, and that is what Patient 7-5 has. About 30% of Alzheimer's patients develop muscle rigidity. *Table 7.11* shows some features distinguishing Parkinson's from Alzheimer's disease.

Remember, the basal ganglia is the 3M Company of the brain: Motor, Memory, Mood.

Table 7.11 Some Distinguishing Features Between Parkinson's and Alzheimer's Disease	
Alzheimer's Disease	**Parkinson Disease**
Typical onset after 70	Onset variable, usually 50-70
30% of patients have rigidity without tremor	All patients have rigidity, most have tremor
Temporoparietal problems occur early with corresponding MRI and SPECT findings	Frontal problems late with corresponding MRI and SPECT findings
Depression uncommon	50-70% become depressed
Motor speech normal	Bradykinesia common and Bradyphrenia may occur
Transcortical sensory aphasia occurs late	No aphasia
Memory not helped by cueing	Memory helped by cueing
Family history of Alzheimer's most common	15% have family history of Parkinson's disease

What is your plan for treating Patient 7-5?

Parkinson's disease is the most common basal ganglia disease associated with dementia (20% of Parkinson's patients). It affects 2% of the general population and 30% of persons over age 65.[19]

If Patient 7-5 has not been specifically treated for Parkinson's disease, he should be. Levodopa or levodopa plus carbidopa is still the standard initial treatment. Because Patient 7-5 has a nonmelancholic modest depression, and because starting two medications or treatments simultaneously is often problematic, the dopaminergic enhancement alone may relieve his depression. Physical therapy and exercise also helps. If the patient is in the early

255

stages of Parkinson's disease or the depression is mild, antiparkinsonian medications, such as bromocriptine, pergolide, or pramipexole are good choices, as these medications have mood elevating properties, as well.[20]

If Patient 7-5 were to have a severe depression, then ECT is the treatment of choice.[21] It is the best and safest antidepressant and it ameliorates Parkinsonian features even in Parkinsonian patients who are not depressed. Some antidepressant drugs with strong serotonergic properties can make movement disorders worse, and may interfere with liver metabolism of the medications. Bupropion can cause delirium in Parkinsonian patients. Venlafaxine, selegiline patch, or low-dose nortriptyline are better drug choices.

Patient 7-6: The Bad Genie in the Bottle

The police bring a 53-year-old chronic alcoholic man to the ER. He has had a "blackout," and is now hospitalized. He has no memory of coming to the emergency room, and says he has had other "blackouts." He is unable to give any cohesive sequential history, often mixing past and more recent events. (Is he a "bad historian"? Patient 7-6 also has difficulty in word finding. Patient 7-6 has trouble with heel to toe walking, poor coordination and decreased reflexes in his lower extremities. (Is he a "bad walker"?) His cognitive exam is in the demented range. However, Patient 7-6 is able to do a three-word immediate recall test, can write and read a sentence, copy a geometric shape (but not without an obvious tremor), and is oriented to year, month and season, but not date. He is not psychotic, depressed, or manic.

> Patients are not "bad historians." A patient who cannot give you a coherent, reasonably detailed story of their illness and life has a cognitive or personality problem. Either way, the "bad history" is a medical sign, not an event requiring condemnation. In fact, the pattern of how the history is "bad" can help with diagnosis. Patients with frontal lobe dysfunction (including primary bipolar patients) can give you details, but often mix up sequences, just like Patient 7-6. You would never characterize a patient with an abnormal gait from leg weakness from stroke as a "bad walker." The brain deserves equal respect.

What is Patient 7-6's syndrome?

Our big picture is memory problems with substantial cognitive impairment, cerebellar motor signs, peripheral nerve signs in legs, chronic alcoholism in a 53-year-old. An alcohol related behavioral syndrome is a good bet. But, which one? *Table 7.12* displays the choices of alcohol-related behavioral syndromes. Assume the first four conditions were ruled out in the ER. So, Patient 7-6 has either Korsakoff's or alcohol dementia.

> Sometimes alcoholics fall and hit their heads. Sometimes they are so annoying that someone hits their heads for them. So always check for a subdural hematoma in these patients. Patient 7-6 does not have one.

Table 7.12 Alcohol Related Syndromes	
Syndrome	**What to look for**
Simple intoxication	High alcohol blood level (but also get a level for barbiturates because that combination can cause respiratory depression and death)
Alcohol withdrawal	Delirium and tremors, a life-threatening condition
Alcohol hallucinosis	A chronic hallucinatory state (classically frightening voices) that usually follows a severe intoxication or withdrawal state
Wernicke's encephalopathy	A delirium with ataxia, nystagmus, ophthalmoplegias (particularly 6th nerve palsy), and peripheral neuropathy
Korsakoff's dementia	Memory deficit that includes new learning (anterograde amnesia), as well as spotty amnesia for past events (retrograde amnesia), other cognitive problems that are frontal or diffuse in pattern, ophthalmoplegias and peripheral neuropathy
Alcohol dementia	A frontal lobe dementia that may occur without other neurologic signs of chronic alcoholism

Because Korsakoff's dementia results from a genetic inability to bind thiamine at low levels, and then not getting enough thiamine to maintain high levels, alcoholism contributes to only 90-95% of patients. Other causes are eating disorders and malabsorption syndromes.

Korsakoff's dementia mostly occurs in persons who are genetically vulnerable to low thiamine levels. This autosomal gene, unrelated to alcoholism, results in low levels of *fibroblast transketolase,* an enzyme needed to bind thiamine. These patients can handle thiamine in high concentrations, but not in low concentrations.[22] Thiamine is a co-factor in glucose metabolism and without it, nerve cells cannot function well and some die, resulting in the syndrome. These patients have gross new learning problems (spotty anterograde amnesia), poor episodic memory, and they forget new information after 1-2 minutes. They may confabulate to fill in memory gaps (a minority of patients), but confabulation may be due to premorbid personality rather than some inherent brain problem, unless frontal lobe dysfunction is also present. Sixth nerve palsy, cerebellar ataxia, and peripheral neuropathy are usually present. Patient 7-6 has dementia, peripheral neuropathy, and cerebellar problems. He also has had mild 6th nerve problems – difficulties looking up and outward. Because of his clear consciousness, he has Korsakoff's dementia and not Wernicke's encephalopathy.

How would you treat Patient 7-6?

Patient 7-6 needs to be on thiamine supplements indefinitely to prevent further problems. You can expect some improvement in his present condition while in the hospital.[23]

What is Patient 7-6's long-term prognosis?

Seventy to 90% or more of alcoholics return to drinking. Most treatment programs require the patient to have adequate cognition, so Patient 7-6 could not participate in any meaningful way in such programs. He may not even have the cognition left to seek and get alcohol on his own. He needs long-term custodial care, good nutrition, and no further alcohol.

Discussion

Patient 7-6 also has some "frontal lobe" features: his mixing up sequences in his history. Some alcoholics who have adequate amounts of fibroblast transketolase nevertheless become demented. This dementia, however, is due to the direct neurotoxic effects of alcohol. The frontal lobes and cerebellum are particularly vulnerable. Fifty to 70% of sober, once chronic alcoholics have cognitive problems. Those who remain sober for two or more years regain some function.

Patient 7-7: Knock, Knock. What's There?

A 38-year-old man is referred to your clinic by his family doctor, who thinks the man is "neurotic." The patient complains of being irritable and having headaches, difficulty concentrating, fatigue, and sensitivity to sounds. He also sleeps poorly. He denies depression, suicidality or features of psychosis. He has no prior psychiatric history. His general medical health is within normal limits. He was seen in the emergency room six months ago following a car accident in which he was "knocked out" (he had a "mild" concussion"). His neurologic examination and a CT scan done at the time were normal.

> In a clinical practice, persons who have had personality problems or an anxiety disorder, or multiple somatic complaints from at least their late teens, are generally referred to as "neurotic," an old term that meant absence of psychosis. When a patient is "normal" and has a substantial change in behavior after maturation, it usually means a brain problem of some sort.

> In war, head injury is usually penetrating, leading to focal syndromes. Most nonwar head injuries are closed, and 90% of patients survive. If the head is in motion when injured, coup-contra-coup is common. If the head is relatively stationary when injured, damage is often to the site of impact. Common causes of head injury are auto accidents (>50%), falls (21%), violence 12%), and recreation (10%).[24]

Is there a link between Patient 7-7's symptoms and head injury? Why is this a bad first question?

It is a bad first question because first you need to identify the syndrome. If he had an ingrown toenail, that syndrome (small and localized but very painful and dysfunctioning, so do not laugh at it) would clearly not be related to a prior head injury, unless he got hit on the head and as he was falling stubbed his toe. So, what is this syndrome if not a mood disorder? Is it a syndrome? Get the big picture items: headache, fatigue, concentration problems, irritability, sensitivity to sounds (hyperacusis).

Although not in the DSM, this syndrome is in the ICD-10[25] and will occur to some degree in 80-100% of persons who have had a head injury. Termed *post-concussion syndrome,* it is characterized by headache, fatigue, dizziness, blurred or double vision, noise and light sensitivity, insomnia, irritability, feelings of anxiety and depression, and cognitive problems with concentration and forgetfulness. Patient 7-7 has a post-concussion syndrome, and also had dizziness for several weeks following his auto accident. But is his head injury substantial enough to account for his present problems? *Table 7.13* displays the characteristics of a closed head injury that is likely to lead to later behavioral problems.[26] The more features, the more likely the link.

Table 7.13 Characteristics of a Closed Head Injury Likely to Lead to Behavioral Problems
Unconsciousness longer than 15-20 minutes
Unconsciousness that is moderate to severe
Anterograde amnesia longer than 48 hours
Neurologic signs (e.g., diplopia, seizure) immediately post-injury
Impaired post-injury functioning longer than several days

Patient 7-7's injury was 6 months ago so he may remember some of the details of his injury and treatment, and his hospital ER records may be available. Some injuries, however, will be years earlier and the patient's recollection of events vague. Nevertheless, you must find out as best you can. Some suggestions are:

1. *Duration of unconsciousness:* "When you woke up from your accident, were you still at the injury site or at the hospital? Could you tell, or did someone tell you how long you were unconscious?"
2. *Degree of unconsciousness:* Emergency rooms sometimes use the *Glasgow Coma Scale* to assess degree of unconsciousness, so getting any records can be helpful. The top score is 15. A score of 12 or less indicates a moderate or worse injury.
3. *Anterograde amnesia:* "During the hours/days you were in the hospital, did it all seem fuzzy, as if you were in a dream? Did people tell you that you seemed 'spacey,' that you were repeating things as if you did not remember saying them?"
4. *Impaired functioning:* "How soon after the accident did you return to your usual activities: work, school, household chores?"
5. *Neurologic signs:* "Did anyone say that after the injury you had a seizure? That you had a skull fracture or a blood clot on your brain? Did you see double? Were you having balance problems or feeling dizzy?"

Patient 7-7 had a mild head injury six months ago. He was only unconscious for several minutes, but was dizzy, and saw double for several more minutes. He had headaches, dizziness, and concentration problems that kept him home for a week.

What can you do to help Patient 7-7?

Treatment of post-concussion syndrome largely remains symptomatic. This patient has fatigue, concentration problems, headaches, and irritability. He may benefit from bupropion, amantadine, methylphenidate, or a serotonin reuptake inhibitor, such as sertraline. The rationale of choosing a drug will depend on the symptom(s) that is most disturbing to the patient. If concentration and fatigue are of main concern, then bupropion, amantadine, or methylphenidate may be used first.[27] If irritability is a major source of concern, then sertraline, which also has dopaminergic action, would be our first choice. Relaxation training may help to reduce overall tension and irritability. Tell Patient 7-7 to avoid situations that cause "information overload," which can further reduce concentration abilities and prompt irritability.

Discussion

Most symptoms of post-concussion syndrome resolve in 3-6 months, but about 6% of patients have symptoms for years. These patients are not malingerers, hysterics, or cranks. They have brain dysfunction that can be demonstrated. Some findings are listed in *Table 7.14*. The underlying pathophysiology is thought to be diffuse axonal injury that occurs during the head injury. This axonal injury leads axon severation and disconnection between the two ends. Disconnected fibers eventually degenerate and result in deafferentation of the target site. In many cases, eventual return of synaptic input to the deafferented site occurs. However, in some cases maladaptive neuroplastic rearrangement can result in less than full recovery.[29] There is no specific lesion location that is responsible for post-concussion syndrome.

Table 7.14 Laboratory Abnormalities in Post-concussion Syndrome[28]
MRI: scattered punctate hyperintensities suggesting axon shearing
SPECT: hypoperfusion during cognitive tasks
EEG: 40% have nonspecific slowing or alpha slowing
Vestibular function: abnormal caloric testing and electronystagomography
Evoked potential: delayed waveforms in brain stem on auditory evoked potential
Cognition: 80% have at least some impairment in attention, reaction time (particularly when faced with choices), and in new learning

Factors that predict poor outcome after a brain injury include persistent pain, poor general health, older age, history of drug and alcohol abuse, history of past injury and presence of APOE4 allele (these patients have increased amyloid deposits).[30] The role of litigation as an impediment to improvement is questionable. There are no clear differences in symptom patterns between those patients that are involved in litigation versus those who are not.[31] Symptoms usually persist even after the litigation is over.

Patient 7-8: The Crude Professor

A 58-year-old college professor who had a severe closed head injury (Glasgow Coma Scale <10) following a fall two years ago is brought to see you by his wife. His wife is angry because he acts inappropriately in social situations. He often makes crude remarks, shows undo familiarity with strangers, and asks inappropriate personal questions. Her repeated attempts to explain this to Patient 7-8 have been unsuccessful, and they often argue about it. In the past they rarely fought.

What has happened to Patient 7-8?

In falls, coup-contra-coup injuries are common, and so frontotemporal injury is most likely because the back of the brain is more protected. Patient 7-8 had a severe head injury, and now he has marked personality changes, typical of frontal lobe damage. He has a modified disinhibited, orbitolateral syndrome. Because the injury is cortical, you should also suspect that Patient 7-8 will have features of some of the other frontal circuits: avolition, perseverativeness, fine motor skills problems, poor finger tapping, poor sequencing. He has these features.

> When a high functioning person has a substantial behavioral change after maturation, it almost always indicates brain dysfunction or disease. Have you read this before? Yup. Will you read it again? Maybe it's important.

How will you treat Patient 7-8?

In treating such patients, we follow a simple rule. We use medications that are used to treat the idiopathic psychiatric syndrome their symptoms most resemble. The only modification is "start slow and go slow." The disinhibition syndrome most closely resembles mania, so Patient 7-8 might be given a trial with a mood stabilizer. Our preference is valproic acid. It is usually well tolerated. We begin at 250 mg BID and target a blood level of 50-100 ug.

What will you tell Patient 7-8's wife?

One of the most important steps in treating Patient 7-8 is making sure his wife understands the nature of his dysfunction. You will need to go into great detail in explaining the effect of brain injury on behavior. This patient's wife needs to know that in her husband's situation, the areas of his brain that normally are responsible for socially appropriate behavior are damaged. Analogies using stroke or diabetes with behavioral change may help. Sometimes findings on SPECT (hypoperfusion), EEG (slowing), or MRI (the injury) dramatically illustrate to the family that the injury is real. Thus, sometimes laboratory tests are helpful, not in choosing a treatment, but in winning over the patient's family so they become your helpers in the patient's care. Traumatic brain injury (TBI) can cause several behavioral syndromes. *Table 7.15* displays these with some clinical tips about each.

Table 7.15 Behavioral Syndromes Associated with Traumatic Brain Injury

Syndrome	Clinical Tips
Post-concussion syndrome	Most substantial injuries cause this. If time, education, and TLC do not help, stimulants or SSRIs may.
Mood Disorder	60% of TBI patients have a subsequent nonmelancholic depression. Large injuries to the nondominant lateral and dorsal frontoparietal cortex cause a dysphoric depression that may respond to carbamazepine. Antidepressants sometimes work for other TBI depressions.
Anxiety disorder	60% of TBI patients develop anxiety symptoms, often a phobic-like response to the injury situation. If this persists past 3-6 months, it tends to generalize. It is often linked to fatigue when cognitive demands upon the patient are high. Do not use benzodiazepines; they cause memory problems. Consider buspirone (5 mg BID to start, 5 mg increases every 5 days to 45 mg daily), propranolol (up to 80 mg BID), naltrexone (50-100 mg daily). Behavior therapy may help.
Obsessive-compulsive disorders	May follow basal ganglia injury. Treatments are the same as for primary OCD
Psychosis	Particularly with temporal lobe or orbitomesial frontal lobe injury. Psychosis is often acute in onset with great emotionality. Antipsychotics sometimes make things worse. Anticonvulsants, lithium, and ECT work best. If an antipsychotic is needed, low dose risperidone may work.
Personality change	Most commonly associated with irritability and, when severe, dyscontrol. Treatment includes avoiding alcohol, hypnotics, or stimulants, while giving rehab and education, anticonvulsants, or lithium, or buspirone.
Epilepsy	5% of mild and 12% of severe closed head injuries are associated with seizure disorder.
Dementia	Usually from widespread axon shearing, so it clinically looks like a white matter dementia: bradyphrenia and bradykinesia without aphasia, apraxia or agnosia.

As antipsychotics may trigger or exacerbate programmed cell death (apoptosis) that can occur around a TBI (or stroke), giving these agents is relatively contraindicated because they may spread the area of damage. If antipsychotics are unavoidable, use low doses, and protect the brain area involved with high doses of vitamin E (2000 u/day), which can prevent apoptosis.[32]

Patient 7-9: If It Looks Like a Seizure, Sounds Like a Seizure . . .

A 45-year-old right-handed woman has had multiple episodes during which she feels as if she is floating out of her body and watching herself. These episodes last about 15-20 minutes, and she remembers these experiences. Patient 7-9 has no history of drug or alcohol abuse. At other times, she falls to the ground, appears unconscious, and shakes. She does not remember these episodes. As a teen, she had a head injury with loss of consciousness of about ten minutes. She had no behavioral or function change after the injury. She had a depression several years ago that lasted two months, but took no medication for it. Her cognitive examination is essentially normal, except for mild deficits in visuospatial processing.[33] Her lab work is normal, except for a right temporal slowing on EEG and reduced right temporal perfusion on SPECT (single photon emission computed tomography).

> Untreated, most depressions will spontaneously resolve. Before antidepressant treatments, 50% resolved within 9-12 months. The fact that Patient 7-9's depression remitted without treatment does not rule out that she had a clinical depression and that she may have a mood disorder.

What is Patient 7-9's syndrome diagnosis? (This is a semi-trick question.)

Episodes of detachment and a feeling of floating sounds like depersonalization, which is a dissociative phenomenon. Dissociation is the disruption of normal integrated function, consciousness, memory, identity and perception of the environment. Patient 7-9 has multiple depersonalization episodes that may meet DSM criteria for dissociative disorder. If so, that is what she has.[34] But, like all DSM categories, it can be primary or secondary. You first determine the syndrome and then the etiology. In Patient 7-9's situation, her lab tests are suggestive. Before reading note 34, see if you can guess their significance.[35]

> The convulsion is paroxysmal, usually stereotyped behavior of rather sudden onset and cessation for which the patient has some amnesia.
>
> The seizure is the electrical storm in the brain that produces the convulsion.
>
> Epilepsy is a condition (70% idiopathic) that results in repeated seizures.

How will you treat Patient 7-9? (This is a semi-trick question.)

Of course, the trick is diagnosis first. So does Patient 7-9 have a seizure disorder: epilepsy? If so, which one? Knowing this will lead to a better treatment plan than the usual psychotherapy formula for dissociative states. Epilepsy has been recognized for millennia. Julius Caesar was an epileptic. Dostoevski and Van Gogh were epileptics. Epilepsy was clinically diagnosed long before Hans Berger, a psychiatrist, invented the EEG machine in 1928. Epilepsy is, therefore, classified by its clinical features, and it is a clinical, not EEG, diagnosis. *Table 7.16* displays a simplification of the present classification system. Can you match Patient 7-9's signs and symptoms to one of the epilepsies?

Table 7.16 The Epilepsies	
Type	*Characteristics*
Generalized (initial electrical discharge originates from all or most centrencephalic structures)	
Absence (petit mal)	15-20 seconds of unresponsivity for which there is no memory
Atonic	Sudden loss of muscle tone, during which the patient collapses (5-10 seconds)
Tonic	Total body spasm with loss of consciousness (5-10 seconds)
Clonic	Generalized flexion-extension movements of all limbs and torso (30-60 seconds)
Tonic-clonic (grand mal)	Combination of initial unconsciousness, body spasm, and then clonic movements (30-120 seconds)
Myoclonic	Generalized muscle jerks (30 seconds)
Partial (initial electrical discharge is focal, cortical or subcortical)	Sudden localized motor stereotypies or sensory experience without alteration in arousal, attention or responsivity (30-60 seconds)
Complex partial (psychosensory/psychomotor) (initial electrical discharge is focal-cortical or subcortical, and with some alteration in consciousness)	Sudden stereotypic episode of behavioral, cognitive or affective phenomena with change in arousal, attention, or responsivity (60 seconds)
Mixed types (begins focally and then spreads to a generalized form)	

Patient 7-9 comes closest to experiencing a complex partial fit. However, most complex partial fits last less than a minute and are associated with an aura, postictal confusion, and substantial amnesia for the event. Patient 7-9 has episodes that last 15-20 minutes, and she can recall the experience. Further, Patient 7-9's EEG is not definitively diagnostic. Rather than showing an epileptic burst of slow waves with some spikes, she just has some localized slowing. However, even after exhaustive study, 10-20% of epileptics cannot be identified by EEG.[36] The absence of spikes and waves does not automatically rule out the possibility of a seizure disorder. So what to do?

Use the diagnostic principles you learned in Chapter 1. If the Duck Principle does not work, try Sutton's Law. Dissociative disorder is very rare. Epilepsy is common and at any point in time 1/200 persons is epileptic and 5 times that many persons are at lifetime risk for seizures. Sutton's law tells you that Patient 7-9 is likely to have epilepsy. The Rule of Parsimony also helps here because Patient 7-9 does have something wrong: 1) Her EEG is not normal and shows a localized problem (always consider localized EEG abnormalities, regardless of pattern, to be abnormal and possibly connected to the cause of the behavioral syndrome). 2) Her SPECT is also abnormal showing hypoperfusion in the same area as the abnormal EEG. 3) Her cognition is abnormal for some visuospatial functioning consistent with a right (nondominant) lesion. And, 4) She had a head injury. Putting it together, Patient 7-9's head injury caused a brain contusion with scarring and the scar has resulted in an excitatory focus that is now producing partial-complex-like fits.

But, wait a minute! Patient 7-9 also has these falling episodes with unconsciousness. Are these also seizures? Are they so-called pseudoseizures?

So called *pseudo-seizures* or *nonepileptic convulsions* can often be distinguished from convulsions due to a seizure. *Table 7.17* shows the differences.

Pseudoseizures or nonepileptic convulsions are convulsions which are not associated with EEG changes. Nonepileptic convulsions are most often associated with epilepsy! The patient (often highly suggestible, dependent, or of low IQ) has epileptic convulsions at other times. The nonepileptic convulsion mimics the typical form of convulsion for that patient, i.e., grand mal-like with grand mal epilepsy, partial complex-like with partial complex epilepsy. [37]

269

Table 7.17 Differences Between Nonepileptic and Epileptic Grand Mal Convulsions	
Epileptic	**Nonepileptic**
Tonic/clonic (flexion-extension)	Writhing or side to side movements
Bilateral, rhythmic, all limbs	Only upper or lower limbs
Unconscious and uncommunicative	Communicative
Tongue biting/urinary incontinence uncommon	Slow onset with safe fall
Post-ictal recovery: slow, no crying, reduced reflexes, orienting behavior, flushed, injected conjunctiva, sleepiness, fatigue, achy	Post episode: quick recovery with tears and uproar, normal reflexes
3-4 fold rise in prolactin	Minimal or no rise in prolactin

Table 7.18 describes characteristics of a complex partial seizure fit.

How will you treat Patient 7-9?

Epilepsy is not only common. It is treatable. Treatment with carbamazepine 1200 mg daily resolved Patient 7-9's dissociative disorder due to epilepsy. Her pseudoseizures also resolved.

Table 7.18   Characteristic Form of a Complex Partial Seizure
Sudden onset (many with a 1-5 second aura)
Brief duration (typically <60 seconds)
Paroxysmal (from onset to peak intensity fast)
Some alteration in attention, consciousness, or responsivity
Some loss of memory (details, clarity of the event, gaps)

270

Patient 7-10: Schizophrenic Until the Insurance Runs Out

A 38-year-old man is brought to the emergency room by his wife. She says she is at her wits' end. She found her husband in their bedroom with a loaded gun pressed to his chest, staring intently out the window. She was able to take the gun away from him. She says he has been psychiatrically ill for eight years since getting out of the Air Force. He was a sergeant and was active for 8 years. His wife also says that over the last several years, her husband has become violent, suddenly shouting and smashing objects. She also says he has been irritable at work and suspicious of his co-workers. His boss has warned him that one more incident and he will be fired. Although he has never harmed or threatened anyone, she says she will leave him if he does not get better because she fears for the safety of their two children. He has been privately hospitalized eight times over the past eight years for hearing voices and having visions, has been diagnosed schizophrenic, and has received antipsychotic medication. Now that his health insurance has run out, he is transferred to a public teaching hospital.

On examination, Patient 7-10 speaks without emotion, almost robotically. He denies wanting to kill himself. He states he was going to kill the demon that has been trying to invade his body. Several times a day, the demon comes from outside his window, and gets closer and closer, and larger and larger, until it stands next to him. Most recently, the demon has been trying to push its way into his body from the right side, and he feels suddenly cold and very scared. During this time, Patient 7-10 says he sees the world like images in a fun house mirror, or through a glass of water. Patient 7-10 decided that once in his body, the demon would be vulnerable. He insists he would have killed the demon without hurting himself.

> The form of psychopathology is almost always diagnostically more important than the content. Patient 7-10 has visual distortions of something increasing in size (dysmegalopsia).

What do you do first? Are there any helpful guidelines for doing it?

As always, try to get the big picture and then determine the etiology. The Duck Principle, Sutton's Law, and the Rule of Parsimony prevail. For Patient 7-10, he is a 38-year-old man

> The definition of violence includes injury to self and others and damage to property. Persons who injure themselves or property are also more likely to injure others, so clinically manage such patients as persons with an increased risk for violence.

with a recurrent psychosis, visual perceptual problems and auditory hallucinations, emotional blunting, delusional ideas, and bursts of violence.

Patient 7-10 is psychotic and would meet DSM criteria for schizophrenia. If his violent episodes were associated with enough features of depression or mania, he might meet criteria for schizoaffective disorder, or even mood disorder with psychosis. He had no such episodes. The problem with his past evaluations was not the syndromal diagnosis "schizophrenia," but that his physicians did not try to determine etiology. There are several clues that his syndrome is likely secondary:

1. Onset of psychosis around age 30 after good premorbid functioning
2. Continues to work despite several hospitalizations
3. Has a family
4. Dysmegalopsia can occur in many psychoses, but because it is a temporolimbic feature, it should be a red flag. One swallow does not a spring make, nor does one temporolimbic feature indicate epilepsy -- but check it out. In fact, when a patient experiences hallucinations in multiple sensory fields (voices, vision of demon, tactile hallucination of a demon pushing into his body), the syndrome is almost always secondary.

What do you do second? Are there any helpful guidelines for doing it?

Among psychotic patients under age 40, the big etiologic suspects are substance abuse, head injury, and epilepsy.

The principles involved are:

1. Not all substance abusers become psychotic, so look for the specific features of the abuse that makes it more likely the abuse has directly led to the psychosis.
2. Not all bumps on the head are permanently brain damaging to the degree of being able to cause psychosis. Look for a substantial head injury.
3. Epilepsy can cause psychotic symptoms in each of its stages: prodrome, ictal, postictal, interictal. The psychosis in each of these stages differ somewhat.

Patient 7-10 fell from a helicopter while landing to deploy troops. He suffered a head injury and was unconscious for several hours.

Although Patient 7-10 eventually recovered from his head trauma, he was discharged from the Air Force and entered civilian life. Several years later he started having episodes of psychosis. Within a year of his injury, Patient 7-10 began experiencing episodes of "missed" time that others did not notice and which he was embarrassed to relate. These were the beginnings of his partial complex fits. His epilepsy-related psychoses began several years later.

In traumatic brain injury a rule of thumb is that if the head is in motion at impact (e.g., auto accidents, falls), the brain injury is likely to be coup-contra-coup. If the head is not in motion and it is hit by a moving object (e.g., iron pipe, falling stone work), the worst of the brain injury is usually at the site of the impact.[38]

Head injuries can lead to brain contusions. If there is sufficient bleeding with cortical irritability at the time of injury, seizures can occur. However, even without these early seizures, as healing takes place (gliosis, a form of brain scarring), an epileptic focus can develop over several years, and delayed seizures can occur.

Once you have decided what's wrong with Patient 7-10, can you devise a treatment plan for him?

Epilepsy is treatable, but it is not easy. You cannot simply give a pill and hope for the best. *Table 7.19* displays the steps to consider in planning treatment. A prerequisite to treatment is to a) be convinced the patient has a seizure disorder (two or more convulsions), and b) decide on the form or forms of the convulsions.

Table 7.19 Steps to Consider in Planning Treatment for Epilepsy

Step	Rationale
Choosing medication	Different forms of epilepsy respond to different medications. When you are unsure, or the patient has more than one form, start with a broad spectrum anticonvulsant (e.g., valproic acid) rather than polypharmacy.
Identifying triggers, reducing exposure to them, and deciding how best to deal with those that cannot be avoided (e.g., life stress)	Like all illness, epilepsy is influenced by environmental factors. Some factors can trigger seizures, and reducing the exposure or managing the triggers can reduce convulsions. Common triggers are drug-drug interactions, alcohol, fatigue, stressful problems of living, exposure to harsh or intense stimuli (e.g., fluorescent lighting, flickering lights), hormonal fluctuations (menses, menopause, variable dose estrogen replacement), viral infection.
Teaching behavioral techniques	Relaxation and rebreathing techniques used as part of the treatment for anxiety disorder, also help with seizure disorder.
Keeping a journal	Some baseline of frequency and types of behavioral change is needed to monitor treatment response. The more infrequent the seizures, the longer it will take to determine if treatment works. Sometimes 6-12 months is needed for a treatment trial.
Suspending high-risk behaviors	Using machinery, driving, working in potentially dangerous settings (e.g., a roofer) are often avoided (driving by state laws) for a period of time until seizure control is established (often 1-2 years of no seizures). Modifying the patient's lifestyle will often be necessary to accommodate these potentially lifesaving measures.
Educating the patient and family	Both need to understand the illness and what behaviors are controllable (not driving until seizure free, not using alcohol) and which behaviors are seizure-related and uncontrollable (irritability). Both need to know the early warnings (if any), how to avoid triggers, and the rationale for the other steps in treatment.
Psychotherapy	All good doctors do psychotherapy; they just call it something else. What we mean is that Patient 7-10 needs regular periodic follow-up visits where in addition to a review of his medication, side effects and seizure control efforts, he will need empathic help in dealing with being a person with a brain disease, interacting with family, friends, co-workers and employers and any difficulties in life.

Discussion

Patient 7-10 was experiencing ictal and post-ictal psychoses. His ictal psychosis was the anxiety and dysmegalopsia and other perceptual changes he experienced for several minutes (ictal psychosis rarely last longer than a few minutes). His continuing experience of delusions, voices, and irritability were post-ictal. He was given carbamazepine and became seizure free. Because he was no longer having seizures, he was no longer having ictal or post-ictal psychosis. He did not need antipsychotic medication.

Epilepsy is a clinical, not a laboratory, diagnosis. If you are convinced a patient has epilepsy, despite the patient having repeatedly nonepileptic EEG findings, the patient is epileptic. Twenty percent of epileptics never have a diagnosable EEG. Their focus is too deep to pick up. *Table 7.20* displays some helpful laboratory tests that you can do for Patient 7-10. They are based, however, on the clinical conclusion from the type of head injury (fall on the back of the head) and his clinical symptoms that a) he has complex partial epilepsy, and b) the temporal lobes are likely involved.

| Table 7.20   Laboratory Tests Helpful in Evaluating Patient 7-10 ||
Test	What to Ask For, what to Look For
EEG	Several standard EEGs or 24-72 hour continuous recordings may be needed. For standard EEGs, tell the lab where you think the focus is so their montage (pattern of electrode connections) will maximize sensitivity. Ask for a sleep- deprived EEG (the patient may doze during the recording, revealing abnormalities in the transition from wakefulness to sleep). Ask for hyperventilation and photic stimulation to stimulate potential foci. Bursts of slow waves or some slowing with spikes or sharp waves over the area you predict clinically is considered "a hit."
MRI	An MRI can reveal structural abnormalities that can cause seizures: stroke, small dysplastic or a bit of ectopic cortex, vascular malformation, injury, space occupying lesion. Also ask for temporal lobe volumes as chronic temporal lobe seizures can result in reduced volume on the side of the focus.
SPECT	A SPECT shows hyperperfusion over the focus during a seizure, and interictally hypoperfusion over the focus.
Prolactin[39]	Although prolactin level is most helpful in distinguishing grand mal epilepsy from nonepileptic seizures, 40-60% of persons with complex partial fits will have elevated prolactin levels (4-5 times normal) 15-20 minutes after a seizure.
Cognitive testing	If you suspect a localized problem ask for or administer cognitive tests that assess functions subserved by that area, as well as doing generalized testing. A specific cognitive deficit that is predicted is "a hit."

Patient 7-11: The Road to Hell is Paved with Good Intentions

A 26-year-old woman is referred to you by a social worker for possible medication therapy for a depression. The patient has been in therapy for years and has also been treated with several antidepressants with no or only modest effect. The patient states she has been depressed over the past three weeks with loss of energy, feeling subdued and tearful and with reduced interest in usually enjoyable activities, including sex. She has no appetite but has not lost any weight. She states that during each episode she has to force herself to concentrate. She feels "fuzzy-headed, as if drunk."

She has had no episodes of mania or hypomania, or soft bipolar spectrum patterns, although her father was diagnosed as manic-depressive and is doing well on lithium. She has had episodes of depression since puberty at age 14. Early episodes lasted a week and occurred 1-2 times yearly. In the past several years episodes have lasted 2-3 weeks. This year she has had two in six months. Each episode begins with sudden moderate anxiety with typical physiologic features, but no panic. She then feels as if she is detached from herself, her thinking is no longer clear, and she feels drunk. Other persons either do not notice any change in her behavior or say she seems "quiet" or "subdued." Recently at work, her supervisor said she was not her usual efficient self. These features last several days and then her depressive features unfold. She says they eventually end "like a cold" tapering off and then she is "Okay" again. During her episodes in the past several years she has also noticed a loss of her sense of smell. After her last episode her sense of smell did not return for six months.

On examination she is alert, neat, and cooperative. She sits calmly and gestures appropriately as she speaks. She has no abnormal movements. She is subdued and says she is a bit anxious. She has no speech or language problems and is not psychotic. A review of cognitive domains indicates that prior to this episode she functioned at a high level, worked steadily and well, and had an active life.

> Always test olfaction - you know, the cranial nerve no one ever tests. Because of their location beneath the frontal lobes and then into the temporal lobes, the olfactory pathways are subject to disruption from frontal lobe injury or mass effects. Unilateral olfactory loss without a clear peripheral explanation is a danger signal for frontal lobe or forebrain pathology.

What medication would you give Patient 7-11 for her recurrent depressive illness? (This is a *big* trick question.)

Patient 7-11 describes episodes that are depressive-like, and she meets DSM criteria for nonmelancholic recurrent depressions. But, she has many atypical features: feeling "fuzzy-headed.....as if drunk," early episodes lasting only a week or so and present episodes being of relatively short duration. Even if you were convinced she had depressions, you would still be obliged to look for etiology.

When diagnosing complicated conditions, do not just get enough information to generate a DSM diagnosis. Get all the information needed to give you a picture of the process. You want to know the story of the illness, not just the cast of characters in the story.

Each episode starts with sudden anxiety of several days (the prodrome) followed by a day of feeling fuzzy headed and drunk (a seizure), followed by a prolonged period of needing to concentrate on how she moves, as if it no longer comes automatically to her. When driving she has trouble judging speed. The experience is then followed by a week or weeks of depression (a post-ictal period?).

Table 7.21 Psychiatric symptoms During Various Stages of Epilepsy			
Prodrome	*Ictal*	*Post-ictal*	*Interictal*
Hours or days	*Seconds or minutes*	*Hours or days*	*Weeks to continuously*
Anxiety Cognitive inefficiency Psychosis (usually with grand mal epilepsy)	Paroxysmal psycho-pathology Altered alertness Psychosensory features Stereotypic behavior Psychosis	Delirium Irritability and violence Depression Psychosis Fatigue and need to sleep	Psychosis Personality changes: adhesive/viscous (perseverative, circumstantial, overly detailed, pedantic) Paranoid personality disorder Psychomotor quartet (hypergraphic, hyposexuality, pseudo-profundity, hyperreligiosity)

Forty percent of epileptics develop clinical depressions, 10% recurrent psychosis, 40% chronic personality change. Table 7.21 displays the stages of epilepsy and some of the classic behaviors associated with each stage. [40]

Epilepsy is a clinical diagnosis, and Patient 7-11's behavioral syndrome is consistent with seizure disorder. Her depressions would then be post-ictal, and preventing the seizures should also prevent the depressions. So, our question's "big trick" is that her depressions should be treated, but with an anticonvulsant, not an antidepressant. Carbamazepine, which has weak antidepressant and some mood-stabilizing properties, was given to Patient 7-11 with initially good results. Valproic acid also has modest antidepressant properties.

Once you learn the trick, what should you do next?

Seventy percent of epilepsies are idiopathic, but you must still search for treatable or life-threatening causes of seizures. No one had done this for Patient 7-11, although she had been having depressive episodes for 13 years. She received several different antidepressants (each new one on the market was tried), and continuing psychotherapy. Her treaters cared about her, but did not follow the principles of diagnosis and management. An MRI now reveals that she has a vascular malformation which, over the years, has grown to involve a large part of her left frontal lobe, with extensions into the anterior parietal lobe and parts of the temporal lobe.

> Because of the uncinate fasciculus' one-way path from frontal to temporal lobe, frontal lobe lesions can produce temporal lobe signs and symptoms, but temporal lobe lesions cannot produce frontal lobe features. [41]

Her vascular malformation is so extensive that she was no longer a candidate for surgery and radiation would make the risk of hemorrhage too great. Carbamazepine controlled her seizures, but the malformation continued its slow growth. Hemorrhage and early death is the most likely outcome for Patient 7-11.

Patient 7-12: Don't Ask, Don't Tell

A 29-year-old woman has a 10 year history of bipolar disorder for which she has received lithium, various antidepressants, and on several occasions, an antipsychotic, all with only modest success. She recovers completely from episodes, but her episodes are frequent (2-3 yearly). She is referred for evaluation for treatment resistant mood disorder.

As part of the evaluation for etiology (she has rather typical manias, but atypical depressions with avolition and apathy rather than apprehension and sadness), she is *asked* about experiences consistent with epilepsy (*Table 7.22*). Her response is surprise and then tears of relief, "No one ever asked me about my spells before. . .I did not want to say anything 'cause I was afraid people would think I was crazy."

Her story: Several times monthly she loses short periods of time, e.g., I get to the parking lot at work and the next thing I know I am at my desk and I have no idea how I got there or where I parked my car. Following

Table 7.22 Screening Questions for Epilepsy
Have you ever had short periods where you lost time or had blackout spells, although you were not drinking (or using drugs)?
Have you ever found yourself in a room in your house and did not know how you got there?
Have you ever lost control of part of your body and it started shaking, or you passed out and people said you were shaking all over?
Do you have intense daydreams during which it is hard for you to respond to people?
Have you ever had experiences that you or someone described as a "fit" or a "seizure?"
Have you ever had brief episodes (seconds or minutes), during which your vision becomes distorted (like a fun-house mirror image)?

these "blackouts" her speech is slightly slurred and co-workers tease her about being "hung-over." She feels fuzzy headed. The slurring and mental change clear by mid-morning.

At other times she has brief, intense experiences where she gets hot and then feels that she is doing things she has done before, and that everything that is happening around her has happened exactly that way before. She experiences a sweet smell of flowers that makes her slightly sick to her stomach. At other times the world seems flat "like a cartoon," and she feels as if she is out of her body watching herself.

Assuming Patient 7-12 has a seizure disorder, what kind is it, and where is the focus?

Patient 7-12's experiences fit best complex partial seizures. Her episodes are sudden, brief, and involve altered awareness followed by some amnesia. Patient 7-12 describes diffuse warmth followed by an olfactory hallucination and visceral experience, déjà vu, and perceptual changes. At other times she has thinking changes and motor speech problems. These experiences are consistent with both frontal and temporal foci. Because speech is involved, the dominant hemisphere is most likely involved. What would you do to determine which hemisphere is dominant? Check the bottom of this page for the answer.*

So, Patient 7-12 has a dominant hemisphere frontal lobe (and perhaps temporal) seizure focus that produces partial complex epilepsy (sometimes termed psychosensory epilepsy). Her EEG confirms this. *Table 7.23* displays the classic psychosensory features.

Psychosensory features are expressions of temporolimbic disease, so they can occur in other temporolimbic conditions, such as mood disorder. Thirty percent of patients with bipolar mood disorder experience several of these features during episodes of illness. The form of the episode, however, distinguishes the mood disorder with psychosensory features from the seizure disorder with mood changes. Seizures are sudden, intense, brief episodes. [42]

*Determine her handedness by having her demonstrate how she uses everyday objects (cutting bread with a knife, pouring water from a pitcher into a glass, brushing teeth, threading a needle). Patient 7-12 is a pure right-hander, so her dominant language hemisphere is likely her left.

Table 7.23   Definitions of Various Psychosensory Phenomenon[43]

SENSORY FEATURES

Autonomic disturbances	Paroxysmal feelings of heat or cold, panic attacks with tachycardia, tachypnea, tremors, diaphoresis, etc.
Depersonalization/ derealization	A subjective sense of estrangement or unreality of oneself (depersonalization) or of one's environment (derealization)
Dsymorphopsia	The perception that objects are changing in shape
Dysmegalopsia	The perception that objects are changing in size
Deja vu/Jamais vu	Familiarity of the unfamiliar/unfamiliarity of the familiar
Gustatory hallucinations	Tasting something that is not there or an illogical taste, i.e., metal
Macroacusia	The illusion of a stimulus sounding louder than it really is
Olfactory hallucinations	Smelling something that is not there or an illogical odor, i.e., smell of death
Tactile (haptic) hallucinations	The experience of the feeling that electricity or insects are on one's body, of being touched
Visceral hallucinations	Such as having a sudden onset of a strange, hollow, or warm feeling in one's stomach; feeling objects in one's body
Complex formed visual hallucinations	Autoscopic, panoramic - - the hallucination of seeing 2 or 3 dimensional images- - could be of oneself (autoscopic) or scenic

EMOTIONAL FEATURES

Disinhibition	Inability to modulate one's social behavior
Emotional incontinence	Exaggerated emotional expression with unintended laughing or unmotivated weeping. The emotion expressed may be completely unrelated to the mood of the patient or may reflect the appropriate feeling but is out of proportion to the intensity of the emotion experienced.
Paroxysmal and transient euphoria	Without obvious cause
Paroxysmal and transient sadness	Without obvious cause

Table 7.23   Definitions of Various Psychosensory Phenomenon (cont'd)

BEHAVIORAL FEATURES

Emotionality	A deepening of all emotions, sustained intense affect
Hyposexuality	Reduced sexual behavior during adulthood
Orality	Tendency to move or stimulate the oral-buccolingual area such as lip smacking, chewing movements, tendency to put objects in one's mouth
Circumstantiality	Inability to directly answer the goal of a question because of added peripheral details
Religiosity/pseudo-philosophical interests	Holding deep religious beliefs, or cosmological or metaphysical interests that are idiosyncratic and out of proportion to educational/social background
Humorless sobriety	Overgeneralized ponderous concerns; humor lacking, over-"intellectualizing" at the expense of humor, i.e. a stuffed shirt
Hypergraphia	Keeping an extensive diary, detailed notes; writing an autobiography or novel out of proportion to one's background
Viscosity	inability to break off communication with subject; "stickiness"; a tendency to repeat (perseverate) on topics, ideas, thoughts

CLASSIC PSYCHIATRIC FEATURES

Auditory hallucinations	Complete voices, extracampine voices (hearing voices from miles away)
Unprovoked aggressive outbursts	Irritability, rage attacks, unprovoked temper outbursts, violent behavior
Delusional mood	The experience of the "feeling" that something is wrong, that things are not right and are sinister, i.e., "Something is going on out there, I don't know what it is, but I feel it and I'm afraid."
Delusional perception	A belief based upon perceiving a real stimulus, making it significant, making it personal and then reaching a conclusion for which the examiner cannot feel a meaningful connection between the real stimulus and the patient's conclusion
Experience of alienation	The experience that one's feelings, impulses, thoughts and actions are imposed by some external agency. One is literally "being controlled," can literally "feel" the controlling force, and must passively submit to the experience.
Thought blocking with derailment	Complete stoppage of one's thoughts with the subsequent jump to another topic
Thought broadcasting	The experience that one's thoughts can literally escape from one's head aloud into the external world

Table 7.23 Definitions of Various Psychosensory Phenomenon (cont'd)	
NEUROLOGIC FEATURES	
Denial and neglect	The tendency to fail to notice, report or respond to stimuli in one-half of space. Included in this definition is the unawareness of one's illness, indifference to one's disability, hatred of one's disability, phantom limb phenomenon, in which the feeling of a third upper or lower extremity has appeared.
Dysrhythmic speech	Rate of speech of at least 100 words/minute with evidence of paraphasic errors, verbal and literal, driveling, neologisms
Compulsive/stereoty pic behaviors	Such as whistling, arranging, etc.
Dressing difficulty	The tendency to dress only one side of the body, don multiple layers or clothing; the inability to correctly orient one's arm to the sleeve or to wear one's shirt on one's leg or put pants on backwards
Poor topographic orientation	Failure to describe the spatial characteristics of familiar surroundings, to tell how one would travel from one part to another in one's environment, and how to indicate the location of major cities on a map one's native country
Pain asymbolia	The patient, although capable of distinguishing the different types of pain stimuli from one another and from touch, makes none of the usual emotional, motor, or verbal responses to pain. The patient seems totally unaware of the painful or hurtful nature of stimuli delivered to any part of the body, whether one side or the other and may actually experience the stimulus as pleasurable.

How can you best treat Patient 7-12?

In addition to following the principles of management for epilepsy described previously, you can get two birds with a single stone here: valproic acid works well for both partial complex epilepsy and bipolar disorder.

Patient 7-13: All That Glitters Isn't Gold, and All Strange Behavior Isn't "Functional"

A 41-year-old man is receiving therapy for "psychogenic spells." He has episodes where he suddenly feels warm and mentally unclear, as if he just woke up. He cannot think clearly during these episodes and feels as if he is slow and almost unable to move. Sometimes he has spells where he collapses and is unconscious for a second or two. At other times he has staring spells that last for 20-30 seconds during which he is uncommunicative. At other times, he has become upset with his treaters and switched therapists. He is short tempered when his "spells" are most frequent. At other times he complains of depression and has made several suicide gestures. This has been going on since he was 30 years old.

Why was Patient 7-13 seen by psychiatrists during his decade plus of illness?

Patient 7-13 was underdiagnosed rather than simply misdiagnosed. His EEG was read as normal, and so it was assumed that he was not epileptic. He was diagnosed as having conversion disorder, and, as his illness led to mood lability, borderline personality disorder. But, regardless of the syndrome, etiology cannot be assumed. This is particularly needed if a patient has either a dissociative disorder or borderline personality. These patients offer an identifiable explanation for their dysfunctional behavior. *Tables 7.24* and *7.25* display the differential diagnosis of dissociative disorder and borderline personality disorder.

Table 7.24 The Differential Diagnosis of Dissociative Disorder [44]

Diagnostic Possibility	What to Look For
Drug and alcohol abuse	Mimics depersonalization and derealization, is associated with personality traits of impulsivity, aggressiveness, novelty seeking, and excitability
Epilepsy	Fugues will be of short duration (minutes) and wandering in feet or rarely several miles. The fugue will be post-ictal. Depersonalization and derealization will be brief and ictal related.
Sleep disorder	Can result in daytime microsleep events mimicking depersonalization and derealization. Both REM and non-REM disorders can cause this.
Multiple sclerosis	Mistaken for conversion or other psychiatric conditions, MS features can quickly resolve. Diagnostically helpful MRIs and evoked potentials are not routinely done in primary care practice. In addition to early adult onset, MS has a second peak in midlife often with cerebellar features that mimic astasia abasia (wobbly gait) and falling episodes.
Migraine	Can produce the transient contralateral Todd's paralysis that is mistaken for a conversion reaction or temporary blindness, particularly in the migraineur with comorbid mood disorder or epilepsy.
Movement disorders	Atypical movement disorders secondary to encephalitis or a drug reaction can be mistaken for "hysteria."
Personality disorder	About 25% of persons with either histrionic and antisocial personality disorder have conversion symptoms. If a patient with a conversion symptom does not have a longstanding dramatic-emotional abnormal personality, then conversion is almost always secondary to some general medical or neurologic disorder.

Table 7.25 The Differential Diagnosis of Borderline Personality Disorder [45]

Diagnostic Possibility	What to Look For
Bipolar mood disorder	About 50% of "borderlines" have a soft bipolar spectrum or a bipolar disorder with a childhood onset (less episodic, more chronic, less severe, drug abuse, often co-morbid).
Drug and alcohol abuse	These patients will also have personality traits of impulsivity, risk taking, and excitability.
Traumatic brain injury	Particularly of frontal or nondominant hemisphere structures Mood stabilizers can help these patients. Antipsychotics and benzodiazepines can make cognition worse.
Epilepsy	Particularly with mesial frontotemporal foci . Mood stabilizing anticonvulsants can help these patients. Some antipsychotics can lower seizure threshold, worsening the condition.
Personality disorder	Borderline may be diagnosed based on the consequences of the behaviors associated with antisocial, histrionic, or narcissistic personality disorders. The validity of these trait disorders is substantial.
Self-mutilation	A stormy life with self-mutilating behavior often generates a borderline diagnosis. More reliable (the DSM reliability of borderline is poor) and perhaps more valid diagnoses to consider are mild mental retardation and associated syndromes, obsessive compulsive disorder, mood disorders, chronic drug abuse affecting basal ganglia (stimulants), epilepsy.

What are the clues that Patient 7-13 is epileptic?

1. Sudden change in behavior and subjective experience
2. Subjective feeling of mental change "as if he just woke up"
3. Being unconscious for several seconds and collapsing
4. Staring spells of 20-30 seconds during which he has altered arousal and responsivity

Patients with several types of seizures typically have subcortical foci in crossroad areas of the brain where the focus location influences more than one pathway. Also typically this will be in frontal circuits. If the location of the seizure focus is subcortical, routine EEG studies are often unhelpful and at most may show only mild frontal slowing. Patient 7-13 had cataplexic attacks (falling), absence attacks (staring), and complex partial attacks (feeling mentally altered). A sudden feeling of warmth is a typical frontal lobe aura. Aura, which literally means "breeze," occurs at the beginning of ictus and lasts a few seconds. *Table 7.26* displays the auras of epileptic sites by cerebral hemisphere region.

Table 7.26   The Auras of Cerebral Hemisphere Regions [46]

Frontal	Temporal	Parietal	Occipital
• *Cephalic* Light-headedness Pressure on top of head Band around head Vertigo, dizziness Drugged feeling Head feeling inflated • *Diffuse warmth* May begin elsewhere and ascend into the head • *Language* Speech arrest Forced speech Garbled speech • *Motor* Side to side head movement Pelvic thrusting	• *Emotive* Sudden intense emotion (sadness, elation, fear) Brief panic attack Sudden violence • *Perceptual* Brief hallucinations or perceptual distortions • *Mnestic* Flashbacks Déjà vu Jamais vu • *Arousal* Derealization Depersonalization • Autonomic Sudden cold Tachycardia Flushing • *Visceral* Epigastric rush Nausea	• *Somatosensory* Sudden intense tingling Electric shocks Burning Unilateral pain • *Body part perceptual distortion* Limb feels odd in shape, composition, weight, location	• *Visual changes* Seeing lights, halos, colors • *Ocular sensations* Electric feeling in eyes Feeling eyes are being pulled out of their sockets (may lead to mutilation of eyeball)

What would you do to try to prove that Patient 7-13 is epileptic?

Epilepsy is a clinical, not a laboratory, diagnosis. You can do all the tests we have mentioned, but in about 20% of patients you will find nothing to confirm your clinical opinion. Your best bet is to get a detailed careful history of signs and symptoms and how they unfold. If you still are convinced the patient has epilepsy, and no other better prognosis condition is likely, treat for epilepsy.

How can Patient 7-13 best be treated?

To treat an epileptic you must be prepared to provide comprehensive management. *Table 7.27* displays the requirement of this treatment. Because of his complex seizure forms, Patient 7-13 would likely do best on a broad spectrum anticonvulsant, like valproic acid.

Table 7.27 Principles of Epilepsy Management
Polypharmacy is usually bad: Poor seizure control and cognitive problems from medication leading to frustration, irritability, and explosiveness in adults, attention deficit hyperactivity disorder-like syndromes in children.

Therapeutic trials will take longer than for other psychiatric patients:
    a. Depends on frequency and seasonality of fits
    b. Behavioral syndrome, e.g., mood or psychotic disorder
    c. Interictal functioning

Identify triggers and avoid them: Alcohol, fluorescent lights, flickering lights, high altitude, and frequent flying.
Reduce stressors: Expressed emotion, fatigue
In women, consider menses, menopause, estrogen replacement as triggers, and that 50% of women epileptics have menstrual/reproductive problems, i.e., hypogonadism, polycystic ovaries, other menstrual/reproductive irregularities.
Avoid antipsychotics: Behavioral episodes are best treated with treatment of choice for primary condition; anticonvulsants and ECT often work best.
Personality changes are unresponsive to treatments.
Psychosurgery for intractable seizures is high tech and works for some patients.

Quick Rounds

1. A 76-year-old man was diagnosed as having Alzheimer's disease 6 years ago. Over the last 3 years the patient has been continuously deteriorating (Min-Mental State Examination is now less than 6). The patient was prescribed donepezil 10 mg 6 years ago, which he is still taking. During one office visit his wife requests that you discontinue donepezil because it does not seem to help at all and is very expensive. Should you oblige?

2. A 78-year-old woman with a diagnosis of Alzheimer's comes to you for evaluation. You detect frontal lobe cognitive problems, but the patient has no difficulty copying geometrical shapes or doing simple arithmetic. What do you do for her Alzheimer's disease?

3. A 70-year-old man is evaluated for dementia. Neuropsychological testing reveals age-related cognitive deficits but no dementia. A SPECT scan shows bilateral temporoparietal hypoperfusion. The patient has a family history of dementia. What do you do?

4. A 35-year-old man with a history of severe traumatic brain injury and depression is currently stable on bupropion. He wants to know if he can stop taking the drug. What should you tell him?

5. A 19-year-old college student with a history of epilepsy and mood disorder comes to the clinic requesting oral contraceptives. She is currently taking carbamazepine 600 mg BID. What do you do?

6. A 14-year-old boy with ADD was diagnosed epileptic. His mother wants to know if he can play sports. What do you advise?

7. Every month before her menstrual period, a 22-year-old woman with epilepsy complains of several episodes of sudden irritability followed by sudden confusion lasting 2-3 minutes. After that she has headaches and complains of a dysphoric mood lasting for a day. What is happening to her?

8. A 44-year-old man continues to have daily complex partial seizures despite treatment with carbamazepine (level 12 ug/ml), valproic acid (level 145 ug/ml), and gabapentin 2400 mg/day. The patient does not want any more anticonvulsants and is not willing to undergo psychosurgery. What should be done?

9. A 26-year-old woman with an 8 year history of tonic-clonic epilepsy is currently stable on valproic acid 500 mg TID. She wants to become pregnant. What should you tell her?

Quick Rounds Answers

1. Yes! The patient is no longer in the early stages of Alzheimer's. A cholinergic enhancing drug such as donepezil only works early on. At this point, it probably has no effect except on their budget. So, you could agree to his wife's request. Selegiline (20 mg patch), however, might offer some benefit.

2. You rediagnose it. Alzheimer's dementia is associated with a temporoparietal pattern of cognitive deficits. The patient is exhibiting a frontal lobe deficit perhaps without any parietal lobe abnormalities. Further assessment is needed to identify the etiology of her problems. Not only is the correct diagnosis important for her, it is important for her family, who undoubtedly are concerned about their risks for Alzheimer's disease.

3. Treat him as if he is in the preclinical stage of Alzheimer's. Because he has a family history of Alzheimer's, and a perfusion pattern consistent with Alzheimer's, we would also start him on a nonsteroidal anti-inflammatory agent and perhaps vitamin E. We would prescribe cognitive and aerobic exercise. We would follow him closely, and, if needed, at some point start a cholinesterase inhibitor. Persons at risk for Alzheimer's in 4 or so years have mild cognitive problems.

4. Although the decision to stop an antidepressant is based on factors such as the number of previous episodes or severity of relapse, for patients with significant brain damage our policy is to continue the antidepressant for life. The only time we would agree to a switch or a trial off medication is if the patient is experiencing significant side effects.

5. Oral contraceptives interact with antiepileptic medications, such as carbamazepine, phenytoin, and primidone. Carbamazepine decreases oral contraceptive efficacy. Epileptic patients should be told this, and the patient may want to use additional contraceptive methods. Alternatively, the patient can be switched to valproic acid, which does not reduce oral contraceptive concentrations, but may cause ovarian problems later on. There is no free lunch.

6. Having epilepsy should not prevent the boy from leading a normal life. A child with epilepsy can play sports that are not of unusual risk, e.g., rock climbing. Patients with poorly controlled seizures should not swim. Even those with good control of seizures should restrict

swimming in a lake or pool and should always be accompanied by a buddy.

7.   This woman is experiencing several seizures before her menstrual cycle. A consistent increase in seizures during and before a menstrual cycle is called *catamenial seizures*. Some open studies in women with catamenial seizures show improvement with medroxyprogesterone. Alternatively, intermittent anticonvulsant therapy is also used.

8.   The odds are that reducing his polypharmacy will help. We vote for the carbamazepine because combined with valproic acid, it is more likely metabolized to an epoxy metabolite, which is a neurotoxin. Gabapentin is not metabolized in the liver. There is some evidence that biofeedback and behavioral conditioning techniques help in controlling seizure frequency in some patients. General relaxation and stress management may also help some patients. Children with intractable epilepsy may respond to a ketogenic diet, as may some adults.

9.   A woman patient with epilepsy needs to consider several factors before becoming pregnant. A discussion of pregnancy and childbearing should occur before initiating anticonvulsant therapy. Epilepsy is familial, and there is evidence that genetic factors play some role. This woman must be aware that there is a chance that her child might also develop epilepsy.

Infants of epileptic mothers exposed to anticonvulsants in utero have a greater risk of developing congenital malformations than nonexposed infants or infants of mothers without epilepsy. The overall risk is about 4-6%. All commonly used anticonvulsants cross the placenta and are present in fetal circulation. All the commonly used anticonvulsants have been associated with congenital malformation, most frequent being cleft lip. However, generalized seizure poses clear risks for maternal injury and miscarriage. For most women with generalized seizures, experts recommend continued anticonvulsant therapy and providing good prenatal care and high serum folate levels. Multivitamins with folate reduce the risk of malformation. Women taking valproic acid should be informed of additional risks of spina bifida. However, changing or stopping an anticonvulsant which effectively controls seizure is not the best policy, because increased risk of seizure may outweigh the risk of teratogenesis. The literature has shown that despite the increased risk, more than 90% of women with epilepsy deliver healthy babies.[47]

Chapter 8

Psychiatric Consultations

Patient 8-1: Each Customer Gets Full Service

A 40-year-old nurse comes to the emergency room complaining that over the past 6 months the doctors at his hospital have been trying to get him fired because of his "great" medical skills, of which they are jealous. He says they have reported him to the Food and Drug Administration for prescribing medications. He has had no prior similar notions and no family history of psychiatric illness. He denies perceptual disturbances. His affect is full, and he is angry. The ER physician calls you.

What is your first step of patient care for an emergency room patient with a behavioral syndrome? (This is a semi-trick question.)

A patient is a patient is a patient. The clinical setting alters the ultimate goals of patient care, but the initial job is still the same: determine the clinical syndrome by getting the big picture. In the ER this needs to be done faster than in other settings, but the concept is the same. Because the ER selects patients of high acuity, part of the first step in the ER is deciding if the patient is likely to die from the syndrome within hours or a few days at most. This is just as true for patients with behavioral syndromes as it is for others. Because Patient 8-1 has been ill for at least 6 months, the likelihood of imminent death is unlikely. Nevertheless, you always ask yourself this question: Is this patient physiologically stable, and is there any evidence that his condition is imminently life-threatening? Does Patient 8-1 have a brain aneurysm ready to burst? Does he have a brain tumor that is now impinging on his homeostatic brain systems? It turns out he does not, but we (you) did a careful general medical and neurologic examination to be sure.

Sometimes delusional patients extend their delusional ideas into their past lives, thus, falsifying their lives. Termed paramnesia, it can sometimes lead to false diagnostic conclusions: maybe the 6 months is really 6 days or weeks. Typically, however, *paramnesia* is easy to spot as the circumstances "remembered" are clearly false and delusional, e.g., I remember the surgery where they put the transmitter into my brain.

Forty percent of acutely hospitalized psychiatric patients have general medical or neurologic problems that either caused their behavioral symptoms or complicate treatment for them.[1]

What are your steps of action from A to Z for emergency room patients, and specifically for Patient 8-1?

1. *Determine acuity and imminent life threatening conditions.* Psychiatrists are consultants to ERs, not primary ER caregivers. Do not go to see a patient until the ER physician has done this first step. When you do go, do not assume the ER physician has done this first step well, so make your own assessment. Patient 8-1 is angry and delusional, but does not appear in any life threatening state. In fact, his general medical health is good. His traditional neurologic examination is within normal limits.

2. *Determine the problem or syndrome.* Patient 8-1 has a delusional disorder with grandiose content. His mood is angry. He has been ill for some time. In fact, his problems at work, to a lesser degree, date back several years. Three categories of syndromes should come to mind. Before you look, think.

Drug induced disorder. Patient 8-1 denies any drugs or use of prescription medication. But you must always consider a *late-occurring psychotic disorder* secondary to chronic drug use. This is a psychosis occurring in a person who years before used hallucinogenic drugs or inhalants, resulting in brain damage and subsequent psychotic episodes.[2] Again, Patient 8-1 says he never used street drugs and rarely drinks alcohol.

> Always get a drug screen on an ER patient who is psychotic or has a major mood disorder. In some ERs intoxication or drug effect either accounts for the patient's behavioral signs or complicates the situation in 70% of visits. If the patient has recently been prescribed psychotropic medication get a blood level if possible to guide further treatment. Does the ER visit represents a relapse due to noncompliance (low blood levels) or break through despite compliance (therapeutic blood level)?

Primary mood disorder. It is common. It is treatable. So, always look for it. Patient 8-1, however, has no past episodes, but began to have behavioral changes at age 36. He also has a negative family history for psychiatric disorder. He does not show any other features of a present mania or depression other than his irritability and grandiose ideas.

Secondary delusional disorder. If not drug related, particularly stimulants or phencyclidine, think of head injury, epilepsy, or a stroke as top choices, followed by less common disorders involving frontal circuitry.

3. *Treatment.* If the syndrome can be resolved or ameliorated in the ER, do it. Patient 8-1 has a long-standing condition that needs to be evaluated to determine etiology. What he needs now is not to have the last three years of illness resolved, but just what happened in the last day or so that got him angry enough to come to the ER. The best treatment for him now is letting him get things off his chest and develop some trust in you, so that you can convince him of step D.
4. *Disposition.* Without adequate follow-up, many ER visits do not resolve the problem. Patient 8-1 needs to be evaluated for the etiology of his delusional disorder. He either needs to be hospitalized voluntarily to do this, or needs evaluation at a specialty clinic within 24-48 hours.

Discussion

The goals of ER treatment are to prevent something bad from happening and then to solve the immediate problem. Definitive care, particularly for behavioral syndromes is typically done at follow-up. Thus, definitive treatments (i.e., antipsychotics, mood stabilizers) are to be avoided in favor of behavioral crisis interventions, antianxiety agents, and sedative-hypnotics. Follow-up appointments should be as specific as possible, preferably to an identified person, e.g., Dr. Jones rather than the mental health clinic.

In presenting the options to Patient 8-1, although he is a nurse, do not assume his knowledge and experience are good. Even if it is, explain important things you are considering and would like to do for him as you would any patient. Professionals deserve and need the full service like any other patient. The more consideration you give in your explanations, the better most patients who are healthy professionals feel, and the more confidence they have in you. The "trick" in doing this with Patient 8-1 is that he is delusional or at least has an overvalued idea, so he will be less likely to accept your idea that he is ill. Nevertheless, he came to the ER with some complaints. Use them to try convincing him of the need for evaluation.

Patient 8-2: The Evil Eyes Have It

A 30-year-old man is brought to the ER after attacking his neighbor. He has not slept well in a week, and is hearing voices telling him to eradicate "all evil forces." He also believes he has the ability to detect evil by looking into people's eyes. The ER doctor calls you.

About 10% of the US population are victims of violence annually. Males between 15 and 25 (like Patient 8-3) are most likely to commit violent acts. Better than half of persons committing criminal violence do so under the influence of alcohol. [3]

What should be your first step in caring for Patient 8-2?

Patient 8-2 has recently attacked a neighbor. He hears voices telling him to "eradicate" evil. Is he an imminent threat? He may need to be restrained to protect the ER staff, other ER patients, and himself. *Table 8.1* displays behaviors associated with imminent violence.

Table 8.1   Imminent Violence Risk Indicators
Irritability in previously violent person
Agitation or psychotic excitement
Shouting, threatening, menacing gestures
Current violent thoughts or statements

Patients like Patient 8-2 with any of the risk factors in *Table 8.1* need to be evaluated with security personnel present and enough trained staff who are ready to restrain the patient. Your job is to 1) protect everyone, 2) decide if the patient has a life threatening condition, and 3) control the patient so he can be hospitalized. Control may require a "show of force" or restraints *and* a sedative. Hospitalization is needed because he is a danger to others. It is likely to be *involuntary*.

In outpatient/ER settings, men patients are more likely than women patients to be violent. Men under 50 with a history of drug abuse (inhalants and PCP are the worst) or past violence, and of lower socioeconomic background are most likely to harm ER staff. [4]

Patient 8-2 is irritable and agitated. He refuses to sit down (getting a patient to sit while you are also sitting at a safe distance may calm the situation). He threatens you and "sees" evil in your eyes. The police who brought him have conveniently disappeared. Security personnel arrive and after a minimal struggle, they subdue and restrain Patient 8-2. When Patient 8-2 is put into hospital clothes, he is found to have two large hunting knives in his jacket.

> Before admitting patients from the ER have them change into hospital clothes. This way any hidden weapons can be diplomatically found and removed.

Patient 8-2 is sedated and examined. Blood is drawn and he is catheterized for a urine sample that among other things will be tested for street drugs. Because he is physiologically stable and his general medical health appears adequate, he is admitted to psychiatry under an involuntary certificate. Although commitment and follow-up procedures vary from state to state, there are some common features. *Table 8.2* displays these.

What is the likelihood of Patient 8-2's attacking someone again?

Table 8.2 *General Procedures for Involuntary Hospitalization and Further Inpatient Treatment*
A petition to start the commitment is filed by someone who has observed the patient's behavior. It should include one of the following: • Patient is a danger to self or others due to a mental illness. • Patient is unable to take care of himself due to a mental illness. • Patient is mentally retarded and is unable to take care of himself.
A qualified mental health professional (usually an MD, but it can be a psychologist or social worker) examines the patient and writes a certificate stating that due to a mental illness, the patient is indeed unable to protect himself or is a danger to himself or others.
Commitment is a legal procedure and only a judge can commit, so after a petition and certificate, the patient is taken to court. Some places require a second certificate by a qualified mental health professional before a patient can be taken to court. The court needs to see the patient and you or a colleague within 72 working hours of the involuntary admission.
A patient awaiting commitment procedures can be detained in the hospital (duration varies) and should follow general inpatient rules. Only emergency medications can be administered to the patient awaiting commitment.

This is really a two-part question. Part one focuses on his inpatient stay. Part two focuses on the months and years following this hospitalization.

If any of the indicators of imminent risk persist once he awakens, then he is an imminent violence risk. If they do not persist (sedation, behavioral controls, and some sleep have helped), then does he still have high risk features? *Table 8.3* displays these.

Table 8.3   Increased Violence Risk Factors
Recent assaultiveness
Involuntary patient or patient stating wishes to sign out of the hospital against medical advice, each with a history of violence
Experiencing angry command hallucinations
Having experiences of alienation or control that cause irritability or anxiety
Having fantastic persecutory delusions (e.g., being possessed by the devil)
Having delusions of being poisoned
Diagnosis of drug abuse, head injury, conduct disorder, or antisocial personality disorder

Patient 8-2 has the first three features in *Table 8.3* and may have others. He will remain a high risk until whatever has caused his psychosis is resolved. Because past behavior is a good predictor of future behavior, he will be a long-term violence risk unless his illness can be remitted.

Patient 8-3: Guilty by Reasons of Bad Behavior

A 24-year-old man is brought to the ER after threatening to kill his girlfriend. Patient 8-3 says he is angry because his girlfriend wants to break up with him. Patient 8-3 has no history of psychiatric illness and currently exhibits no psychopathology, other than some irritability. General medical examination is essentially normal except he has slightly reddish sclera and alcohol on his breath. He admits to consuming a six-pack of beer during the course of the evening. Patient 8-3 has a history of provoked and unprovoked aggressive behavior. The ER doctor calls you.

Should Patient 8-3 be hospitalized?

Patient 8-3 has recently threatened violence and has a history of violence. He is irritable and perhaps still somewhat intoxicated from alcohol. He is potentially violent, and that is one criterion for psychiatric admission.

However, to be admitted, the violence or risks of it must be felt to result from disease, i.e., he is violent because he is an irritable manic. The concept here is that the violence will not be criminal violence and it will also be treatable. For example, when mania resolves, the irritability and violence proneness of the patient also resolves. The information you have is that Patient 8-3 is not psychiatrically ill. He may have antisocial personality, but as far as we know, that is not an illness and legally not an excuse for bad behavior. Intoxication is not an illness and does not mitigate criminal violence. Thus, Patient 8-3 might go to your local jail, but not into your hospital.

What ER treatment is appropriate for Patient 8-3?

Patient 8-3 is a patient in your ER. His behavior has gotten him there, and into trouble. You are obligated to give him your best evaluation. If you find no illness, that is good news. You tell him so. If you think he is likely to leave the ER and kill his girlfriend, you are legally obligated to notify her and the police. You may need security to hold Patient 8-3 until the police arrive, but the police may choose not to arrest him. That is their

> In 1974, the California Supreme Court ruled that therapists have a legal duty to warn the victims of foreseeable violence against them, even if they (intended victims) are not therapist's patients (Tarasoff vs. Regents of University of California). [5]

decision and responsibility, not yours. Life isn't a TV show. If you think Patient 8-3's threats are not serious, he, nevertheless, has a problem with violence, probably alcohol, and maybe a personality disorder. If you know of treatment programs for these problems that you think work, you enthusiastically offer these as referrals. Not admitting Patient 8-3 and giving him an excuse for his bad behavior is therapeutic. Offering him a real choice of getting his act together may be the best treatment he can get.

Patient 8-4: It's Easy to Admit

A 28-year-old accountant is brought to your ER semi-comatose. Over the next hour she gradually awakens. She says she took an overdose of diazepam (prescribed for back spasms) after breaking up with her boyfriend. She says she wants to leave the ER, and the ER doctor calls you.

Should Patient 8-4 be discharged from the ER or admitted to the hospital?

Administratively, and because of the time and effort spent, it is almost always less work to admit a patient than to try to treat the patient in the ER and then send the patient home. Hospitalization, however, is not always in the patient's best interest because it can reinforce behaviors leading to the ER visit. For Patient 8-4, the problem in admitting her is that it will reinforce whatever manipulative quality there was to her suicide attempt, making it more likely that she will repeatedly deal with problems of living by dramatic maladaptive responses. The danger of not admitting her is that she may be seriously depressed and suicidal, and will kill herself in the next few days. So, resist any tendency to take the easy route, which is   admission. However, because discharge may be dangerous also, do not automatically discharge her from the ER. Think about it first. See the next question.

What additional information do you need, if any, to make your decision?

You know the answer to this because it is all in the depression chapter about suicide. We know that Patient 8-4 is at a higher risk for suicide than an average citizen, but not whether this risk can be lowered by a good interaction with you and a good referral. So what to do. (Think of an answer before you turn the page.)

What? You want us to tell you what to do? Well, you have all the information, so you must decide – admit and be safe, but maybe make her a chronic patient. Send her home with a good referral and perhaps she kills herself. This is why they pay you the big bucks.

Anxious, agitated melancholics are at greatest risk to kill themselves. Nonmelancholic patients with family to watch and support them over the crisis, are less likely to do so.

Patient 8-5: You Blow My Mind

A 35-year-old man is brought to the ER by the police because he was threatening strangers in the street and shouting at passing cars. He said people were "ray gunning" him and stealing his mind. He then attacked the policemen. In being subdued he suffered several bruises to his head and face. He bit and kicked one policeman.

There are three immediate concerns in this situation. What are they, and what do you do about each?

A. *Is Patient 8-5 still imminently violent, and does he need sedation and restraints?* In most situations like this, the patient will arrive handcuffed. If he remains agitated, angry, shouts, threatens or makes *any* display of irritability or uncooperativeness, he needs to remain in restraints. If so, with the help of the police and hospital security, transfer him to four point restraints. Then decide if he can be evaluated without sedation (the best choice). If he needs sedation, and you have not yet made a specific diagnosis, try 0.5-1 mg lorazepam IV. If held down and in restraints, most patients can safely be given single-dose IV medication, and a tourniquet may not be needed as veins are often prominent when a patient is restrained and held.

B. *Did Patient 8-5 suffer a subdural hematoma in his struggle with the police? Were the bruises to his head and face inflicted with night sticks?* A CT scan is needed, as it is most sensitive to recent hemorrhagic brain lesions. This will be done under full sedation in most hospitals.

C. Now for "out of the box": *Did the bite expose the policeman to deadly pathogens, particularly HIV?* The policeman's wound needs to be expertly treated and blood drawn from the patient to determine what "bad things" he might be carrying. The policeman also needs blood drawn to establish a baseline. Every hospital has a universal precautions policy that involves step-by-step procedures in the event of contact with blood, tissue, or body fluids. This involves administration of first aid and then notifying the appropriate people or departments.

With additional information do you need to formulate a management plan for Patient 8-5? What important areas do you need to think about in formulating the plan?

For any acutely violent psychotic patient, always think of drug intoxication. Drug screens can be definitive, but take time, so a good history and examination is needed to permit more immediate treatment. If the patient is in restraints, pulse and blood pressure will likely be up, so *sympathomimetic drug effects* will be confounded. If the patient has *rotary nystagmus*, has decreased sense of pain, and is described by the police as having some alteration in gait consistent with *ataxia*, then phencyclidine is the likely culprit. If the patient continuously scans the room as if searching for danger, and is described as "jerky" in movement with stereotypes or repetitive, compulsive-like behavior, then stimulants are the likely culprit. Cocaine intoxication can also produce tactile hallucinations of bugs crawling on or under the skin (ask and look for excoriations) and hallucinations of geometric shapes. Anticholinergic drugs in younger persons will also produce dry skin, dilated pupils, a tachycardia (under these circumstances, unhelpful) and low grade fever. In older persons only the delirium may be present.

> Drug screens are helpful if you know how to order them and interpret the results. Ask the lab to report even traces of a drug because the period from use to detection varies. Cocaine can be undetectable or in only trace amounts after 5-12 hours of a dose. Marijuana can be detected after up to 6 weeks or more of abstinence. Other detection limits in days are amphetamines (1-2), barbiturates (3-5 short-acting, 10-14 long-acting), benzodiazepines (2-9), opiates (1-2), phencyclidine (2-8). Immunoassay is the preferred lab method.[6]

In this case, Patient 8-6 has the signs of cocaine intoxication. He has stereotypic grimacing and shoulder and head tics. His arms and legs are excoriated from scratching (presumably in response to tactile hallucinations). A drug screen is positive for cocaine.

Treatment for drug states follows the same rules as treatment for other conditions. So management is divided into acute, continuation, and maintenance phases. *Table 8.4* displays the concerns of treatment. In planning *detoxification* for patients like Patient 8-5, *violence, excitement, and sympathetic nervous system overarousal* are the first concerns. Restraints, sedation and blood pressure and cardiac rhythm control may be needed. Acidification of the urine to help with excretion has no proven benefit.

Table 8.4	Concerns in Formulating Treatment of Cocaine Abuse
Acute Intoxication	Violence, excitement, sympathetic nervous system hyperarousal, psychosis, co-morbid stroke, arrhythmia, placental abruption
Detoxification	Prolonged psychosis, craving
Continuation of recovery	Reduce craving, avoid stimuli triggering psychological dependency response
Long-term treatment	Personality factors predicting risk of relapse

If a patient remains *psychotic* after detoxification, treatment may be with valproic acid, antipsychotics, or ECT. If detoxification is prolonged and *craving* a management problem, craving may be moderated with dopaminergic agents, such as bromocriptine, methylphenidate, carbidopa/levodopa, pergolide or amantadine. Rapid detoxification may lead to the "crash," an atypical, dysphoric depression that needs no specific treatment other than for craving. Let the patient sleep and eat as much as needed (usually a lot for both).

Once detoxification is fully completed (1-4 weeks), continuation of recovery follows (3-6 months) using dopaminergic or serotonergic drugs to reduce craving. Desipramine, imipramine, bupropion, fluoxetine, sertraline, and phenelzine have all been found modestly helpful in their typical antidepressant dosage. Naltrexone (100 mg Monday and Wednesday, 150 mg used Friday) and carbamazepine (200-800 mg) daily have also been used. Long-term management includes an anticraving drug, counseling, and rehabilitation and random urine screens. Success rates are not great.

Cocaine intoxication can cause fatal strokes (both hemorrhagic and ischemic) and arrhythmias, placental abruption, and direct brain damage from a neurotoxic metabolite, 6-hydroxyclopamine.

If the patient's cocaine level is high and he is in an excited psychotic state, he is at greater risk for NMS if exposed to an antipsychotic. So, try sedating the patient first with a benzodiazepine. If an antipsychotic is still needed, you can use an atypical antipsychotic. [7]

306

Patient 8-6: I've a Pain in My Back, But Not Because I'm a Pain in the Neck

A 40-year-old married woman is referred by a primary care physician to your clinic for evaluation. The patient reports feeling depressed for the last five years. However, she claims that this is because of her back injury and the pain she experiences. She suffered the injury while lifting a heavy box at work. According to the patient, severe back pain has kept her from doing any work. On good days, she is able to do household chores, but on bad days she has to stay in bed. Albeit a little shy and anxious, she has had no psychiatric problems prior to this injury. She has no history of general medical or neurologic problems. According to her primary care physician, her general medical and neurologic examinations are within normal limits.

What condition does Patient 8-6 have?

Patient 8-6 continues to complain of incapacitating pain, although her primary care physician thinks "it's all in her head." The key information here is the onset of illness after age 35, and the occurrence of her problems during a strenuous task at work. The patient may have chronic pain due to several factors. She may have a general medical condition that does explain her pain, e.g., a herniated disc, degenerative arthritis secondary to the injury. If her doctor prematurely assumed her pain was "mental," he may have only done a bare minimum search. Depression must also be considered. Depressed patients often complain of somatic symptoms. Anhedonic mood, vegetative signs, suicidality, and altered cognition are the ducks of depression. A repeat general medical and neurologic evaluation should rule out any herniated disc or arthritic changes. Don't assume these were done well.

Malingering and *factitious disorders* are official DSM diagnoses. Patients with these conditions actually fake symptoms. In malingering the gain is materialistic (e.g., insurance money, avoiding prosecution). In factitious disorder, the gain is presumed psychological (e.g., to reduce anxiety, to bolster self-esteem). To rule out malingering, you need to find out about any pending lawsuits against an employer, other legal situations, and a prior history of antisocial behavior. *Table 8.6* lists the behaviors to assess for antisocial personality.

> When a patient fakes signs and symptoms and even laboratory test results in their child, it is termed *factitious disorder by proxy*. It is child abuse and, if suspected, you need to inform child welfare agencies about it.

Antisocial personality is not an exclusive diagnosis of the poor or gang member. Think of all the medical fraud, national accounting and business scandals, insider trading, etc. Leather jacket and a three-piece business suit are not diagnostic signs.

To rule out a factitious disorder you would need to inquire about the consequences of the injury. For example, has the patient received additional attention from a family member?

Table 8.6   Checklist for Antisocial Personality
Childhood enuresis, fire-setting, and cruelty to animals
Childhood aggressiveness and using weapons in fights
Truancy and poor school behavior
Running away from home
Manipulative interpersonal style, unconcerned for the rights of others
Selfish, narcissistic
High risk taker and thrill seeker
Impulsive
Cold and calculating, often behind a veneer of affability and glibness

Somatization disorder is another consideration. Symptoms are not limited to a single organ system and often involve many.[8] When a patient has excessive pain that cannot be explained by the extent of any pathology, and has other unexplained symptoms reflecting other organ disease, the patient has somatization. When excessive pain occurs without other features, the patient is said to have *somatoform pain disorder*. Assuming patient 8 is not faking, her most likely diagnosis is somatoform pain disorder.

Patients with somatization disorder have increased family history of criminality and alcohol abuse and criminality.

Somatoform disorder is more common in women and often there is a family history of pain disorders. These patients often develop secondary dependence on analgesics or benzodiazepines. These patients often go from one doctor to another because they do not get adequate pain relief. In order to reduce pain, they take invasive amounts of painkillers and/or muscle relaxants. Many of them develop secondary dependence on narcotic analgesics or benzodiazepines.

How would you confirm the diagnosis? (This is a trick question.)

This is a trick question, because there is no laboratory test that will confirm this diagnosis. Somatoform pain disorder is a diagnosis of exclusion. Although neurologists often make the distinction between central neuropathic pain and psychogenic pain, we believe that the distinction is rarely helpful.

> Even after psychiatric disorders are excluded, 20-40% of primary care patients have physical symptoms that cannot be explained medically or neurologically.

How would you treat her?

Pain disorder patients often have a history of doctor shopping and use of multiple pain medication and surgeries for pain control. To treat Patient 8-6, use the following guidelines:

1. Patients should be informed of their diagnosis. Patients should be told they have a condition that can be helped, but not cured. They should not be told, "It's all in your head" or "It's due to stress." There is no evidence supporting those remarks.
2. The realistic goal of the treatment now is not to cure the disorder, but to manage the illness and prevent complications.
3. Regularly scheduled office visits, physical examinations, and listening to the patient's complaints in a sympathetic but nonreactive manner is helpful.
4. Unnecessary tests and surgeries should be avoided. New complaints should always be evaluated.
5. Narcotic analgesics should be avoided. These patients are at risk of becoming dependent.
6. Co-existing psychiatric syndromes, such as depression, should be treated.
7. Antidepressants, such as amitriptyline, serotonin uptake inhibitors, and anticonvulsants, such as gabapentin, may help and can be tried.

Discussion

The distinction between "neuropathic" and "psychogenic" pain is rarely helpful. If the patient's complaint of pain is not due to depression, somatization, or malingering, then treat it as a chronic pain syndrome, regardless of etiology. Do not label this patient with somatization disorder. In chronic pain disorder the specific pain predominates and is of sufficient severity to warrant treatment.

The sensation of pain is a product of neural networks of the brain. Noxious (painful), mechanical, thermal, or chemical stimuli activate specific peripheral nerve endings, and impulses are transmitted to the spinal cord or brain stem. These impulses are then transmitted to neurons that convey the information to the thalamus and ultimately to the cortex. Pain is classified based on underlying pathophysiology as nocioceptive or neuropathic pain. Nocioceptive pain is caused by ongoing activity of nocioceptors (pain receptors) as a result of painful stimuli. Here the pain is proportional to injury, and the nervous system is functioning properly. Neuropathic pain is caused by abnormal signal processing in peripheral and central nervous system. This pain reflects impairment or injury of the nervous system. This pain is often disproportional to the injury. There are many theories regarding development of chronic pain. Abnormal or persistent pain can occur if a) nonnoxious stimuli are perceived as noxious by the central nervous system; this occurs due to loss of inhibition produced by myelinated neurons, and by sensitization of central nervous system; or b) the thalamus is generating ectopic impulses without any stimuli; or c) peripheral nerve damage leads to hypersensitivity of the neurons. Descending pathways from the brain attenuate the transmission of pain. Multiple brain regions (e.g., cortex, thalamus) contribute to descending inhibitory pathways. Nerve fibers from these pathways release inhibitory substances, such as serotonin, opioids, GABA, etc. This explains why antidepressants are helpful in alleviating pain.[9]

Patient 8-7: Where the "Psyche" Lurks

A 39-year-old woman is referred by her primary care physician for psychiatric evaluation. He wants to know if her symptoms are "psychogenic." Patient 8-7 was seen initially for weakness of both her legs, tingling and unsteady gait. There was no history of injury or recent flu-like symptoms. Prior to that episode Patient 8-7 was in good general medical health, with no prior psychiatric or neurologic history. A neurologist, who saw her before you made the following observations. "During the examination she is cooperative but seems anxious about her condition. Deep tendon reflexes are 4+, equal bilaterally, and muscle strength is normal. Her sensation to pinprick is somewhat decreased but the rest of the neurologic examination is normal." Patient 8-7's general medical examination and labs, including CBC and electrolytes, are normal. Her MRI shows one small area of periventricular hyperintensity, which was read as "inconclusive." The neurologist did not think the woman's problem was neurologic.   He called it a *conversion disorder* and recommended that the primary care physician get a psychiatric evaluation for the patient.

What additional information is needed to seriously consider the conversion disorder diagnosis?

Although claiming to be empirical and not theoretical, the DSM *conversion disorder* criteria require the clinician to conclude that "psychological factors" are "etiologically related to the symptom because of a temporal relationship between a *psychological stressor* that is apparently related to a *psychological conflict or need* and initiation or exacerbation of the symptom." The patient cannot be faking and the symptoms not culturally sanctioned.

So, at the very least, Patient 8-7 would have to be under some substantial stress that directly perturbs her psychological make-up. However, despite this theoretical requirement, the DSM structure of dividing syndromes into primary (idiopathic psychiatric) and secondary (secondary to medical or neurologic etiology) is a good one. so to consider conversion disorder or a diagnosis, all medical and neurologic disorders that can give rise to these symptoms must be ruled out. So, on to the next question.

What might account for Patient 8-7's behavioral syndrome?

Step 1. The first step in your evaluation is to define the syndrome. The big picture here is that of a not too old – not too young – woman with acute onset vague neurologic symptoms. There is no history of acute injury or infection, no personal or family history of previous neurologic illness, and no other symptoms.

Persons with syndromes that are believed "psychogenic" are supposed to already have problems because of some underlying psychological situation, e.g., they are overly dependent, have poor self-esteem, or a definable personality disorder. Patient 8-7 has none of this and no acute stress or injury or illness to explain her symptoms. It rules out a lot. It tells us what she has is likely going to be a big deal as opposed to just stress or another outburst in a long line of outbursts. If we were Patient 8-7, we'd also be anxious.

Step 2. The next step is to consider the neurologic exam findings. Because the findings are essentially normal, an upper or lower motor neuron lesion is less likely. Myopathy is also unlikely, as is a neuropathy. The only abnormality is reduced pinprick to pain sensation. This finding alone is nonspecific.

Because of her weakness and tingling, electrolyte imbalance is possible, especially hypo- or hyperkalemia, but she has a normal CBC, electrolytes, liver, and kidney function. Electromyography (EMG) might be helpful in assessing peripheral nerve or muscle problems. These were done and were normal. The only other peg to hang a diagnosis on is her MRI. Even that was dismissed. But it is the only peg on the wall, so far.

Step 3. Consider any other psychiatric disorder. The usual suspects, i.e., depression, mania, and psychosis are not here. This review leaves us again at the doorstep of conversion disorder: a patient with some neurologic symptoms that cannot be explained.

But!!! The diagnosis of conversion disorder should be made with caution because it has been demonstrated that 20-30% of patients diagnosed with conversion disorder have later discovered neurologic illness, and not counting psychiatric disorder, at least 20-40% of patients in general medical practice have some unexplained symptoms. We are at a crossroad: one path leads to psychogenic

"La belle indifference" total unconcern for one's condition (considered pathognomic of conversion) could be a manifestation of parietal lobe dysfunction. Also, many patients with "conversion disorder" are not indifferent to their symptoms.

conversion while the other leads to rule out some neurologic disease that could produce the MRI findings and her symptoms. Patients in the early stages of autoimmune and demyelinating diseases may have neurologic findings similar to Patient 8-7. More work on that road.

Although MRI is currently the most useful tool for diagnosis, a single lesion is not conclusive. Enhancement with gandolium may help detect new lesions. When clinical evidence is less strong, CSF and evoked potential responses are studies that can help. The CSF will show oligoclonal bands or increased production of immunoglobulin G in more than 90% of MS patients. Visual evoked potentials are abnormal in more than 75% of the patients.[10]

How would you treat Patient 8-7?

If you take the road marked psychogenic conversion (let us hypothesize that you do this after deciding Patient 8-7 does *not* have an autoimmune or demyelinating disease). What should you then do?

No specific treatment is recommended. Reassure the family and continue to observe the patient for a development of neurological findings. Psychotherapy (focusing on neurologic deficits to establish a link between emotional stress and conflicts) is unnecessary and may be counterproductive. There are no controlled studies that prove the efficacy of psychotherapeutic techniques. At least half of the patients with acute and uncomplicated "conversion" improve with a combination of anxiolytic or antidepressant medication and emotional support and education. There appears to be some benefit to counseling that all symptoms may not have a general medical or neurologic explanation, reinforcing the belief that improvement will occur, and providing understanding and support regarding any stressor present at the time of the episode.[11]

If you take the road marked conversion disorder due to a still unidentified brain process, what should you do? Let us hypothesize that you do all the diagnostic steps above, and still you cannot find the cause of Patient 8-7's symptoms. Then *follow* the patient.

The neurologic mechanism underlying conversion is unknown. It is hypothesized that symptoms of conversion are generated by induction of an altered state of consciousness. Some patients with conversion respond to sodium amytal or lorazepam. Reversible ischemia induced by sudden release of vasopressors could also cause neurological symptoms akin to a TIA or RIND.

Follow-up

The story does not end here. Because of her anxiety and worry about her weakness, Patient 8-7's primary care doctor gave her lorazepam 1 mg PO TID. Later, fluoxetine 20 mg was added because she complained of sadness. She then had an episode of dizziness and tremors that were thought to be due to fluoxetine, and her dose was reduced to 10 mg daily. A few months later, she again complained of dizziness and tingling, which again was attributed to fluoxetine, and the fluoxetine was discontinued. Patient 8-7 did well for the next few months, but then again complained of depression. At this time the primary care physician decided to again refer her to a psychiatrist. Her neurologic examination was essentially similar to the first examination. MRI was repeated. This one showed several hyperintense areas of demyelination, confirming a diagnosis of multiple sclerosis. Patient 8-7's course is typical of many patients with MS.[12] In our experience, multiple sclerosis, because of its waxing and waning course and presentation, is a common culprit of "conversion."[13] If patient 8 did not have any psychiatric symptoms in the beginning, she would not have been put on fluoxetine and probably would have been diagnosed earlier. *Table 8.7* includes factors that suggest neurologic etiology in conversion symptoms.[15]

Table 8.7   Signs Suggesting Neurologic Etiology
Previous history of neurologic symptoms
Family history of neurologic disease
No prior personal or family history of psychiatric illness
An abnormal neurologic examination, laboratory testing even if it is not consistent with the typical neurologic illness [14]
Age over 50

Treatment of Multiple Sclerosis

Treatment of multiple sclerosis can be divided into three categories:

1. *Treatment to modify the cause of illness*. The main focus of treatment here is immunomodulating drugs. Subcutaneous injections of interferon B are helpful in some patients. Immunosuppressives such as cyclosporine is also helpful in high doses, but often side effects are too cumbersome.
2. T*reatment to control relapse*. Steroids are accepted in the treatment of relapse. Methylprednisolone given intravenously is effective, so is prednisone. ACTH can also be given (80-100 IM daily over a week).

3. *Symptomatic treatment to control the debilitating symptoms of progressive MS.*

Because Patient 8-7 is still in the early stages of illness, interferon B injections are recommended to prevent progression. Forty percent of patients receiving interferon B develop depression. Some reports indicate that starting paroxetine before the interferon trial reduces this rate to 10% or less.[16] General supportive measures, such as avoiding excessive fatigue and maintaining good general health and nutrition are also beneficial.[17]

High dose steroids can induce depression. Patients with a family history of mood disorder may be at greatest risk. Some Glucocorticoid receptor antagonists can block the limbic affect of the steroids without affecting overall efficacy. Mifepristone 600 mg daily is helpful.[18]

Patient 8-8: Same Old Psychosis or Something New?

You are on night call and are paged by the nurse on duty because a 62-year-old patient admitted in the evening for chronic psychosis "has been talking out of his head and has not left his room." His pulse is 130 beats/minute and his temperature is 105° F. His speech is rambling[19] and dysarthric. It is hard to keep his attention. He does not know where he is and why he is in the hospital.

What is his problem?

The patient obviously has both a behavioral problem and a general medical problem. His behavioral problems are a) he has been "talking out of his head," b) his speech is rambling and dysarthric, c) it is hard to keep his attention, and d) he is disoriented. His general medical problems are: a) tachycardia, and b) high fever. Applying the Rule of Parsimony, we look for a single cause. Applying the Zebra Principle (i.e., common things occur more commonly), we can assume the syndrome is delirium. The prevalence of delirium is high.

1. *Evidence for delirium:* fever, tachycardia, rambling and dysarthric speech, disorientation
2. *Confirming the diagnosis of delirium*

   a. A behavioral assessment for a reduced sensorium (cannot focus attention, delayed reactions, signs of lethargy)
   b. Administering tests of concentration and continuous performance (e.g., Serial 7's, Letter Cancellation)
   c. EEG looking for diffuse slowing (almost always present in delirium)

What more must you do?

Patient 8-8 is seriously ill and needs teamwork and a prompt response. Look for physical exam and historical evidence of the common culprits that induce delirium. These include infection, drug toxicity, metabolic disorder, hypoxia.

For Patient 8-8, examination reveals a severely stiff neck (nuchal rigidity). With the patient lying supine and the right hip flexed to a right angle, it is impossible to extend the leg at the thigh (i.e., to "straighten" the right lower extremity). Crackling sounds are auscultated in the left-mid-lung zone posteriorly. No other signs of infection are found. The working diagnosis is meningitis. The patient was transferred to medicine. Lumbar puncture reveals cloudy (purulent) cerebrospinal fluid (CSF) with pressure of 220-mm. water and 200 polymorphs per high power field. The CSF was sent to the laboratory for culture and sensitivity. Gram stain revealed gram-positive diplococci.

How will you treat him?

There are two answers to this question. Answer 1 is, "I don't treat his meningitis; infectious disease specialists do that!" Obviously Patient 8-8 needs intravenous antibiotic to achieve prompt response. The antibiotic chosen for his gram-positive diplococci was penicillin intravenously. The second part of the answer is that while the infection is being treated, Patient 8-8 is still delirious and needs some treatment for that. *Table 8.8* lists the environmental management of delirium.

Nonspecific pharmacotherapy may be used if a) diagnostic efforts do not yield a specific etiology and a specific effective treatment, and b) the environmental management cannot

Table 8.8   Environmental Management of Delirium
Someone should be with the patient all the time (ideally a relative or friend, but a sitter or nurse is okay, too) to ensure that the patient does not injure himself accidentally.
The patient's room should be lighted and with a nightlight and a window to facilitate environment cueing.
Persons entering the room must introduce themselves and explain what they are doing.
The bed should have side rails.
The bathtub or shower should have side rails.

reduce problem behaviors. The most recommended nonspecific medication is parenteral (intramuscular or even intravenous) haloperidol. Do not do this unless all behavioral approaches have been ineffective. If an antipsychotic is needed and the patient will take oral medication, low-dose risperidone can work. Oral dissolving olanzapine may be helpful. If haloperidol is used – use very low doses.

Discussion

Delirium is extremely common. It is easy to diagnose, and curable in the majority of cases, yet it is often underdiagnosed and in many cases that proves to be fatal.[20] It is a syndrome of multiple etiologies and varied presentations and diffuse cognitive dysfunction, which is probably why it is difficult to diagnose. *Table 8.9* lists features of delirium.

Any generalized metabolic, toxic, or infectious process that affects all parts of the brain directly, any space-occupying lesion that can cause brain edema or a focal process that affects alertness (e.g., brain stem or thalamic involvement) profoundly can cause delirium. So, the bottom line is applying the rule of parsimony. If you identify delirium, then the co-existing general medical condition or drug the patient is taking is the most likely culprit for causing the delirium.

Table 8.9 Common Features of Delirium [21]

Reduced alertness

Disturbed sleep-wake cycle

Language impairment
- Dysarthria
- Rambling speech
- Aphasia

Perceptual disturbances
- Illusion
- Hallucination in any sensory modality

Delusion
- Often in response to surroundings

Intense mood
- Anxiety
- Irritability
- Lability

Motor abnormalities
- Asterixis – flapping tremor
- Gait disturbances
- Other tremors
- Catatonia
- Myoclonus

Cognitive dysfunction
- Anterograde amnesia
- Impaired reasoning
- Disorientation specifically to time of day
- Dysgraphia
- Dysnomia
- Dyspraxia

Uncooperative behavior
- Yelling
- Pulling out IV lines

Patient 8-9: Over the Counter, Under the Weather

You are asked to evaluate a 70-year-old woman because she took an unknown number of capsules of an over-the-counter "cold remedy." She says she cannot see well. She is flushed. Her tongue is dry. Her pupils are enlarged. She has trouble paying attention to what you are saying. She does not know where she is, nor the date. She seems apprehensive and fidgets during the exam. At times her speech rambles.

What syndrome does Patient 8-9 have?

Patient 8-9 has behavioral and general medical symptoms. The behavioral symptoms include disorientation, trouble paying attention, agitation, and anxiety. Her general medical symptoms include dry tongue, flushed skin, and blurred vision with dilated pupils. She gives a history of taking some medication. Applying the Rule of Parsimony, we can assume the over-the-counter medication had something to do with all of her symptoms. The common adverse effect of hundreds of medications is delirium. Unless proven otherwise, she is delirious due to the "cold remedy" she took. *Table 8.10* displays some red flags warning of delirium in a hospitalized patient.

Table 8.10 Red Flags of Delirium in a Hospitalized Patient
Fluctuating behavior across nursing staff shifts
Unable to perform activities of daily living without an adequate general medical explanation
Any confusion about the time of day (off by several hours)
Newly expressed perseverative speech, speech content, or motor behavior
Nighttime agitation or uncooperativeness (so-called "sundown syndrome")

How would you confirm this diagnosis?

Delirious patients cannot concentrate. Tests of attention and concentration are typically abnormal. Except for the EEG of alcohol withdrawal (DTs) which shows diffuse fast activity, all other deliria are associated with EEG slowing. However, delirium is a clinical diagnosis and so that is what Patient 8-9 has; a lab test is not needed.

How would you treat Patient 8-9?

Before you treat, you still need to determine etiology, and then treat the specific cause, if possible. Patient 8-9 has exhibited all the signs of anticholinergic toxicity. She has skin flushing, blurred vision with dilated pupils, mucosal dryness and delirium. Reading the ingredients on the label of the cold medicine should confirm the diagnosis.

> Anticholinergic delirium: Dry as a bone, red as a beet, blind as a bat, and mad as a hatter.

To treat Patient 8-9 you must first determine the time she took the pills. If she took the overdose within a couple of hours, lavage her stomach with a nasogastric tube and administer activated charcoal to stop further absorption of the drug. Then administer physostigmine 1-2 mg intravenously or subcutaneously. Patient 8-9's condition should improve within 20 minutes. If not, repeat again. Up to 8 mg over the first 6-8 hours may be needed to resolve an anticholinergic delirium. Because most anticholinergic agents have half-lives longer than physostigmine, additional dosing for another 24-36 hours after resolution of the delirium may be needed to avoid relapse.[22]

Discussion

Anticholinergic delirium is extremely common in the elderly, mostly because of the number of medications they take. Even if each drug is being taken in therapeutic doses the cumulative anticholinergic effect may be toxic. The elderly are also more susceptible to the CNS effects of drugs, and so can become delirious even before peripheral signs are obvious. Educating patients as well as doctors about the possibility of causing anticholinergic delirium by polypharmacy is an important aspect of overall treatment.

Patient 8-10: Long-Distance Wake-Up Call

A 43-year-old woman is seen by her generalist for irritability and apathy. She complains of poor memory. The generalist diagnoses depression and starts Patient 8-10 on fluoxetine 20 mg PO daily. Patient 8-10 continues to complain of irritability and memory problems. Fluoxetine is increased to 40 mg PO daily. Several weeks later, she is brought to the hospital because she is disoriented, has difficulty speaking, and is staggering.

> Under every patient's bed there is a lawyer! The primary doc is shooting Prozac from the hip and is likely to eventually get in deep doo-doo.

What happened to Patient 8-10?

Look at the big picture. Patient 8-10 is a 43-year-old woman with no prior psychiatric or neurologic history who has developed symptoms suggestive of central nervous system involvement. Unless proven otherwise, this is a secondary syndrome. The first step is to obtain a careful history and a thorough neurologic examination. When she first came to the primary care physician, she was given an antidepressant without a careful examination – a big no-no.

What diagnostic steps must you follow, and why?

Patient 8-10 is not depressed. Patient 8-10 is apathetic. She has difficulty speaking, memory problems and a gait disturbance. She could have some involvement in a dorsolateral frontal subcortical loop. She could have a fluoxetine overdose to boot. Her symptoms before fluoxetine at her age might reflect a) a space occupying lesion, and 2) demyelinating illness, and 3) brain trauma, among a number of other possibilities. Evaluation reveals no evidence of any infection, head injury, or exposure to heavy metals. Her MRI is normal. In short, none of the usual suspects are there. We now need to look for those diseases outside the brain that affect the brain. Applying the Sutton's Law, look for the most common cause of what is left that affect women of Patient 8-10's age that can affect the brain – malignancy, i.e., cervical, breast, ovarian.[23] This patient obviously does not have overt signs of malignancy, i.e., palpable tumor or lymph node, so we must look for occult malignancy.

What syndrome does this woman have?

At this time you may say – wait a minute. There is no mass in the brain, no metastasis. Why would we want to look for malignancy? Cancerous tumors have distant effects by nonmetastatic, sometimes immune related mechanisms. These distant effects are called *paraneoplastic syndromes*. They are not rare and their recognition can lead to detection of the primary tumor. Usually malignancies of the breast and ovary are associated with the presence of antineuronal nuclear autoantibodies, such as anti-Hu (more common with small cell carcinoma), anti-Ta (also called auto-Ma2), and auto-Yo (often seen with cerebellar degeneration).[24] A positive anti-Yo titre confirms the diagnosis of paraneoplastic syndrome, and the search for the primary revealed a small ductal carcinoma of the right breast. Based on her clinical symptoms, Patient 8-10 has cerebellar degeneration, which is a paraneoplastic syndrome characterized by apathy, speech and memory problems, irritability, and occasionally dementia. These symptoms often precede the diagnosis of cancer. Although most of the types of antineuronal antibodies are specific for specific malignancies, there are several case reports to the contrary.[25] So, the absence of these antibodies should not automatically rule out the diagnosis of paraneoplastic syndrome.

Discussion

The most important lesson this patient teaches us is that disease in one organ of the body can affect another without any obvious relationship.

Paraneoplastic syndromes often precede the clinically recognized tumors by 1-2 years. Diagnosing this syndrome will lead to the search for the occult cancer. These syndromes are often associated with small cell lung carcinoma, renal cell carcinoma, prostate carcinoma, breast and ovarian carcinoma. Common paraneoplastic syndromes of the CNS are listed in *Table 8.11*.

Table 8.11 *Common Paraneoplastic Syndromes of the CNS* [26]
Limbic encephalitis
Cerebellar degeneration
Progressive multifocal leukoencephalopathy
Polyneuropathy
Dermatomyositis
Eaton Lambert type of myasthenia gravis

When evaluating patients with behavioral changes, once the usual suspects are ruled out, search for neoplasms of the lung, kidney, prostate, and breast. Successful treatment of the primary can stop the progression of the paraneoplastic syndrome, as well as extend the life of the patient. Would you like to be in the legal shoes of Patient 8-10's primary doc?!

Patient 8-11: More Than Meets the Eye

A 50-year-old internist is referred to you for management of behavioral problems associated with cognitive decline that one clinician has characterized as dementia. Patient 8-11 also has disturbed sleep at night, with periods of drowsiness during the day. She was practicing medicine until three months ago when she quit because of continuing memory problems. She was evaluated at a major medical center and diagnosed as having probable Alzheimer's disease. The neurologist's note reads as follows: "Patient is disoriented to time, place, and persons, appears perplexed, at times tearful, unable to answer most questions, could not do Mini-Mental State." Patient 8-11's EEG shows diffuse slowing. SPECT shows bilateral parietal hypoperfusion and MRI was normal. Patient 8-11 has no psychiatric or neurologic history, and family history is negative for dementia. Her general medical condition is unremarkable, except for chronic back spasms and a restless leg syndrome that was diagnosed four months ago. She also dieted and lost about 20 pounds in 5 weeks (25% of her body weight).

> On licensure and specialty board exams the question must include the information needed to answer it. If a clinical feature or a lab test is not mentioned, the rule is, it is normal or not present. So too, if something is mentioned, it is likely relevant. So what's this weight loss all about? A red herring? Hint: It is helpful in an important diagnostic way.

Is Patient 8-11 demented?

Dementia is what the neurologist at the academic medical center diagnosed. Isn't that diagnosis good enough? No! If your name appears on the chart, you need to be personally assured that so momentous a diagnosis is correct. If you apply the Duck Principle to Patient 8-11's condition, her age of onset is atypical, her course is sudden, her family history is negative, her sensorium is not really clear. Her lab findings are not specific. All the pieces do not fit. All doctors, even our most esteemed academic colleagues, are human and, therefore, make errors. Inattentiveness, distractibility, disturbances of the sleep-wake cycle, all lead to one Duck. Yes, you guessed it. *Delirium*.

What is your next step?

You next need to determine the etiology of Patient 8-11's syndrome. Obviously, there is no evidence of any infectious or metabolic etiology, and the most common causes of delirium is drugs. What drugs?

There is something in the history that should tip us off. Restless leg syndrome is often treated with clonazepam, which is what Patient 8-11 was taking (about 4 mg). She was also taking 45 mg of diazepam for her back spasms. Two long-acting benzodiazepines together can cause encephalopathy leading to delirium. But, what about that SPECT hypoperfusion? Remember the weight loss? Well it has been documented that sudden weight loss can have starvation-like effects and parietal hypoperfusion is observed both in starvation and anorexia. Although biparietal hypoperfusion is an early feature of Alzheimer's disease, it is not pathognomonic, and in the clinical setting of weight loss, Patient 8-11's SPECT finding is a red herring.[27] Her weight loss, not common in the early stages of Alzheimer's, caused her SPECT changes.

How would you treat Patient 8-11?

You need to gradually taper the benzodiazepines. You do this by determining the total benzodiazepine dose (4 mg of clonazepam is equivalent to 40 mg of diazepam): total dose is 85 mg equivalents of diazepam. The weekly tapering dose is determined by dividing the total dose by five and rounding up. Each week the dose should be reduced by that amount.[28] For Patient 8-11 that means 20 mg per week. An alternative method would be to reduce the dose by 40% on the same day and reduce 10% each day. By this method the patient would be given 50 mg on the first day and those would be reduced by 5 mg every day. *Caution:* This second taper could precipitate depression, anxiety, and lability.

Patient 8-12: Heart is the Reason

A 55-year-old man with a history of two myocardial infarctions and associated mild congestive heart failure complains of feeling tired all the time. He is not able to sleep at night because of shortness of breath. He has lost weight because of the diet he has been put on, and he does not enjoy food anymore. During an office visit he expresses frustration at this situation and says that he frequently thinks of taking his own life. Patient 8-12 remains sad throughout your examination.

Is Patient 8-12 depressed?

Diagnosing depression in a medically ill patient can be difficult if you focus on DSM criteria. For example, is his insomnia due to heart failure or due to depression? Is he not eating because he is depressed, or because he truly hates that low fat diet? Who would not be frustrated at being practically housebound? Is he tired because he is depressed or because his heart cannot pump blood adequately?

Underdiagnosis and not treating depression in a cardiac patient not only makes the patient suffer but also makes the cardiac disease worse.[29] Thus, treating his depression also treats his heart disease. The first step is to determine reactivity of the patient's mood. Even the most ill patients will have a reactive mood if they are not depressed and you are a sociable examiner. Some patients will smile if you crack a joke, or if you let them reminisce about happy events in their lives. Another important feature is cognition. Depressed patients will often blame themselves and feel worthless. Patients who are subdued because of illness but not depressed, blame the illness. When depressed, everything seems futile. Frequent suicidal ideation suggests depression. It is also helpful to correlate the patient's medical disability to his depressive symptoms. Vegetative signs that are much more severe than the general medical condition would predict also suggest depression. Let us say that you decide based on the history and your observations that Patient 8-12 is depressed.

What should you do now?

Treating Patient 8-12 is a three-step affair. Step 1 is to treat his congestive heart failure vigorously, making sure that his cardiac status is as best as it can be. Improving oxygenation will improve his mood. Step 2 is to make sure that his cardiac medications (e.g., digoxin, B blockers) are not making his depression worse, as depression is a frequent side effect of many cardiac drugs. Step 3 is choosing an antidepressant. It is best to choose an antidepressant with the least cardiac effects. In studies of the effects of antidepressant drugs on cardiac function, the balance is as always between efficacy and safety. Nortriptyline in low doses has been found safe despite the bad press that it will adversely affect the Q-T interval.[30] But, if higher doses are anticipated, other drugs are preferred. In rare instances, venlafaxine has been associated with induced infarction and conduction disturbances and can cause hypertension in some patients.[31] Bupropion increases blood pressure, and cardiac patients tend to stop treatment when on it.[32] In contrast, paroxetine, sertraline, and citalopram have been found relatively safe in cardiac patients.[33] If the patient is melancholic, however, those drugs are likely to be minimally effective and will need to be given at the higher end of their dose range. For apathetic syndromes, psychostimulants, such as methylphenidate, can also be used, but pretreatment EKG and careful monitoring are needed.

ECT is not contraindicated in cardiac patients. It can be used initially or if the depression does not respond to medications or if suicide is an imminent risk. A cardiologist should be present during ECT if the patient is in the acute phase of cardiac treatment. The important thing is to remember to treat with adequate doses for adequate duration (see Chapter 3).

Discussion

Depression is associated with increased mortality in patients with coronary artery disease with or without infarction. About 40-65% of patients with a myocardial infarct have symptoms of depression, and about 20% meet DSM criteria for major depressive disorder.[34] Coronary artery disease or stroke accounts for more than 60% of deaths in mood disorder patients, usually from fatal arrhythmias, because in depression normal EKG variability is reduced. In addition, the presence of depression worsens the outcome of cardiac disease. Depressed patients are less likely to adhere to their treatment plan or remember to take their medications. Strong mood states with anxiety also can directly affect cardiac rhythms, and vagal-vagal responses can lead to asystole. Vigorously treating depression in all cardiac patients also treats their heart.

327

Patient 8-13: The Wallflower

A 39-year-old woman is referred to you by her primary care physician. She has had two previous major depressive episodes that required treatment, but she says to you she is now frequently "down" and anxious. She says she is a shy, overly cautious person, a "worry-wart," and generally pessimistic about events or situations in her life. She says she is afraid of her own shadow, is unable to assert herself, even when she knows she is right. She has few friends and trouble making new ones. She divorced after her second nonmelancholic depression and has one son, age 15. She also tells you that people think she is good-hearted. She thinks she is a loving person (likes to be demonstrable with close friends and family and craves affection), but has difficulty establishing relationships because of her shyness. She tells you depression runs in her family and so does drinking. She believes she is empathic, hard working, and loyal. Your colleague has requested your opinion regarding the need for switching antidepressants.

How many DSM diagnoses does Patient 8-13 have, and what are they?

Assuming the referral is a good one, Patient 8-13 has a history of recurrent major depression. In real-world terms she is *unipolar*. But, she also has long-standing behavior patterns that appear problematic for her. Most definitions of *personality disorder* (including the DSM) define it as long-standing, unchanging, maladaptive behavior that pervades one's life.

> Personality traits are habitual, characteristic of the person, develop in the formative years, and are mostly unchanging. A dramatic personality change after age 30-35 almost always means brain disease. Table 8.12 displays the conditions most likely to alter personality. [35]

Based on the above definition of personality disorder, Patient 8-13's anxious-fearful behavior traits satisfy DSM criteria for cluster C personality disorder. See *Table 8.13* for a description of DSM personality disorders.

Table 8.12   Conditions Most Likely to Alter Personality

Condition	Common Associations	Personality Change
Epilepsy	Temporal lobe foci	Adhesive or paranoid (like DSM Cluster A subtype)
Head injury	Large right hemisphere or frontal injuries	Irritable and coarsening, respectively
Stroke	Large or multiple anterior strokes	Avolitional or disinhibited frontal lobe syndromes
Drug abuse	Chronic use of cannabis, inhalants, cocaine	Avolitional, irritable/paranoid, viscous/adhesive, respectively
Bipolar mood disorder	Chronic form	Adhesive
Degenerative brain disease	White matter dementias, Pick's disease, basal ganglia dementias, chronic metabolic disorders	Avolitional or disinhibited frontal lobe syndromes

Table 8.13 DSM Personality Disorders

Cluster A	Cluster B	Cluster C
Paranoid • Distrust and suspiciousness • Unforgiving and bears grudges • Perceives threat Schizoid • Detachment and restricted range of emotional expression • Paucity of interests, activities, friends Schizotypal • Schizoid plus cognitive or perceptual distortions and eccentricities	Antisocial • Disregard for and violation of rights of others • Nonconforming to social and legal norms • Deceitful, impulsive, aggressive • Reckless, irresponsible, remorseless Borderline • Unstable relationships, self-image, moods • Impulsive, fear of abandonment • Suicidal, self-mutilating, anger • Intense, reactive, unstable moods Histrionic • Excessive emotionality and attention seeking • Seductive, dramatic, suggestible • Unstable and shallow emotions and vague speech Narcissistic • Grandiose sense of self-importance • Sense of entitlement and need for excessive admiration • Interpersonally exploitative • Lacks empathy	Avoidant • Social inhibition, feelings of inadequacy, hypersensitive to criticism • Avoids interpersonal contact and risks • Views self as inept, inferior, unappealing Dependent • Submissive, clinging, fears separation • Indecisive, unassertive • Low self-confidence, follower Obsessive-compulsive • Preoccupation with orderliness, perfectionism, and mental and interpersonal control • Decrease in flexibility, openness, and efficiency • Stubborn, miserly, hoarding • Cannot delegate, overly conscientious • Scrupulous, workaholic

How do her diagnoses interrelate?

Persons with personality disorder are prone to also having a DSM Axis I condition.[36] Persons with anxious-fearful personality are prone to nonmelancholic depression, anxiety, obsessive-compulsive disorders, eating disorders, and sedative-hypnotic substance abuse. Having a comorbid personality disorder makes treatment of a patient with an axis I condition more complicated. Patient 8-13 has two DSM diagnoses. One is nonmelancholic depression and the second is cluster C personality disorder.

How does the interrelationship of her diagnoses guide your treatments (that's right, plural) for Patient 8-13?

Because of her previous depressions, personality, and family history, Patient 8-13 is at risk for developing future depressive episodes. She would benefit from continued antidepressant treatment. The standard procedure in selecting an antidepressant is to first decide on which drug is theoretically best for the type of depression the patient has (see Chapter 3 for details). The second step is to select from the choices from step 1 those drugs that have a side-effect profile that best matches the pharmacodynamic, pharmacokinetic, and other general medical and neurologic factors that play a role in the patient's overall health. Superimposed on these steps is the principle that the quality of therapeutics generally increases with your increased experience with the drug. So, knowing a few drugs very well is better than knowing a bunch more superficially. If you adhere to the above method for choosing an antidepressant, you will end up with either a single drug of choice, and you will prescribe it; or you will end up with a few choices. Trying to pick one drug from the remaining choices based on the patient's personality may now help if the patient has a nonmelancholic depression like Patient 8-13. Patient 8-13 has an anxious-fearful personality. So our preference would be sertraline; it is serotonergic, can be titrated and is supposed to be more effective in Premenopausal women (see pearl).

Discussion

More than 50-60% of patients seen in psychiatric clinics have personality disorder diagnosis.[38] The presence of a personality disorder makes the primary axis I disorder more difficult to treat. Patients with a

> A recent study also suggests that gender affects antidepressant response.[37] Men and post-menopausal women do better on the older compounds, such as desipramine or nortriptyline, and premenopausal women do better on the newer antidepressants.

personality disorder are also at greater risk for developing Axis I psychopathology. Therefore, you should always determine a patient's personality traits. However, a diagnosis of primary personality disorder needs to be made with caution. Many patients exhibit changes in personality due to Axis I conditions that would lead to an erroneous diagnosis of personality disorder. For example, a patient with chronic depression may avoid any contact with strangers, be unable to initiate conversation, and you may mistake this behavior as cluster C avoidant personality disorder. Other cluster C personality disorders are dependent and obsessive compulsive. Psychotherapy aimed at personality change is often time-consuming and labor-intensive. Assertiveness training in individual and group setting is helpful for anxious fearful persons[39] and should be recommended to improve socialization. Because deviance in personality may have underlying neurotransmitter abnormalities, psychopharmacological intervention based on these deviations may also be helpful, but no data exist to support this hope.

Patient 8-14: To Eat or Not to Eat – That is the Question

A 16-year-old girl is referred by her internist for evaluation. The patient's mother is concerned about her daughter's refusal to eat with her family, and looking "too thin." On reviewing the internist's notes, you find that the girl is 22 pounds underweight. She is about 101 pounds and is 5'7" tall. Her skin is pale, and she has not had a normal menstrual period in three cycles. Her blood glucose is 50 mg/dl, Hgb is 10 mg/dl, albumin is 2.5 gm/dl, and potassium is 3.5 mg/dl. She denies any problem and complains that her mother is overprotective.

What is the first step in taking care of this young woman? (This is a semi-trick question.)

The first step in care is diagnosis, defining the syndrome. The big picture is that of a teenage girl whose parents are concerned about her weight loss. The semi-trick, however, is regardless of anything else, if a young woman previously menstruating stops, it's a pregnancy test. She is not pregnant. With the information you now have, you look for the most likely causes of unexplained weight loss (Sutton's Law strikes again) (see *Table 8.14*). Of all the possibilities listed in *Table 8.14*, the most likely causes in a young woman are a) systemic infections, b) Crohn's disease, c) nausea/vomiting/ diarrhea due to inflammatory bowel disease or infection. Hyperthyroidism increases metabolism and can also cause weight loss. Mood disorder and an eating disorder are also possible. A detailed history of the patient's food intake to determine if the weight loss is intentional or

Table 8.14 Differential Diagnosis of Weight Loss in a Young Woman[40]	
Reduced Intake	
Structural abnormalities	
Pharyngeal	Pharyngitis Tumor
Esophageal complication	Inflammation Stricture Obstruction
Gastric complication	Pyloric outlet obstruction
Loss of appetite	Depression, anorexia nervosa
Reduced/altered absorption	
Small intestinal disease	Infection Crohn's disease
Nausea/vomiting/ diarrhea	Infection Inflammatory bowel disease
Increased metabolism	
Endocrine disease	Hyperthyroidism Diabetes
Hematologic malignancy	Leukemia Lymphoma
Solid tumor	Gastric tumor Pancreatic tumor
Infection	AIDS Tuberculosis

unintentional is always needed. It appears that the weight loss for this girl is due to reduced intake and, most likely, is intentional.

> Although eating disorders are more common in women, when both partial and full syndromes are considered, there is no difference in the prevalence for younger men and women.

> Eating disorders run in families. Family members of patients with eating disorders also have an increased prevalence of other psychiatric disorders, such as depression, bipolar disorder, alcohol or drug use.[41]

The next step is to rule out any psychiatric disorder that can lead to reduced food intake. The girl is presently not depressed, so a diagnosis of eating disorder is likely.

How are her symptoms different from other disorders of eating?

Table 8.15 compares anorexia and bulimia nervosa. Based on the terminology, one would assume that anorexics restrict food and that bulimics binge and purge. However, both patient groups binge and purge. The term *anorexia* is a misnomer. Anorexics do not lose their desire to eat; they purposefully restrict food. The main difference between anorexics and bulimics is age of onset and body weight. Typically, patients with anorexia nervosa tend to be younger and 10% below their ideal body weight. In contrast, bulimic patients tend to be older with normal body weight. Leptin, a neuropeptide secreted by

Table 8.15 Comparison of Diagnostic Features of Anorexia and Bulimia	
Anorexia Nervosa	**Bulimia Nervosa**
• Refusal to maintain minimum body weight for age and height (less than 85% of what is expected) • Intense fear of gaining weight or becoming fat even though underweight • Denial of seriousness of weight loss; disturbances of body image • Absence of three menstrual cycles • Either restricting or binge eating/purging type	• Recurrent episodes of binge eating • Recurrent, inappropriate compensatory behavior to prevent weight gain • Self-evaluation unduly influenced by weight and body shape

adipose tissue cells, which regulates fat stores and correlates with fat mass, is low in anorexics, whereas bulimics have normal leptin levels.[42] Cholecystokinin (CCK) is secreted by the gastrointestinal system and transmits satiety signals. Bulimics have low plasma and CSF CCK, whereas anorexics have high basal and post-prandial CCK. Severely underweight anorexics show cerebral brain atrophy, whereas bulimics have normal brain size. In addition, anorexics tend to have obsessive temperaments, whereas bulimics have explosive personality traits. *Table 8.16* summarizes laboratory abnormalities associated with anorexia.

Table 8.16 Clinical and Laboratory Abnormalities in Anorexia Nervosa	
Hematology	Leukopenia with a relative lymphocytosis Reduced bactericidal capacity in leukocytes Low erythrocyte sedimentation rate
Serum electrolytes	Hypokalemic alkalosis-elevated serum bicarbonate Hypochloremia, hypokalemia Low fasting blood glucose Enzymes-elevated serum SGOT, LDG, alkaline-phosphatase and amylase Osteoporosis Carotenemia Elevated serum cholesterol Low FSH, LH
Cardiac	Bradycardia and hypotension Arrhythmias
Neurological	EEG-6 per second spike and wave 6-14 per second spikes
CT scans	"Cerebral atrophy" in some patients; findings return to normal with immediate weight restoration in some, but not all, patients
PET scan	Hypermetabolism in caudate, right parietal hypometabolism

Should this girl be hospitalized?

The decision to hospitalize an anorexic depends on the severity of weight loss, the patient's cooperativeness, and secondary complications. The normal weight range for a small built 5'7" 16-year-old is about 123-136. At 101, she is less than 85% of her expected weight, and her potassium, albumin, glucose and hemoglobin are all low. In view of these findings and the fact that the patient does not recognize the weight loss, inpatient hospitalization should be recommended.

Once hospitalized, the patient needs to gain weight. However, sudden feeding can lead to complications, such as gastric rupture, edema, or congestive cardiac failure. The patient, therefore, needs to be evaluated by a nutritionist for a refeeding program and nutritional education. Anorexic patients often have erratic eating patterns and need training in choosing healthy meals. Refeeding is initially done at the rate of about 25 cal/kg/day and gradually increased to about 50 cal/kg/day.

Medications. Overall, medications are of limited help. Treating an anorexic as a variant of OCD offers guidelines. SSRIs may help in the long-term, however they are not often useful during the weight restoration phase. Other medications that have been used with some help include cyproheptadine (a serotonin agonist) up to 32 mg/day or naltrexone (opioid antagonist) 100 mg BID (reduced bingeing).[43]

Behavior modification programs where patients are rewarded for maintaining the weight gain, are often helpful.

Family therapy. Some form of family education, as well as understanding how family interaction affects the eating pattern are essential in treating eating disorders.

Treatment as an outpatient: The patient should be discharged after she gains weight and resumes menses. Amenorrhea in anorexia occurs as a result of severe weight loss and subsequent increase of FSH/LH to prepubertal levels. Weight gain reverses these findings, and menstruation resumes. A monthly follow-up to monitor eating/exercising patterns is helpful. *Table 8.17* includes factors predicting poor prognosis.

Table 8.17   Factors Predicting Poor Prognosis of Anorexia Nervosa
Later age of onset
Duration longer than 2 years
Extremely low weight
Purging behavior
Alcohol and drug abuse
Poor premorbid adjustment

Patient 8-15: Mr. March: He Came in Like a Lamb and Left Like a Lion

Mr. March, a 58-year-old man, suddenly experienced shortness of breath, tachycardia, and dizziness while on a business trip. He developed congestive heart failure, and was admitted to a cardiac care unit. He was in atrial fibrillation with multiple PVCs. He had an enlarged left atrium and ventricle. He was not diabetic and did not have a seizure disorder. He had been diagnosed as hypertensive 10 years earlier. He was given an internal pacemaker. Several days later, he suddenly experienced left hemiparesis. CT scan revealed small vessel ischemic changes with no focal infarct, hemorrhage, or mass effects. The patient recovered and was discharged home on anticoagulant medication.

Anterior Circulation	*Posterior Circulation*
(serves most of the cerebral cortex, subcortical white matter, basal ganglia, and the internal capsule)	(serves the brain stem, cerebellum, thalamus, and portions of the occipital and temporal lobes)[44]
Aphasia Headache Hemiparesis Hemisensory deficits	Diplopia and other cranial nerve signs Vertigo Drop attacks Altered consciousness

Mr. March's wife immediately notes a change in his behavior. In the past, he was quiet and reserved, and rarely spoke unless spoken to. Now he is hypertalkative, outgoing, and energetic. He wants to go out and shovel the snow against his doctor's advice. He ruminates about past business deals gone sour, and how he wants to pursue legal action against others. He is also incessantly writing details in a new diary. Although his wife does not notice any memory problems, he constantly complains about not being able to remember people's names.

> Personality, particularly temperament is very stable after maturation (by age 15-20). Dramatic changes in personality after age 30-35 almost always means brain illness.

About a month later, Mr. March is hospitalized for a thumb hematoma. He has a prolonged prothrombin time. Upon his discharge, his wife notes further changes in his personality. He appears somewhat more irritable. One day he suddenly decides to drive to the hospital. He went to his original general medical unit and insists on being admitted. He was wearing only his underwear. When he is reminded that he needs to go through admissions, he becomes loud, angry, and argumentative.[45] He is agitated and suspicious. He speaks rapidly and his train of thought is difficult to follow. His general medical and traditional neurologic examinations are within normal limits. The patient is transferred to psychiatry.

Apply the Duck Principle, Sutton's Law, and the Rule of Parsimony to Mr. March's problems. What are your conclusions?

There are several Ducks here:

Ischemic vascular event. Following his pacemaker implant, Mr. March had a sudden neurologic event with most features resolving. This could qualify as a RIND -- a reversible ischemic neurologic deficit. However, Mr. March had a CT, scan, which is good shortly after a stroke for detecting hemorrhagic conditions, but less helpful in detecting small ischemic strokes. Eighty percent of strokes are ischemic. Immediately following a suspected stroke in a patient, get a CT scan and look for hemorrhagic strokes and calcified and bony lesions. MRI is best for everything else and will show the extent of the damage, which may not become clear until 7-10 days post-stroke. A RIND can last for a week with apparent full recovery. A stroke can involve the same signs and symptoms, but lasts longer than 2 weeks. A transient ischemic attack (TIA) lasts several hours to less than a day with apparent full recovery (25% of patients with TIAs go on to have a stroke within 3 months of the TIAs).

Ischemic heart disease. His heart failure, fibrillation, enlarged left heart are consistent with this.

Personality disorder. There has been a dramatic change in his typical behavior and temperament that appear maladaptive (poor judgment in wanting to shovel snow, becoming litigious).

Mania. Driving to the hospital in his underwear, being irritable and demanding, probable flight of ideas, rapid speech.

Sutton's Law suggests the Ducks above are indeed present because they are all too common.

The Rule of Parsimony suggests Mr. March's mania is secondary to a likely ischemic stroke in the right hemisphere near the internal capsule or motor cortex. His personality change is part of the same process and suggests a frontal lobe dysinhibited syndrome. So, heart disease directly or as part of a generalized cardiovascular system problem, plus its treatment have led to brain lesions that have resulted in his change in personality and mood regulation.

What are the areas of assessment you will use to decide if a behavioral syndrome is primary or secondary?

1. Typicality of the acute episode and course of illness
2. Which came first, the episode, past similar episodes, or the evidence of the etiologic process you have in mind?
3. Family history of a similar behavioral disorder

What behavioral co-morbidities do you look for in patients like Mr. March?

Strokes that produce bipolar mood disorders can produce other action brain syndromes. These include obsessive compulsive disorders, including kleptomania, trichotillomania and pyromania (right basal ganglia); episodic dyscontrol syndrome (right frontal), personality changes (dorsolateral avolitional syndrome, orbitomedial disinhibited syndrome); and paraphilias and other sexual aberrations or sexually inappropriate behaviors (basal ganglia and frontal lobe).[46]

What are the treatment guidelines for such patients?

1. The more the secondary syndrome looks like the primary form, the more likely the patient will respond to treatments for the primary form.
2. Psychotropics with motor side effects are more likely to produce those side effects in patients with defined brain lesions, so either avoid these drugs or start low and go slow.
3. Psychotropics with substantial anticholinergic properties and all benzodiazepines can make cognitive function worse in these patients.
4. Anticonvulsants may provide the broadest therapeutic spectrum in these patients. Lithium can exacerbate stroke symptoms.
5. ECT is often the safest treatment, particularly in patients who do not respond to anticonvulsants.
6. Efforts to prevent future strokes include 1) good diet, exercise, and weight control, 2) antiplatelet agents for noncardiogenic vascular events and anticoagulation for atrial fibrillation, and 3) antihypertensive agents for hypertension.

Quick Rounds

1. A 35-year-old married woman with no psychiatric history is brought to the ER after an accidental overdose of a painkiller. She was prescribed these analgesics after she suffered a sports related injury. She denies any depression or intent to die. She says she did not realize that the dose she took would be too much. She has been happily married for the past 13 years, has two children, works as a gym teacher and volunteer for her children's teachers. The ER doctor wants a psychiatric evaluation. What do you do?

2. A 23-year-old single woman with a history of recurrent agitated depression comes to the emergency room for a refill of her medication. During the assessment you notice severe bruises on her four-year-old son's arm and around his neck. He has been sitting quietly in the room while you are talking to his mother. What should you do next? What would you do if this woman was a regular patient of yours and after several visits now has a good relationship with you? (This is a trick question.)

3. A 42-year-old patient with a history of chronic psychosis comes to the ER. The patient says he is hearing voices that tell him to kill himself. The patient has had 8 hospitalizations in the last 3 years, mostly between November to February. All of his admissions were for the same complaint. The patient has no history of any suicide attempts. He has been hallucinating continuously. At present his mood is euthymic and he is calm. He has no family and no place to live. Should you hospitalize this patient, and what would be the optimal treatment for him?

4. A 39-year-old woman with a history of recurrent anxiety attacks and dependent personality disorder comes to the emergency room with complaints of worsening symptoms. Because of her psychiatric history, the nurse sends the patient to you. The patient reports palpitations, difficulty in breathing, and dizziness. She appears restless, her voice sounds low and labored. She is sweating. What should you do?

5. A 50-year-old man with a diagnosis of lung carcinoma declines all medical treatment and wishes to leave the hospital against medical advice. You are called to determine if he is competent. The patient has no past psychiatric illness. What do you do?

6. A 62-year-old man who was hospitalized for an appendectomy refuses to eat hospital food and screams at the nurses for not allowing him to order food from outside. The patient has no past psychiatric illness or history or any personality disorder. What do you do?

7. A 36-year-old homeless man is found wandering in the streets and is brought to the ER by the police. He says he prefers the streets to shelters. He is alert, talks reluctantly, and makes minimal eye contact. His speech is monotonous and stilted. He is vague and elliptical in his conversation. He says his mood and creativity are influenced by the planets and stars. He is not depressed or manic. There is no evidence of hallucinations or delusions other than his astrological ideas, but as we know, those notions are shared by many people. He is not currently intoxicated. Does this man have an illness, and how would you treat him?

Quick Rounds Answers

1.   You evaluate! If your observations confirm that this patient is not depressed and that her overdose was accidental, and if her family confirms this, then there is no Duck here. She and her family need further education about her medications, but she does not need admission. Also, keep in mind that you are a consultant to the ER doctors, so you advise the ER doctor to send her home, educate him about your reasoning so that next time a patient like this comes to the ER, the ER doctor will feel more comfortable in handling the situation himself.

2.   Multiple bruises on a child should make you suspect physical abuse, especially if the bruises are around the neck or on the abdomen. After your evaluation, if you suspect child abuse, you must report it to your local equivalent of Child and Family Services. It's the law. Even if you know the patient and could be wrong, the benefit of the doubt should go TO reporting the situation. So the answer to both questions is evaluate the situation and report it to the DCFS if you still have the slightest concern. The child's welfare supercedes your relationship with his mother.

3.   The decision to hospitalize any patient is based on the need to a) stabilize the patient in a protective environment, b) further evaluate an acute episode, or c) protect the patient from immediate harm to himself or others. None of these reasons exist for this patient. The fact that all his ER visits are during the winter months suggests that he may need a place to stay. A good solution for him would be for you to find a temporary place for him and ask a social worker to find an appropriate group home for him.

4.   Psychiatrists are routinely called to the ER to see patients with prior psychiatric history. Psychiatric history, however, does not protect anyone from other illnesses. Some of this patient's symptoms could be due to an anxiety attack, but her low and labored voice should concern you. You also need to ask the patient if these symptoms are any different from her usual anxiety attacks. If the answer is yes, she should be treated as any other patient coming to the ER. Acute medical problems such as heart attack, pulmonary embolism, and stroke must be ruled out.

5.   A psychiatrist does not decide on *competency;* that is a legal decision. However, you need to evaluate the patient for the presence of any psychiatric illness that may interfere with his ability

(*capacity* is the technical term) to decide his treatment. For example, depression, dementia, and psychosis will interfere with judgment, and a court might, on that basis, declare the patient incompetent. However, because this patient does not have any such illness, he has the right to choose his treatment, especially if he understands the consequences of his action.

6. Psychiatrists are often called to see medical/surgical patients who are acting badly. If these behavior problems are not the result of an Axis I or III illness, then it is up to the primary physicians and nursing to solve the problem. Psychiatrists are not negotiators or solvers of problems any more or less than any other healthcare workers. Do what you are trained to do, not what others think you should do. Personally, we'd let him order any outside food appropriate to his surgical condition. What's the big deal. In fact, not wanting hospital food tells you he is cognitively OK and not psychotic.

7. The first step in evaluating this man is identifying the problem. Why was he brought to the emergency room? Does he have an Axis I illness? Is there any environmental or interpersonal problem? Or both? Based on the history, it appears that he has no mood disorder, delusions, or hallucinations. The patient does not appear to be anxious or intoxicated. Based on this, you can conclude that an Axis I illness is unlikely. Next, you need to make sure that the patient is medically stable and there is no evidence of a brain injury that led to his wandering the streets. If he does not have either an Axis I or II illness, then the question remains why was he brought to the ER? Obviously he is not normal. He is odd in his behavior and in his thinking. In the absence of a primary or secondary Axis I disorder, these features suggest an axis II illness, specifically cluster A. He has the cardinal features of schizotypal personality disorder (see Chapter 6 on psychotic disorders). He is emotionally detached, has restricted interests plus mild thinking problems, vague speech, and odd ideas. In the general population the lifetime risk of schizotypal personality is 2-3%. However, there is no specific reason to hospitalize this patient. He was brought to the ER by the police because he has no place to live and he is odd. Offer him a place to stay. State your concerns about his condition and offer outpatient follow-up.

Because many clinicians consider schizotypal a chronic, low-grade form of psychosis, they choose to treat, and this man might benefit from low doses of an antipsychotic. Our preference will be to choose one of the atypical antipsychotics, and offer him treatment.

If the patient is exhibiting several perceptual disturbances, then we first try an anticonvulsant.

Chapter 9

Child Psychiatry

with

P.S.B. Sarma, MD

Patient 9-1: Sometimes Hoofbeats Ain't Horses

A 4-year-old boy is brought for consultation because of a year-long decline in his language. This started after the birth of his sister, when he stopped talking in sentences and began pointing at instead of naming objects. He also has begun to have severe temper tantrums which start rather abruptly, and at times in response to minimal frustrations. He has started bedwetting two to three times a week, although he had been dry at night for about two months. On examination, he is of average size and right-handed. He has fleeting eye contact, is not able to sit still in his chair, and jumps on the furniture. He has some echolalia.[1] When asked his name or his age, he does not respond.

His mother wants to know if "Concerta," which she saw advertised on TV, might help his hyperactivity.

Just because the patient is short, it doesn't mean he gets "short shrift" when it comes to diagnosis. It's the "full Monty" for him -- to mix images. Diagnosis first, treatment afterwards. Thus, although the boy is hyperactive, the use of attention deficit hyperactivity disorder (ADHD) as a diagnostic label may be against the rules. If his hyperactivity is due to something more fundamental, then that's the diagnosis, not ADHD. So does he have something else? Does he meet the criteria for ADHD?

ADHD is characterized by inattention and hyperactivity-impulsivity that results in significant difficulty in school and home. These features must occur in the absence of other behavioral disorders, such as pervasive developmental disorder, depression or substance abuse. He is not depressed and does not use drugs. He is not psychotic. Whatever he has is not trivial because while enuresis (bedwetting) can be a temporary response to stress, his affect and language problems are bad news. His decline and problems in multiple areas of functioning is also bad news. Pervasive developmental disorders are characterized by impairments in social interaction and communication and abnormal patterns of stereotypical behaviors. The patient's language skills and general functioning deteriorated significantly, he has poor eye contact, echolalia and abrupt temper tantrums.

Although some of his symptoms are suggestive of either pervasive developmental disorder (PDD) or autism, the rather late onset (at 3 years of age) is atypical for autism. The sudden onset of temper tantrums associated with language disturbance and bedwetting is suggestive of seizures. This presentation is very similar to the "syndrome of acquired aphasia with convulsive disorder in children" originally described in 1957 by Landau and Kleffner and is known as LKS or Landau Kleffner syndrome.[2] LKS is a rare disorder with unknown etiology. It first appears in children between ages 3 and 10 and is associated with deterioration of cognitive function, especially expressive and receptive speech, and abnormal EEG with spike and wave discharges. Although most have EEG seizures, many do not have convulsions.

Patients with schizophrenia spectrum disorders or pervasive developmental disorders can become quite agitated with a dopaminergic agent that can be very good for ADHD. So "Concerta," which is a long-acting methylphenidate product, with a primary action of increasing synaptic dopamine by blocking dopamine transporter, is not an appropriate medication for Patient 9-1.

What investigations are indicated?

Many patients with seizure disorder are misdiagnosed as PDD. So get an EEG.[3] If a sleep EEG shows paroxysmal discharges, it would further strengthen the LKS diagnosis. An MRI will be helpful in ruling out a space occupying brain lesion. A urine amino acid screen will rule out a disorder of protein metabolism.

How would you treat him?

Antiepileptic drugs treat the seizures, but have no effect on aphasia. Language impairment tends to be permanent. Treatment with corticosteroid ACTH or nifedipine has been reported to improve language skills.[4] It is important to educate the mother about this disorder and assure her that it is unlikely that her other children may get it. Behavioral intervention targeted at reducing temper tantrums is often helpful.

Discussion

Although general principles of diagnosis and treatment remain the same for children and adults there are some differences between the practice of child and adult psychiatry.

1. *The historian needs to be evaluated as well as the patient.* The parent or teacher is the historian. Sometimes, an adult brings a child for imagined illnesses the child does not have. Always evaluate the reliability and validity of the statements

made and the conclusions drawn by the historian. Also, assess the functioning of the historian.

2. *What is normal or abnormal is often contextually determined.* Some behaviors (e.g., auditory hallucinations) are abnormal in any context. Some may be normal in certain situations but not so in others (e.g., urinating in one's undergarments if a toilet is unavailable for long time may be normal for a 6-year-old, but the same behavior is abnormal if done regularly). Some may be normal in an earlier level of development, but would be immature or inappropriate in others (e.g., baby talk in front of people in a 2-year-old as compared to an 8-year-old).

3. *Normality can be a function of frequency of occurrence.* The frequency of a behavior may be the criterion of normality or abnormality. For example, looking at one's hand or shaking one's head occurs only occasionally. However, if the same behavior occurs every 2-3 minutes, it is abnormal. Normally, speech is a frequently occurring behavior in a group of children. However, if a child rarely talks in the presence of peers, it is abnormal.

4. *Abnormal behavior in children may be triggered by new circumstances or may only occur in certain situations.* Abnormal behavior may result from the arrival of a new sibling, the mother feeling depressed and overwhelmed, a new bully moving into the neighborhood, or a favorite teacher leaving work to get married. In these contexts children may become restless, importunate, and irritable, and be disruptive and hyperactive in school. This situation becomes more complicated if the mother and the new teacher give the child more attention when he is symptomatic (albeit in the form of scolding and punishment) and give no attention when he is quiet and depressed.

5. When prescribing treatment, special attention needs to be paid to the size of children, their developing nervous system, whether or not a given medication is approved for use in children.

Patient 9-2: Sometimes You Can Tell a Book By Its Cover

A 3 ½ -year-old boy is brought to you for evaluation because "he is still not talking clearly." His parents say that his gestation and delivery were uncomplicated. His birth weight was 7 pounds, and there were no problems in early behavioral development. His motor development was slightly behind schedule. He is affectionate but gets easily frustrated and has tantrums. He makes gestures and sounds to communicate, but his speech is not as clear as that of a 2 ½-year-old. He is quite active and in good general medical health.

On examination, you find that Patient 9-2 initially hides behind his mother, but gradually becomes comfortable after you bring out some toys. He is of normal size. His head is normal in size. He has rather large ears that seem to fan out, and he has bilateral epicanthal folds. He is overactive, seems easily distractible, and is unable to point to a red, green or yellow block on the Denver Developmental Screening Test (DDST).[5] He does not seem to understand the concepts of "on the table and under the table," but responds to "give this to your mom."

What is Patient 9-2's most likely diagnosis?

The Duck here is that of a toddler with broad developmental delays, particularly in language skills (both receptive and expressive). Developmental delay in a toddler can be due to 1) perinatal brain damage, 2) chromosomal abnormalities, or 3) endocrine changes. *Table 9.1* describes the main causes of mental retardation. The delay in Patient 9-2 is not explained by any evidence of early brain damage. The presence of minor physical anomalies (epicanthic folds, large ears that fan out) suggest a chromosomal abnormality. In the absence of any evidence of metabolic disturbances (seizures, hepatosplenomegaly, vomiting, or urine with a strange smell), amino acid disorders such as phenylketonuria are unlikely.   Because his height is normal, the chance of hypothyroidism causing the developmental delay is low. His hearing is normal. He does have features of ADHD, but these are very common in children with language and developmental delays.

Although Down's syndrome is the most common chromosomal abnormality, it is usually diagnosed at amniocentesis or soon after birth. Because of Patient 9-2's large ears and epicanthal folds combined with normal head size, fragile-X is more likely. If his mother has facial features associated with fragile-X (large head with prominent ears and mandible), the index of probability is heightened. Family history of mental retardation

When you are faced with a blond haired, blue eyed child with autistic features, the most important laboratory investigation to order is urine amino acid serum. Even though we have newborn screening for phenylketonuria in all 50 states, there are occasional lapses of identification and/or communication leading to a missed diagnosis of phenylketonuria.[6]

or learning disabilities on the mother's side can further increase the index of probability. These are your horses; zebras follow.

If a child has a cognitive developmental delay combined with a history of aortic stenosis and also seems overactive and repetitive in questions, the rather uncommon Williams syndrome is the answer. These children often (not always) have hypercalcemia and are excessively talkative (like medical school faculty). They have macrostomia (large mouth) and short stature. If an obese child, who has a history of hypotonia and poor sucking at birth, is eating voraciously at age 2, and also exhibits tantrums, hyperactivity and cognitive delay, Prader Willi syndrome is the likely diagnosis.

Table 9.1   Disorders Causing Mental Retardation (MR) [7]

Cause	Example	Physiology	Clinical Features and Associated Medical Complications
Metabolic disorders: lipid	Tay-Sachs disease	Deficiency of hexosaminidase A with neuronal accumulation of sphingolipids	Progressive MR, paralysis, blindness, retinal "cherry red spot," death by 3-4 yrs.
Mucopoly-saccharide	Hurler syndrome (MPS I)	Deficiency in iduronidase activity; autosomal recessive; rare	Early onset, short stature, hirsutism, corneal clouding, death usually before 10 yrs.
	Hunter syndrome (MPS II)	Chr X; rare	MR by 2 yrs, hyperactivity, hearing loss, ataxia, hernia common, enlarged liver and spleen by 2 yrs.; symptoms absent neonatally; later development of seizures, hyperactivity, rash

			Clinical Features and Associated Medical
Cause	Example	Physiology	Complications

Table 9.1   Disorders Causing Mental Retardation (MR) [7]

Cause	Example	Physiology	Clinical Features and Associated Medical Complications
Amino acid	Phenylketo-nuria	Defect in phenylalanine hydroxylases (PAH) or co-factor (Biopterin) with accumulation of phenylalanine; 1/10-20,000 births	Failure to thrive, vomiting and seizures after protein intake; musty odor; severe MR and often autistic features; more blondish than unaffected siblings.
Carbohydrate	Galactosemia	Defect in galactose-1-phosphate uridyltransferase or galactokinase; rare	Vomiting in early infancy, jaundice, hepatomegaly, later cataracts
Purine	Lesch-Nyhan syndrome	Defect in hypoxanthine guanine ribosyltransferase with accumulation of uric acid; Chr X ; recessive; rare	Ataxia, chorea, self-biting, kidney failure, gout
Other genetic disorders: neurocutaneous disorders	Tuberous sclerosis complex	Benign tumors (hamartomas) and malformations of CNS, skin, kidney, heart; Chr 9,11; dominant; 1/10,000 births	Epilepsy, autism, hyperactivity, impulsivity, aggression, spectrum of MR from none to profound
	Neurofibro-matosis	Neurocutaneous tumors and malformations; Chr 17,22; dominant; 1/3,000 births	Cafe au lait spots, infrequent MR depending on CNS tumor location and size

Table 9.1   Disorders Causing Mental Retardation (cont'd)

Cause	Example	Physiology	Clinical Features and Associated Medical Complications
Chromosomal disorders	Fragile X syndrome	Inactivation of FMR-1 gene on xq27 due to excessive CGG repeats, methylation. Dominant with reduced penetrance in females. 1:1,500 males/1:4,000 females. Most frequent cause of inherited mental retardation. Unaffected carriers have 50-200 repeats.	Long face, large ears, macroorchidism in males at puberty; hyperactivity, anxiety, stereotypies, learning disorders; carrier females often have the facial features. - Phenotypically normal carriers with repeat size of 50-200 are called premutation carriers (normal repeats are 6-50). - Female carriers with a premutation or full mutation have an increased risk for affected offspring. - Male carriers with a premutation (repeat size of 50-200) will transmit this, usually unaltered, to their daughters. - 33% of female carriers are retarded
	Klinefelter's syndrome	47 XXY or greater number of X chromosomes; 1/1,000 male births	Delayed puberty, low testosterone, elevated gonadotrophin and depression, testosterone replacement of some value
	Homo-cystinuria	Autosomal recessive disorder with gene located on chromosome 21, cysthionine B synthetase deficiency; rare	Tall stature, lens dislocation, propensity for blood clotting and cognitive delay. Patients do better with pyridoxine supplementation.
	Down's syndrome	Trisomy 21, 14/21 translocation (4% of cases); 1/1,000 births	Hypotonia, upward-slanted palpebral fissures, midface depression, flat nasal bridge, simian crease, passivity, dependency, hyperactivity in childhood, stubbornness, mild to severe MR

Table 9.1 Disorders Causing Mental Retardation (cont'd)

Cause	Example	Physiology	Clinical Features and Associated Medical Complications
Chromosomal disorders	Prader-Willi syndrome	Deletion in 15q12 of paternal origin; dominant; 1/10,000 births; frequency unavailable	Hypotonia, failure to thrive in infancy, polyphagia and obesity, small hands and feet, micro-orchidism, almond-shaped eyes, compulsive behavior, hoarding, impulsivity, mild to moderate MR
	Angelman syndrome	Deletion on 15q12 of maternal origin; dominant; frequent deletion of GABA B-3 receptor subunit	Happy disposition, paroxysmal laughter, epilepsy (90%), hand flapping, clapping, profound MR, large facial features, hands, and feet
	Cornelia De Lange syndrome	Absent pregnancy-associated plasma protein A (PAPPA) linked to CHR 9q33; similar phenotype associated with trisomy 5p; ring Chr 3; rare	Continuous eyebrows, thin down-turning upper lip, microcephaly, short stature, small hands and feet, self-injury, severe to profound MR
	Williams syndrome	Chr 7; 1/20,000 births	Attention deficit hyperactivity disorder, poor peer relations, loquaciousness, excessive anxiety, sleep difficulties, short stature, hypercalcemia, thyroid abnormalities
Acquired disorders: Intrauterine infections	Rubella, CMV, toxoplasmosis, HIV, syphilis	Chronic intrauterine infection; rare	Sensory loss (auditory, visual), hyperactivity, mild to profound MR
Toxic Substances	Fetal alcohol syndrome	Maternal alcohol consumption 1/1,200 births in the U.S.	Microcephaly, short stature, mild MR, midface hypoplasia, short palpebral fissures, thin upper lip; cardiac defects; hyperactivity.
	Maternal heroin addiction	Frequency – variable	Low birth weight; withdrawal symptoms starting within 48 hours after birth (tremors, hyperreflexia, irritability)

Table 9.1 Disorders Causing Mental Retardation (cont'd)

Cause	Example	Physiology	Clinical Features and Associated Medical Complications
Toxic Substances	Maternal methadone addiction	Frequency – variable	Weight better than heroin babies; seizures higher incidence; later onset of withdrawal -- even 2-6 weeks
	Maternal cocaine addiction	Frequency – variable	Premature labor, growth retardation, microcephaly, intracranial hemorrhage, congenital anomalies of the urinary tract; developmental delays and learning problems.
	Heavy metals (lead, mercury)	Congenital exposure to heavy metal; rare	Irritability, seizures, sensory impairment, choreoathetosis, mild to profound MR
Later pregnancy problems; Perinatal difficulties	Birth anoxia, extreme prematurity		
Acquired childhood diseases; brain injury	Meningoencephalitis; trauma; severe malnutrition; lead intoxication		No minor physical anomalies. There may be residual features of the offending process or offending agent.

What should you do about Patient 9-2's diagnosis?

In the absence of a seizure or a metabolic disorder, symptoms of ADHD can be treated with either an alpha agonist (clonidine) or a stimulant (dextroamphetamine). It is much safer to use an alpha agonist like clonidine to manage the hyper-activity in developmental disorder patients, than to use a dopaminergic agent like methylphenidate or dextro-amphetamine. A dopaminergic agent has a reater risk of producing further agitation in developmental disorder.[8] With his improvement in hyperactive/impulsive behaviors, Patient 9-2 might cooperate better with etiological investigations.

A karyotype study or more specifically, evaluation for excessive CGG repeats on the FMR-1 gene is the first step. In fragile-X the repeats will usually exceed 200. Since this is a condition with a dose-effect relationship between the CGG repeats and phenotype, in individuals with minimal cognitive delay, there can at times be repeats in the 60-200 range.

Patient 9-2 has Fragile-X syndrome with ADHD and mild mental retardation. He responds well to a combination of clonidine, folic acid, and the later addition of methylphenidate. Providing a structured, supervised setting for learning appropriate social behaviors is helpful. It is also helpful to provide counseling to parents regarding the long-term outcome and vocational training opportunities tailored to the child's intellectual ability. Patient 9-2 was placed in a special education program because of his mental retardation and will continue to require special education placement throughout his school years.

Patient 9-3: Just a Shy Boy?

A 9-year-old, the youngest child of Chinese parents who immigrated to the US 1½ years ago, is noted by his teachers to be shy and quiet during the first year at school. They assume that he needs time to adjust to the US. After returning to school from summer vacation, the boy does not speak to any adults or children. After a month, he is referred for evaluation.

According to the parents (who were interviewed with the help of an interpreter), Patient 9-3 has always been rather quiet and shy. He does not present any problems at home. He talks to his parents and to the two older sisters. The sisters have adjusted well socially and are fluent in English. Developmental history is unremarkable, except for several earaches during his preschool years.

What should be done next?

The short answer is the rest of the examination! This means a thorough general medical and neurologic examination, and a careful neuropsychiatry evaluation. The boy's family and other environmental situations also need to be considered. Patient 9-3 is right-handed and of rather small stature (like his parents). His general appearance is unremarkable. He has poor eye contact and does not initially show any interest in the toys. When shown a sketch of a house, the boy picks up the pencil and adds a chimney to the house. He does this without any affective expression and without eye contact.

He sits quietly. After ten minutes the examiner turns on a video monitor, so Patient 9-3 can see himself on the screen. The boy suddenly became animated. He tries to hide from the camera by going to different parts of the room. He makes faces at the camera, dances, and clearly enjoys himself (all without any verbalizations). He shows one of the toy cars to the camera. The examiner asks him, "What is that?" The patient answers, "Car." The examiner asks the boy to say his name to the camera. The boy complies with obvious pleasure! He draws an appropriate sketch of the examiner, indicating age appropriate visual-motor skill. However, he does not make any spontaneous verbalizations for the rest of the evaluation.

What is a reasonable differential diagnosis?

Thirty percent of child psychiatric patients have speech and language problems, either as a primary diagnosis or comorbid with other psychiatric disorders. Children who have speech and language (S/L) impairments at age 5 have increased rates of ADHD and anxiety disorders. Because S/L impairments are closely related to brain dysfunction and probably also because early S/L impairments have a significant impact on social relations, their presence before age 5 predicts a significantly increased risk for emotional-behavior disorders during adolescence and young adulthood. The risk is particularly high for social phobia, and in males for antisocial personality. Language impairments strongly predict reading deficits.[9] Language disorders in children, although they have a neurologic basis, do not have the same localizing lesions as in adult aphasias. Child psychiatrists, therefore, prefer to use the term *language disorders* to *aphasia*.[10]

Language disorders in children can be associated with prenatal exposure to drugs and alcohol and severe abuse and neglect. Children with language problems are more likely to experience maltreatment.

Patient 9-3 has a classic pattern of social phobia[11] presenting as *selective mutism*. This disorder is more common in children from immigrant families, probably because they are faced with the double challenge of adapting to a new social setting as well as to a new language. Although there is some response to treatment with selective serotonin reuptake inhibitors, chronicity is not uncommon. For the majority of patients, the onset is gradual, although occasionally a child can develop selective mutism after a traumatic experience. A majority of patients like Patient 9-3 have an underlying expressive and/or receptive language disorder.

What can be done to help Patient 9-3?

A good assessment of hearing is an important first step in any S/L impairment in a young child. Patient 9-3's history of ear infections requires this early on. This can be easily done informally by obtaining an audiotape recording of the child's speech at home, with the person that the child is comfortable speaking to. If that speech shows poor clarity of sounds for the child's age, then formal audiologic evaluation is needed.

Assessment of the child's academic skills that do not require speech will help assess some nonverbal and brain functions, and will help to identify those who are broadly impaired (spelling, mathematics,

357

graphomotor skills). The Peabody Picture Vocabulary Test (PPVT),[12] which is a test of receptive vocabulary, is an easy, quick (5-10 minutes), and reliable indicator of receptive language. These three steps help differentiate patients with reasonable language skills, but who are paralyzed by social anxiety (and who might respond to a combination of pharmacotherapy and behavior modification) from those who are severely impaired in receptive and expressive language and are using silence as a compensatory strategy (i.e., not talking instead of making errors) and will, thus, be reluctant to give up that behavior.

Some studies have found fluoxetine to be more effective than placebo in treating social anxiety in children.[13] However, pharmacotherapy alone is unlikely to produce significant improvement in overall functioning. Speech therapy is necessary for those with significant problems of phonation or articulation. Behavior therapy can focus on desensitizing the child to his anxiety in social settings, using "in vitro" or "in vivo" procedures.

Patient 9-4: Every Shut Eye is Not Asleep, and Every Teen is Not a Rebel

A 13-year-old boy is brought to you by his mother for evaluation. For the last 6 months he has been irritable with his mother and is argumentative when asked to do chores. According to his mother, this behavior started after the parents divorced 6 months ago. He does not sleep well and is tired during school. He has received several detentions for not paying attention. He has also stopped spending after school time with his friends.

What should you do now?

We hope you said "diagnosis." We cannot do anything before making a diagnosis. What is the Duck here? Altered mood and behavior, inattentiveness, sleep disturbance in a teenager. The mnemonics MISERI will help us with a differential diagnosis.

> For nonmelancholic depression, children may have more somatic complaints, and adolescents more impulsive behavior than nonmelancholic adults. Melancholia is about the same in these age groups.

M - Missed secondary depression due to drug abuse conduct disorder, ADHD, and medication. Alternatively, primary depression can be missed if it occurs with the above disorder.
I - Infectious mononucleosis and other viral infections
S - Somatic symptoms (general medical complaints) can be due to depression.
E - Endocrine disorders (such as, hypothyroidism and epilepsy) can cause secondary depression.
R - Reaction to stress (divorce, moving, family illness) can cause adjustment disorder with mood symptoms). However, recurrent adjustment problems actually may be due to subsyndromal depression.
I - Illness pattern in the family. Family history of attention deficit, anxiety, mood disorder.

Based on this and applying Sutton's Law (go where the money is), we first need to determine if Patient 9-4's behavior change is secondary to drug abuse, seizures, endocrine and other medical illness. Applying the Duck Principle is not always helpful because compared to adults children exhibit a higher rate of co-morbid disorders, such as anxiety disorder and substance abuse; conduct disorder and ADHD occurs more

commonly in children than in adults.[14]
Major depressive disorder without any
co-morbidity occurs in less than 15% of
males and 30% of females. Typical
symptoms such as guilt (excluding
adolescent girls), psychomotor
agitation or retardation, appetite
change, and hypersomnia occur in less than 50% of patients.[16]

> Depression in mothers results in a six-fold increase and depression in fathers results in a three-fold increase in the likelihood of depression in children.[15]

Family history is helpful since first and second degree relatives of depressed children have high rates of psychiatric disorder. Adult criteria can be used to diagnose depression in children. Many depressed children have poor social skills and few friends. The neurobiological features seen in adult patients with melancholic depression (short REM latency, failure to suppress cortisol secretion or escape from suppression after oral dexamethasone) have also been found in children with major depression.[17] Based on available information, it would give us more bang for our bucks if we treat this child as depressed – assuming, of course, that we have ruled out secondary causes.

How should you treat Patient 9-4?

This is a semi-trick question. The answer is based on the diagnosis after taking into account Patient 9-4's age, size, and environment. Children and adolescents metabolize many medications rapidly. For example, tricyclic antidepressants (TCAs) are metabolized more quickly in children, which results in a higher ratio of desmethyl metabolites.[18]

> Suicide is rare in young children, but it is frequent in depressed children by age 11, and is the third leading cause of death in teenagers.

The treatment of depression in children involves 1) management of symptoms, 2) family education, 3) family's active participation in treatment, and 4) reducing stress at school by altering the school environment. (This is done by reducing workload if needed and improving social skills.) The efficacy of tricyclic antidepressant medication in children and adolescents has not been demonstrated, and there are high incidences of side effects with noradrenergic drugs. There are several randomized placebo controlled studies of SSRIs in children and adolescents that have shown efficacy of SSRIs over placebo. These studies include fluoxetine, sertraline, and clomipramine. While clomipramine is technically a TCA, it has high specificity for serotonin receptors.[19]

ECT is an important treatment option for adolescents with mood disorder.[20] At present, there are no systematic studies of ECT in children and adolescents. There are several anecdotal reports of successful use of ECT in adolescents and children with mood disorder. ECT should be considered in adolescents if they have a) severe depressive disorder requiring hospitalization, especially if associated with suicidality and weight loss; failure to respond to two trials of alternative treatment; b) manic delirium requiring hospitalization, unresponsive to lithium or an anticonvulsant plus neuroleptic; c) catatonia or neuroleptic malignant syndrome; and d) acute psychosis unresponsive to neuroleptic.

What is his long-term prognosis?

Most depressed children recover from an episode of depression within one year. However, depressed children and adolescents have a high rate of recurrence (50-75%). Often childhood depression progresses to adult depression. It is unclear if factors predicting recurrence and chronicity in adults (multiple episodes, psychotic symptoms, earlier onset, psychosocial stress) also predict recurrence and chronicity in children.[21]

Patient 9-5: School-Time Blues

A 6-year-old only child is brought by her mother to see you in October because "lately the child is becoming very clingy and tearful when it is time to go to school." Patient 9-5 had missed a few school days in early first grade due to abdominal pains and vomiting. Then in late September, she was way from school for a week because the family had to go out of town due to her maternal grandfather's heart attack and subsequent death. During the time they were away, the child shared a bed with her mother. When they returned home, her mother noticed that Patient 9-5 insisted on sleeping with her because of "scary nightmares of monsters." She also complains of abdominal pains, frequently in the morning. These pains go away by lunchtime when she stays home. Twice she has had to be picked up early from school because of abdominal pains that made her cry.

What is the first step in treating Patient 9-5?

As always, this is a trick question. There is no treatment without diagnosis, and there is no diagnosis without a thorough evaluation. On examination, Patient 9-5 is a child of average size, dressed neatly. She initially insists on her mother coming into the office with her. After about 10 minutes of a drawing game, she is willing to let her mother go back to the waiting room. She periodically sucks her thumb. Her ability to deal with numbers and letters is at about age level. In the drawing game, she draws pictures of monsters. The monsters "eat people." They look like dinosaurs. She denies seeing them when she is awake. She does not seem to understand the concept of worrying, but admits that she is scared to go to school. She cannot explain why. Patient 9-5's general medical health and neurologic functioning are normal. Did you remember to think about that? You must not forget that the behavior, the brain and the rest of the body are interrelated.

Patient 9-5's mother tells you that she too has been somewhat anxious in the last three months because of her father's ill health and death. She says she has been sad, cries at times, and wishes she had spent more time with her father before his death. There is no psychiatric illness in the family. Patient 9-5's father is in the Navy and is currently on sea duty.

What condition does Patient 9-5 have?

The pattern here is that of acute of onset of physical symptoms and behavioral change in a young child with resistance to go to school. The abdominal pain and cramps could be due to a general medical condition, such as a GI infection, and a thorough physical examination and appropriate laboratory investigations must be done. The other possibilities include major depression, generalized anxiety disorder (overanxious disorder), panic disorder or truancy. In simple truancy the child is somewhat older and does not exhibit clingy behavior. Isolated panic disorder rarely occurs before puberty. It is often associated with depression. Depression, although frequently comorbid with anxiety disorder, is present every day. Children with overanxious disorder often have multiple sources of anxiety, are not limited to anxiety about school.

Patient 9-5's pattern of problems (i.e., refusal to separate from his mother, physical symptoms that remit by noon) is characteristic of separation anxiety disorder (see *Table 9.2*). Some children with separation anxiety disorder worry about being kidnapped on the way to or from school and develop a marked school phobia. Even when they manage to stay in school, they worry about their caregivers and are unable to concentrate effectively on the school work. Patient 9-5 is probably unable to verbalize all of her fears and preoccupations because of her age.

Table 9.2   Separation Anxiety Disorder
Inappropriate, excessive anxiety concerning separation from home or from caregivers
Duration more than 4 weeks
Onset before age 18
Disturbance causes significant distress or impairment in functioning.
Disturbance is not due to a medical or psychiatric disorder.

Separation anxiety disorder co-occurs with other conditions, such as generalized anxiety disorder, specific phobia, and nonmelancholic depression. In some children the first sign of the disorder is the inability to sleep in their own bed, or anxiety about visiting the other parent (if the parents are divorced). Chronic abuse is a risk factor.

What treatments would be best for Patient 9-5?

Mild degrees of separation anxiety are treated by cognitive-behavioral therapy. More severe conditions that affect school attendance require additional treatment, including pharmacotherapy. The immediate goal for Patient 9-5's treatment is to decrease her anxiety sufficiently to prevent the "withdrawing from school" response from becoming chronic.

The family should be told that the key to successful treatment is for Patient 9-5 to experience separation, and for her to discover that her catastrophic fears are unfounded. Patient 9-5 has to become accustomed to temporary separation (the fancy term is *in vivo desensitization*). She should be praised and given rewards for her courage in spending the previously arranged time (short periods in the beginning) in school. The first day it may be just 5 minutes. Duration is then gradually increased until she can spend all day in school.[22]

If this behavioral strategy is not effective or the separation anxiety severe, or there is "anxiety contagion" in the family (in this situation her mother's anxiety), medication can be used.

Imipramine in the dose of 3-5 mg/kg/day has been shown to improve school attendance. The dose should be increased very slowly and a pretreatment EKG and follow-up EKG should be ordered. SSRIs have a better cardiac profile and may be considered as first choice. Further research is needed to confirm efficacy of the newer antidepressants. Efficacy data are better for benzodiazepines than tricyclics. Alprazolam 1 mg/day in a divided dose can be used. Buspirone may also be helpful and can be used.[23]

Stress events or situations in the family can contribute to a child's anxiety. Young children often are very susceptible to the anxiety and depression in parents.[24] In Patient 9-5's situation, her mother's bereavement may have exacerbated the separation anxiety. If so, Patient 9-5's mother may need evaluation and some treatment.

> Fifty to 75% of separation anxiety disorder (SAD) children come from low socioeconomic status. Seventy-five percent of SAD children have school refusal, and about 80% of school refusals is due to SAD.[25]

A short-term hospitalization may help the patient who continues to be symptomatic despite the above measures.

Patient 9-6: He Really Makes an Effort

Patient 9-6 is a 7 ½-year-old boy living with his parents. His parents, who have some college education, are concerned about Patient 9-6 not doing well in school and his risk of repeating the first grade. Patient 9-6, although not oppositional or malicious, is disorganized and immature for his age.

Patient 9-6's mother smoked about a pack a day during the first two months of pregnancy and then stopped. The delivery was unremarkable. He weighed about 6 pounds at birth (2 pounds less than his sister). His milestones were within the normal range except for continued occasional bedwetting until 6 years of age. He fell a lot, but had no major injuries. During kindergarten, because of his sister's birth, he spent about 2 months at his maternal grandmother's home, about 100 miles away. His parents decided to have him repeat kindergarten in order to "help him feel in sync with the other children when he goes to first grade." That seemed to help him socially because he is now one of the taller children in his class. However, Patient 9-6 feels bad about not being "smart" in his school work. The family is stable. Both parents work outside the home, and the maternal grandmother, who lives nearby, babysits. The patient's general medical examination and routine laboratory tests, all done by his pediatrician, are within normal limits.

On examination, Patient 9-6 relates well and is not hyperactive. On a circle-the-letter task (involving finding 20 A's on a sheet with about 60 letters), he makes one error of omission. He is able to do one-digit additions and one digit subtractions with two errors, which he is able to correct when given a second chance. His height and weight are at the 70th and 80th percentiles, respectively, for his age. He wants to do well in school and to become a "football player" when he grows up.

What Ducks might be waddling around this vignette?

Patient 9-6 is exhibiting mild deficits in attention and concentration. *Table 9.3* lists the causes of poor attention.

Table 9.3 Causes of Poor Attention	
Diagnosis	Associated Features
Epilepsy	Periods of daydreaming, history of febrile convulsions, birth problems
Mania	Hyperactivity, irritable mood, pressured speech
Depression	Irritable or sad mood, sleep and appetite changes, conduct problems, hallucinations, delusions, odd behavior
Psychosis	Generalized reduced intellectual function
Hypothyroidism	Abnormal TSH, cold intolerance, tiredness
Attention deficit disorder with or without hyperactivity	Poor attention, impulsivity, hyperactivity, normal intelligence

Patient 9-6 is not hyperactive. He has no features of psychosis, epilepsy, mood disorder, or thyroid dysfunction. He does not appear to have a generalized developmental delay because he is able to do math computation at his age level and grade level. He made one error of omission on the circle-the-letter test. He is able to correct his errors on the math computation test on a second attempt. These are examples of the top DSM IV criterion for attentional dysfunction, "makes careless mistakes." So, ADHD (attention deficit hyperactivity disorder) – predominantly inattentive type is likely, although petit mal (absence) epilepsy must be ruled out. A careful history about antecedents, such as birth trauma, febrile convulsion, will be of enormous help.

Attention deficit-hyperactive disorder is familial. Fathers of children with ADHD also have attentional problems. Maternal smoking is a risk factor for ADHD.[26]

What do you need to do to find the likely Duck?

Patient 9-6 needs to be referred to a neuropsychologist for further evaluation of his attention problem.   Auditory and visual continuous performance tests (CPT)[27] can give baseline data on errors of omission and commission. This can be helpful in periodic assessments of response of ADHD to the treatment.[28]

When monozygotic twins who are discordant for ADHD are compared on brain MRI, only the affected twin has significantly smaller caudate volume. There is hypermetabolism of the prefrontal cortex and caudate.[29]

Since his growth is good (70-80th percentiles) and he does not have any symptoms of thyroid dysfunction, a screening of thyroid function is not needed. However, if the child is hyperactive and small for his age (below 10th percentile) and the parents are of normal size, T4 and TSH levels should be done (particularly in children who have features of general developmental delay associated with ADD), because generalized resistance to thyroid hormone frequently manifests with ADD as a comorbidity. An EEG should be considered if the child's attentional functions are extremely variable. Patients with petit mal epilepsy exhibit a typical 3 Hz/sec spike and wave pattern.

What can you do to help Patient 9-6?

The most effective treatment for ADHD-inattentive type is pharmacological. Stimulants like methylphenidate (MPH) or amphetamine products are effective in the majority of these children. Starting with MPH dose of 0.3 mg/kg/day and dividing that dose into AM and lunchtime doses can help establish the lowest effective dose. Close attention to the child's behavior, as well as academic performance (task completion, rate of accuracy) are important. There is good evidence that the effects of treatment for ADHD appear quickly in math computation performance[30] as well as in behavior. In some children, due either to faster metabolism or other factors, higher doses may be required. Although many clinicians recommend a weekly titration upward for adequate control of ADHD symptoms, in a child like Patient 9-6, who is not disruptive, titration upward can be done every two to four weeks, after doing a continuous performance test in the area where the greatest weakness was evident (auditory or visual). An increase by 0.2 mg/kg/day is generally well tolerated. After an effective dose is reached, switching to a long acting, once per day preparation leads to greater stability of attention and better compliance with medication. Long-acting preparations have two peak concentrations. First are 5 within 1-3 hours and second within 4-7 hours.

> When an ADHD patient who is responding well to the medication during the daytime, complains about inability to fall asleep, melatonin (sublingual) can be very helpful as an adjunct at bedtime. Melatonin has been found useful to promote sleep in children with Asperger disease. Asperger's disease is a pervasive developmental disorder in which the patient has poor social skills with relatively preserved language skills.

If MPH is ineffective, or if it becomes ineffective after working for awhile, even with adequate dosing, switching to an amphetamine product can often lead to a good response. If these are ineffective, the new noradrenergic agent atomoxetine can be also tried. *Table 9.4* lists medications used to treat ADHD.

Table 9.4 Medications to Treat ADHD [31]

Drugs	Dose Range	Comments
Stimulants		
Methylphenidate*	.3-.7 mg/kg/day (10-60 mg)	Sustained release preparation can be used once per day. Stimulants cause insomnia, weight loss, headache, anxiety, tics, exacerbation of Tourette's, hypertension, psychosis (rare), hepatitis,** terrors,** choreiform.**
Dextroamphetamine*	.15-.5 mg/kg/day (5-40 mg)	
Amphetamine salt *	.15-.5 mg/kg/day (5-40 mg)	
Pemoline*	.5-2.5 mg/kg/day (37.5-112.5 mg)	
Nonstimulants		
Bupropion*	3-6 mg/kg/day	Contraindicated in patients with seizure and bulimia; can cause headache, insomnia, GI disturbance
Clonidine	3-4 mcg/kg TID (.3-.4 mg/day)	Sedation
Venlafaxine*	25-150 mg/day	Nervousness, insomnia
Atomaxetine	.2 mg-1.8 mg/kg/day	Causes anorexia, increase in pulse and BP, sedation, nausea
Tricyclics		EKG is needed before starting; may be reasonable alternative in patients with tic disorder (see page 375); causes anticholinergic side effects
Imipramine	1-5 mg/kg/day	
Nortriptyline	1-8 mg/kg/day	

*Sustained release preparation available
**Only with pemoline

What is the pathophysiology of Patient 9-6's condition?

The exact etiology of ADHD is not known. A single etiology can account for the syndrome only in a small group of children. The syndrome most likely represents a CNS dysfunction that results in difficulties in regulatory control, such as organization of information processing, attention, appropriate inhibition and social responses. Only 50% of variance of cases is explained by genetic factors. Environment (e.g., gestational events, parenting, family functioning and temperament) may influence the other 50%.

Functional MRI has been used to delineate the "brake system of the brain." Functional imaging studies in ADHD patients show bilateral reduced perfusion in both frontal lobes and basal ganglia. In most studies structural imaging shows reduced cerebral especially frontal and striatal volumes. Other brain regions such as temporal and cerebellar, are also affected.[32] Unmedicated patients with ADHD had significantly smaller white matter volumes than controls and medicated individuals with ADHD. Rubia et al (1999)[33] found that when adolescent boys with ADHD are engaged in a "stop task" (one that requires the inhibition of a planned motor response,) they manifest a lower power of response in the right inferior prefrontal cortex and in the left caudate. Other functional MRI studies have found abnormalities in the putamen in ADHD subjects.

Frontal lobes exert inhibitory influences on lower striatal structures which are mediated by neurotransmitters, such as dopamine and norepinephrine. Neurochemically, dopaminergic function may be abnormal in ADHD. There are very few dopamine transporters in the frontal cortex, which allows the dopamine to diffuse away from the synapse after it is released. Dopamine has a key regulatory role in cognitive functions, such as the working memory and attention.[34] A norepinephrine transporter is said to have an even higher affinity for dopamine than it does for norepinephrine. Dopamine hitches a ride on the norepinephrine reuptake pump, gets co-stored in synaptic vesicles with norepinephrine in noradrenergic neurons. Both dopamine and norepinephrine get released when frontal cortex noradrenergic nerves fire.[35] Thus, medications that increase dopamine and decrease peripheral noradrenergic activity can help improve attention and decrease distractibility. Noradrenergic agent atomoxetine exerts its effectiveness through an indirect impact on the extracellular dopamine levels in the prefrontal cortex.

Patient 9-7: The Little Engine That Wouldn't Stop

A 10-year-old boy with a diagnosis of attention deficit disorder is brought for consultation because of a recent worsening of his "hyperactivity." He has also become more aggressive and is having problems at school.

Patient 9-7 was diagnosed with ADHD at age 7 and was treated with pemoline by his primary physician with good results. A year later, he needed an increase in dose. After two annual dose increases at age 10, his parents became concerned about the potential for liver failure associated with pemoline and requested a change of medication. The physician discontinued pemoline and started methylphenidate 30 mg/day in two doses (about 0.6 mg/kg/day). Within a week, there was an increase in hyperactivity, decrease in sleep to 4 hours per night (from 7 hours per night), and Patient 9-7 was becoming aggressive with his 6-year-old brother. To add to the parents' concerns, his school work deteriorated dramatically, and he was suspended from school for fighting. The methylphenidate was discontinued, and you get a shot at figuring out what's happened.

You see Patient 9-7 four days after the discontinuation of methylphenidate. He has lost 2 pounds in the last two weeks. In the office, he is fidgety, but rather jovial. His current goal is to "Get out of that stupid school." When you ask him what he would like to do when he grows up, he says, "Maybe I will become a mercenary." He admits that two years ago he wanted to become a fireman, but not anymore. He denies hallucinations, obsessive compulsive rituals, or imaginary friends. When given a sheet with math computation items to work on, he loses interest after doing 5 of the 25 items, stating, "This is baby stuff." When asked about his aggression towards his younger brother, he says, "He used to be an all right kid, but now he bugs me too much." Patient 9-7 does not mind his lack of sleep because "I can listen to the Grateful Dead and plan on becoming a mercenary in Iraq."

What is the diagnosis?

The marked and immediate change in behavior after methylphenidate (a dopaminergic agent) was started suggests that the drug has something to do with Patient 9-7's irritability, aggression, lack of sleep, and violent preoccupations. Primary hypomania or mania is uncommon in prepuberty, but secondary hypomania or mania can occur with some drugs,[36] dopaminergic agents (methylphenidate, amphetamines), or guanfacine.[37]

Irritability (extreme, often physical response to frustration and other negative emotional stimuli) is common in juvenile bipolar disorder.[38] Geller et al (1994) found that children who become hypomanic from stimulants are over sixfold more likely to have relatives with mood disorder. These children are more likely to be bullies. Thus, knowing the Duck leads you to getting this information and worrying about the long-term course for Patient 9-7. Stopping the drug may resolve the hypomania. But will he have future episodes, or worse, anyway? Can these be prevented? Stay tuned.

What is the treatment strategy?

The first step is stopping the offending agent. That was done but Patient 9-7 is still symptomatic. Waiting another week if practical might be the least intrusive course. If treatment is needed, it will be with a mood stabilizer to treat the mania. *Table 9.5* lists mood stabilizers for bipolar disorder. Lithium is the oldest mood stabilizer and has the most studies supporting use in adults with bipolar illness. In children and adolescents, studies have shown a response rate of 33-80% reflecting the heterogeneity of the sample and need for careful diagnosis. Lithium is especially helpful in bipolar children with comorbid drug abuse.[39] Because childhood mania is frequently associated with dysphoric mood, using valproic acid (15 mg/kg/day in 3 doses) is more effective compared to lithium or carbamazepine.[40] However, approximately 50% of adults and adolescents with mania do not respond to monotherapy and the same may be true in children.[41] If necessary, a second mood stabilizer or a novel neuroleptic as adjunct can improve the response rate.

After the acute mania has subsided, we still need to treat the ADHD. Pemoline is not advisable because there have been reports of 15 cases of acute liver failure, probably associated with pemoline.[42] Low dose stimulant treatment has been reported to be effective in children with bipolar disorder without serious adverse effects.[43] A new noradrenergic agent, atomoxetine, can be another consideration for treating the ADHD features.

Table 9.5 Mood Stabilizers and Atypical Antipsychotics for Bipolar Children and Adolescents

Generic Name	Starting Dose	Target Dose	Cautions
Carbamazepine* Carbamazepine XR	Outpatients: 7 mg/kg/day 2-3 daily doses	Based on response and serum levels	Monitor for drug interactions.
Lithium*	Outpatients: 25 mg/kg/day 2-3 daily doses	30 mg/kg/day 2-3 daily doses	Monitor for hypothyroidism.
Oxcarbazepine	150 mg BID	20-29 kg 900 mg/day; 30-39 kg 1,200 mg/day; >39 kg 1,800 mg/day;	Monitor for hyponatremia.
Valproic acid* Divalproex sodium	Outpatients: 15 mg/kg/day 2-3 daily doses	20 mg/kg/day 2-3 daily doses	Monitor liver functions and for pancreatitis.
Clozapine	25 mg BID	200-400 mg/day	Monitor WBC weekly. Seizures possible at higher doses.
Olanzapine	2.5 mg BID	10-20 mg/day	Monitor weight, cholesterol.
Risperidone	0.25 mg BID	1-2 mg/day	Monitor for EPS and galactorrhea.
Ziprasidone	20 mg BID	80-120 mg/day	Check baseline EKG.
Aripiprazole	5 mg QHS	10-15 mg/day	Monitor for drug interactions.

*Therapeutic serum levels are the same as for adults. Teratogenic, so avoid in pregnant adolescents, especially in first trimester.

Patient 9-8: Twitches 'R Us

A 13-year-old boy is referred to you because of twitching in his eyes and repeated coughing in his classroom. He has just started in a new school. Although he has always been a shy kid who is described as a "neat freak" by his sister, the boy had no psychiatric or neurologic history. His mother has been diagnosed as having OCD.

Does this child have a psychiatric or a neurologic disorder?

We hope by now you have it in your procedure memory that just because stress precipitates symptom(s) that does not mean psychologic. Stress is bad, period. All sorts of illness are precipitated by stress. This child is exhibiting sudden, rapid recurrent stereotypic movements and vocalizations. These are called tics. Tics usually occur before age 18 and are not caused by substances such as stimulants or neurologic condition, such as Huntington's. *Table 9.6* lists different types of tic disorders. The difference between chronic tic disorder and Tourette's is that in Tourette's both motor and vocal tics have to be present, whereas in chronic tic disorder either vocal or motor tics must be present. Tics and Tourette's disorders are characterized by fluctuating course and preceded

Table 9.6 Tic Disorders
Transient tic disorder
Single or multiple motor and/or vocal tics occurring many times a day nearly every day for at least 4 weeks but not longer than 12 consecutive months.
Criteria for Tourette's disorder or chronic motor or vocal tic disorder have never been met.
Chronic motor or vocal tic disorder
Single or multiple motor or vocal tics, but not both, have been present at some time during the illness.
Tics occur many times a day nearly every day or intermittently for more than 1 year, without a tic-free period of more than 3 consecutive months.
Criteria for Tourette's disorder or chronic motor or vocal tic disorder have never been met.
Tourette's disorder
Both multiple motor and one or more vocal tics have been present at some time during the illness, although not necessarily concurrently.
Tics occur many times a day (usually in bouts) nearly every day or intermittently for more than 1 year, without a tic-free period of more than 3 consecutive months.
Autosomal dominant with 99% prevalence

by tension and worsened by stress, excitement, and fatigue. Tics often occur involuntarily although they can be suppressed voluntarily.

Transient tics are seen in up to 10% of children. Chronic tics are less common, and Tourette's disorder has a community prevalence of 0.1 to 0.8%.

PANDAS (pediatric autoimmune neuropsychiatric disorder after streptococcal infection) should be considered when tics present abruptly with upper respiratory tract illness. A throat culture and antibody titers for group A hemolytic streptococcal infection will rule out PANDAS.

What other problems are likely to occur?

Tic and Tourette's disorders rarely occur in isolation. About 11-80% of tic disorder patients have obsessive compulsive disorder. About 50-90% have ADHD and about 40-45% have major depression.[44] Although this young man does not seem to have OCD, you still must assess him for presence of OCD as his sister did refer to him as "neat freak." In addition, these Tourette's disorder children also exhibit poor impulse control and have rage attacks. Many also have learning disability. It is essential to assess his functioning at school as the tics may have worsened because he is having difficulty academically.

Tic disorders are thought to occur due to disinhibition and dysfunction of dopaminergic and serotonergic pathways of cortico striatal thalamic cortical structures -- specifically the sensory motor circuits.

Table 9.7   Keys to Managing Childhood Tic Disorders
Assess for comorbid illnesses; then prioritize and treat the most troublesome symptoms.
Aim to decrease rather than eliminate tic-related discomfort.
Medicate only if tics cause distress and dysfunction.
Use one agent when needed at the lowest effective dosage to minimize side effects and drug interactions.
Involve the family and school to monitor progress.
Reassess treatment efficacy often. [46]

How would you treat him?

Table 9.7 lists the general approach to treating a patient with tic disorder. In Patient 9-8, the first thing is to establish severity of his symptoms, including frequency of tics and functional impairment. If his symptoms are mild, then medication may not be needed and psychoeducation and supportive behavior therapy may suffice. If symptoms are moderate to severe, then clonidine which is an alpha 2 agonist (.1-.3 mg/day) or guanfacine (.5-4 mg BID) which is an alpha 2 agonist can be used.[45]

An atypical antipsychotic such as risperidone (.5-6 mg) is one of the most often used atypicals followed by olanzapine (2.5-10 mg). If atypicals show no response, then typical antipsychotics, such as haloperidol (2-10 mg) or pimozide (1-8 mg/day), can be used.

Comorbidities must be treated appropriately when treating ADHD. Stimulants cannot be used as it will increase the tics. Clonidine has been shown to improve both ADHD and tic symptoms and thus can be used alone. Otherwise, atomoxetine, a nonstimulant ADHD medication, can be used.

Parents often ignore a child's repeated nose twitching or throat clearing as due to "colds" or "allergy." However, these might be the first signs of a motor or vocal tic disorder in a child. So it is important for the clinician who is treating a child pharmacologically to observe the child carefully for signs of movement disorders.

Quick Rounds

1. A 10-year-old boy with a history of ventricular septal defect is brought to you for consultation because of severe oppositional and fearful behaviors of one-year duration. The onset of these behaviors appears to be preceded by his parents' divorce, which was relatively sedate. The parents still talk to each other. On examination, the boy has a high arched palate, small ears, small mouth with receding chin. He has no friends. What particular syndrome is suggested by the physical features, and what psychiatric disorders are known to be associated with this syndrome?

2. The mother of a 13-year-old boy calls you saying that lately her son has been acting defiant, skipping school, and doing poorly in his grades. She does not know of any sleep disturbance but has noticed that the boy receives many phone calls at night from people whom she does not know. He is relatively unsupervised because the mother, who is divorced, usually works until 8:00 p.m. Your next available appointment is in two weeks. In the meantime, what will be the most advisable thing to do?

3. A 7-year-old boy was recently diagnosed by you as having ADHD (attention deficit hyperactivity disorder). You started methylphenidate 5 mg a.m. and at noontime. After he responds well for about a month, there seems to be some loss of effect. You increase the dose to 7.5 mg BID with no benefit and then to 10 mg BID with a significant improvement. However, now the boy is having difficulty falling asleep at night until almost midnight. What is the best way to combat the insomnia?

4. A 9-year-old boy who lives with his parents has in the last 3 months experienced a deterioration in his school work and has started bed-wetting about twice a month. His general medical health is fine. The family system seems harmonious and stable. He denies any traumatic experiences and feels bad about his recent poor grades. What investigation would be important to do before any treatment decision can be made?

5. A 13-year-old boy is brought to you because in the past year he has often been truant from school. When in school, he often picks on children who are smaller than himself and demands that they bring candy or money for him if they do not want to be beaten up. At home, his mother frequently finds money missing from her purse. She suspects he is taking it without her permission. When she asks him

about it, he always denies taking it, but is unable to explain how he obtained the three comic books that she found in his room. What is the most likely diagnosis?

6. In the middle of the night, a 4-year-old boy wakes screaming. When the parents come to his room, they find him still screaming, sitting in his bed. He doesn't seem to recognize them initially. After they hold him and hug him and reassure him for a few minutes, he stops screaming and goes back to sleep. The next morning he has no memory of what happened the previous night. What is the most likely diagnosis?

7. A 10-year-old boy with attention deficit hyperactivity disorder was started on dextroamphetamine 5 mg a.m. and noontime about three months ago. During the first follow-up visit, the mother and child were pleased with the response. Now, during the second follow up visit, the mother reports that the medication is still working well, but she is concerned about her son's frequently clearing his throat and twitching his nose as if he has some allergy. There is no past history of allergies. There is no nasal discharge or inflammation of the pharynx. He does clear his throat often and twitch his nose. What is the most likely diagnosis, and what is the best treatment strategy at this time?

8. A 7-year-old boy is brought to you with a history of never having been dry at night. Currently, he wets the bed about three times a week even after his parents regularly wake him up to go to the toilet at about 10:00 p.m. There is a family history of nocturnal enuresis on the mother's side. The child wishes he could stop bed-wetting so that he can go to sleepovers at friends' homes. Urinalysis is within normal limits. What is your first-line treatment plan?

Quick Rounds Answers

1. In the last 10 years, there is increasing recognition of the association between chr 22 deletion syndromes and childhood onset psychiatric disorders. The first description of velo-cardio-facial syndrome (VCFS) was in 1978.[47] This boy fits the description of the 22q deletion syndrome, which occurs in about 1 in 4000 births. There is a high incidence of schizophrenia and bipolar disorders in these individuals during and after childhood. The chromosomal pathology can be confirmed by FISH (fluorescent in situ hybridization).

2. Teen years are the period when the child becomes as big as the parent physically and at the same time begins to manifest intolerance of the parent's authority figure status. The male teen's ability to critically evaluate adults from many perspectives interacts with high testosterone levels and leads to hostility and impulsivity, which is often directed at the primary attachment figures. Although this is normal to some extent, when the teenager skips school and his grades head south, it is clearly indicative of psychopathology. The psychopathology can be a pure oppositional defiant disorder, or more frequently, a combination of a mood disorder and oppositional features. A frequent comorbidity is substance abuse. When the parent is faced with the constellation of the features described above, a psychiatric consultation is very important. While waiting for the psychiatric consultation, a urine drug screen would be the most appropriate immediate step to take.

3. Methylphenidate is one of the first-line agents for the treatment of ADHD and almost 60-70% of properly diagnosed and dosed patients. Clinicians generally start with about 0.3 mg/kg/day in two doses and titrate the dose upward as needed to normalize the child's attention and activity, particularly in school. About 2 to 5% of the patients will develop significant insomnia and/or anorexia due to the dopaminergic and noradrenergic effects of methylphenidate. When the daytime behavior is responding well to a particular dose, if insomnia is the primary unwelcome effect, it can be remedied by adding melatonin (1-2 mg) or clonidine (0.05-0.1 mg) at bedtime. Although no systematic long-term studies are available, there is considerable clinical experience with the above agents in the pediatric age group to combat the side effect of insomnia.

4. In the absence of any traumatic or stressful experiences, the development of bed-wetting and poor academic functioning at age 9 is suggestive of brain dysfunction. The peak incidence of seizure

disorders in childhood is before 10 years of age. So, one of the most important investigations for this child is a 24- or 48-hour EEG to unequivocally establish the presence or absence of a cerebral dysrythmia.

5.   The behavior that this patient is exhibiting, i.e., persistent truancy, stealing, lying, and interference with other people's right to live peacefully together, all called conduct disorder. DSM-IV lists 15 behaviors ranging from lying and stealing to sexual assault, setting fires and fighting with weapons. To be diagnosed as having *conduct disorder*, only 3 of these 15 behaviors must be present in a year. Because of these criteria, the patient may have a mild form or a very severe form in which he is exhibiting antisocial behaviors, such as damaging property, fighting with weapons or sexual assaults.

6.   This is a typical description of pavor nocturnus (night terror), which is different from a nightmare in which the child is able to describe a frightening dream that preceded the awakening. This is a non-REM sleep disorder.

7.   The Duck is motor and vocal tic disorder. Occasionally, children develop a tic disorder after being placed on dopaminergic agents like methylphenidate and dextroamphetamine. There is a continuing controversy regarding the role of the dopaminergic agent in the precipitation of the tic syndrome. The predominant evidence from several studies indicates that there is a dopamine system overactivity in Tourette's syndrome.[48] So, it is not advisable to continue treatment with dopaminergic agents like amphetamines or methylphenidate when motor and vocal tics appear in the patient. Discontinuation of such agents sometimes leads to remission of tics. Both the ADHD and the tics can be effectively treated by clonidine or guanfacine. Otherwise, atomoxetine (a nonadrenergic agent) can be used for treating the ADHD. However, there are also some reports of patients with Tourette's syndrome having a good response to low dose methylphenidate when they have a comorbid ADHD.

8.   DDAVP (desmopressin acetate) in tablet form is the medication of first choice in primary nocturnal enuresis. It can be used alone or in conjunction with behavioral conditioning. After a significant improvement has occurred, a gradual weaning of the dosing over a period of one to two months is advisable.

APPENDIX I

DIAGNOSING PSYCHIATRIC DISORDERS

I. History

A. Original 19th and early 20th century nosology of mental illness assumed a biological bases for syndromes, but there was no consensus on the organization of psychiatric disorders.

B. Statistical manual used by institutions for the insane (1918) was the first consensus document.

C. DSM-I (Diagnostic and Statistical Manual, 1952) was the American Psychiatric Association's first classification system. It and DSM-II (1968) were based on psychodynamic concepts.

D. DSM-III was introduced in 1980 as the first "empirical" system. It was advertised as representing science and professional consensus, and having good reliability and no bias.

1. Reliability reflects consistency of observations.
2. Validity reflects accuracy of observations.
3. DSM-III and subsequent versions (DSM-III-R, and DSM-IV) claim both reliability and validity.

E. DSM-IV corresponds to part of the Tenth International Classification of Diseases (ICD-10), the World Health Organization's document on all medical diagnoses.

II. The DSM Structure

A. *Specific criteria-based (some operationally defined).* Criteria-based means that each syndrome is defined by a set of diagnostic criteria rather than just by a descriptive paragraph. If a patient meets all criteria, he has the syndrome. If he does not meet all criteria, but does meet many, he is said to have the category diagnosis (e.g., mood disorder), but as it cannot be pinpointed, it is termed "not otherwise specified," or NOS. Here are DSM criteria for major depressive disorder:

1. More than 2 weeks
2. Change from previous function
3. Depressed mood or loss of interest/pleasure
4. Five of the following:

   a. Depressed or irritable mood
   b. Diminished pleasure
   c. Weight loss or gain more than 5% of body weight
   d. Insomnia or hypersomnia
   e. Agitation or retardation
   f. Fatigue or loss of energy
   g. Feelings of worthlessness, or excessive guilt
   h. Diminished ability to think or concentrate, or indecisiveness
   i. Recurrent thoughts of death, or suicide

The criteria are a list of items and all four must be met. Some criteria are "operationally defined," as is 4c, weight loss. Greater than 5% of body weight is specific. Other criteria are poorly defined as is criterion 4h. What exactly comprises diminished concentration or indecisiveness is not specified. Each clinician must figure it out for himself.

B. *Axis-based: (Axis I, II, III, IV, V).* The DSM is organized into several strata of conditions termed axes.

C. *Hierarchical-based:* Like the "rock-paper-scissors" game, some categories take precedence over others: a person with sad mood, daily anxiety, and panic attacks is considered as having major depression, not has having panic disorder. The more serious conditions get first billing. The hierarchy is necessary because many patients meet criteria for more than one DSM condition. Thus, co-morbidity is common, and the clinician must prioritize the conditions to decide what gets treated as the primary condition, or what gets treated first.

III. Axis I: Clinical Disorders

Represents categories considered "states" of illness. The person is well, then gets sick (e.g., depression), then he recovers and is well again until the next episode (state).

A. The "psychotic disorders"

1. Schizophrenia
2. Delusional disorders
3. Other "psychotic" disorders

B. Mood disorders
C. Anxiety disorders
D. Obsessive compulsive disorders
E. Somatoform disorders
F. Dissociative disorders
G. Factitious disorders
H. Eating disorders
I. Impulse control disorders
J. Adjustment disorders
K. Sleep disorders
L. Sexual and gender identity disorders
M. Substance-related disorders
N. Cognitive disorders
P. Disorders usually first diagnosed in infancy, childhood, or adolescence

IV. Axis II: Personality Disorder/Mental Retardation

Represents categories considered "traits" that deviate from the norm, but not necessarily deviant because of pathology. Traits are long-lasting, relatively unchanging characteristics like eye color, personality, and personality disorder.

A. *Cluster A.* Odd and eccentric personality disorders
B. *Cluster B.* Dramatic and emotional personality disorders
C. *Cluster C.* Anxious and fearful personality disorders
D. In the hierarchy, axis I takes precedence over axis II.

V. Axis III: General Medical Condition

A. Represents general medical and specific neurologic disease.

B. These conditions can co-occur with an axis I or II condition or they can cause the axis I or II condition.

C. When they are the cause (e.g., the patient has generalized anxiety disorder because of hyperthyroidism), the axis I or II condition is said to be *secondary* to the identified general medical or specific neurologic condition. Correcting the axis III problem , may be the most direct, specific, and effective treatment of the axis I or II condition.

D. When the general medical or specific neurologic condition co-occurs, it is listed as a separate axis III diagnosis. Although not causing the axis I or II condition, the co-occurring axis III condition can complicate treatment of the axis I or II condition.

VI. Axis IV: Psychosocial and Environmental Problems

A. Psychosocial and environmental problems that may affect diagnosis, treatment and prognosis of mental disorders.

B. These problems may either cause the mental problem (loss of job causing depression) or may be the consequence of one (e.g., patient losing job due to depression).

C. Multiple stressors may contribute to the problem.

D. if the psychosocial problem is the primary focus of clinical attention, then it is listed on Axis I, e.g., a couple coming to the ER only because of a fight.

VII. Axis V: Global Assessment of Functioning (GAF)

A. It is the reporting clinician's judgment of individual's function.

B. It is useful in measuring outcome and planning.

C. GAF scale ranges from 0-100.

VI. The DSM Procedural Steps

A. *Step 1:* Make the syndromal behavior diagnosis (axis I, II, or both)

B. *Step 2:* Decide if the behavioral syndrome is due to (secondary to) a known neurologic or general medical condition, or if it is idiopathic (primary). This decision helps plan treatments and may lead to very specific treatments, (such as treating the secondary depressions with thyroid [T_4] rather than an antidepressant).

C. *Step 3:* Determine co-morbidities (any co-occurring conditions) pharmacokinetic and environmental factors that can effect treatment and management.

VII. Example of Using DSM Procedural Steps

A. *Step 1:* Use the behavioral examination and the entire general medical evaluation to decide what the patient's chief complaint represents: A 48-year-old Euro-American man says in a shaky voice "Doctor, I don't know what to do, help me, I can't figure things out, I feel terrible, there's no hope for me." Your conclusion is melancholia (in DSM-IV, "major depression with melancholic features").

B. *Step 2:* Except for mild diabetes, there is no evidence that he has any general medical (e.g., Cushing's disease) or other neurologic condition (e.g., stroke) that could produce melancholia. His condition, therefore, is primary.

C. *Step 3:* there is no evidence that this man had a premelancholia personality disorder or other psychiatric problems. He is not an alcoholic or a street drug user. His only co-morbidity is mild diabetes.

D. *Step 4:* The patient is having difficulty concentrating at work and he has fought with his wife.

E. *Step 5:* Patient is still functioning, is not suicidal; GAF is 5.

VIII. Weakness of DSM System

A. No proven validity, especially with personality disorder.

B. Disorders with the same criteria may have different etiologies and disorders with the same etiology may present with different features. For example, catatonic symptoms are seen in schizophrenia, mania, depression, and other neurologic disorders.

C. Many neuropsychiatric diagnoses (e.g., frontal lobe syndrome) have no DSM label.

IX. Diagnostic Principles

Most clinicians diagnose by pattern recognition, the hallmark of residency training: see a few, remember what they looked like and what treatments worked, and if you see it again reach the same conclusion and do the same thing again. As long as the patient has a typical syndrome or is well known to you, using pattern recognition to diagnose can be very accurate. However, it has only modest reliability (e.g., the degree to which a group of clinicians would agree on the diagnoses of a group of patients).

A. The Duck Principle, i.e., "If it looks, walks and quacks like a duck, it most likely is a duck," underlies pattern recognition. For example, a 60-year-old woman complains of concentration and memory problems. Her husband says she is not herself and that she is losing her mind. She is also despondent and apprehensive, is having trouble sleeping, is not eating and has lost substantial weight. She says she wants to die. This "duck" is melancholia.

B. Sutton's Law is based on the vignette that Willy Sutton, a famous U.S. bank robber in the 1950s, when asked by a reporter why he robbed banks, said "because that's where the money is!" Sutton's law tells you that the most likely condition under the particular circumstances of the situation is probably the correct diagnosis. A corollary to this is, when you hear hoof beats in the United States it is horses, not zebras. The above melancholic woman also had problems with concentration and memory. Her husband said she was losing her mind. She is 60. Alzheimer's disease is a reasonable consideration. Sutton's law, however, also favors melancholia because in persons under 70, depression is four times as common as Alzheimer's disease which typically does not fully express itself until the mid-seventies.

C. The Rule of Parsimony tells you to try to explain the patient's many complaints and clinical features by as few underlying pathophysiologic processes as possible – one being the best. Looking for parsimony is looking for the common underlying theme. In the melancholic woman above, you might find out that she has some cortical atrophy and ventricular enlargement on MRI and diffuse cognitive impairment. You could conclude she has both depression and dementia, but the MRI and cognitive findings are also consistent with depression and so all her problems can be explained by that single pathophysiologic process. Parsimony facilitates good treatment.

Appendix 2
Psychopharmacology at a Glance

Some Commonly Used Antipsychotics

Class	Primary Indication(s)	Pharmacokinetics		Pharmaco-dynamics	Side Effects	Adverse Effects
		Half-life/ Dose (mg)	Usual dose range (mg)			
Typical Antipsychotics - Low Potency						
Chlorpromazine (Thorazine)	Psychosis	1-2 days	400-600	D2 nonselective blocker	Sedation Orthostatic Anticholinergic Quinidine-like	Skin discoloration Sudden unexplained death
Thioridazine (Mellaril)	Psychosis	1-3 days	400-600	D2 nonselective blocker	Same as chlorpromazine	Retinal pigmentation with loss of visual activity Hip fracture and anticholinergic delirium Prolonged QT interval
Typical Antispychotics - High Potency						
Haloperidol (Haldol)	Psychotic excitement Psychoses Stimulant psychosis Tourette's syndrome	1-2 days	20-80	D2 nonselective blocker	EPS Dystonias Akathisia	Tardive dyskinesia NMS

Some Commonly Used Antipsychotics

Class	Primary Indication(s)	Pharmacokinetics		Pharmaco-dynamics	Side Effects	Adverse Effects
		Half-life/ Dose (mg)	Usual dose range (mg)			
Fluphenazine (Prolixin)	Psychotic excitement Psychoses	1-2 days	20-80	D2 nonselective blocker	EPS Dystonia Akathisia	Tardive dyskinesia NMS
Thiothixene	Psychoses	1-2 days	20-80	D2 nonselective blocker	EPS Dystonia Akathisia	Tardive dyskinesia NMS
Pimozide (Orap)	Tourette's syndrome Delusional disorder	2-4 days	10-30	D2 nonselective blocker	EPS	Tardive dyskinesia NMS Liver failure
Atypical Antipsychotics						
Risperidone (Risperdal)	Psychotic depression Psychosis with dementia Psychotic with TD Young persons with positive symptom nonmood disorder psychoses	1-2 days	2-8	Selective D_2 blocker less than 8 mg/day $5HT_2$ blocker	EPS at higher doses Sedation Orthostatic hypotension	No major short term adverse effect TD unknown

D2 = dopamine
5HT = 5 hydroxytryptamine

388

Some Commonly Used Antipsychotics

Class	Primary Indication(s)	Pharmacokinetics		Pharmaco-dynamics	Side Effects	Adverse Effects
		Half-life/ Dose (mg)	Usual dose range (mg)			
Olanzapine (Zyprexa)	Schizophrenia	1-2 days	10-30	Higher $5HT_2/D_2$ ratio complicated	Sedation Orthostatic Dizziness Weight gain Constipation Excitement	No major short-term adverse effect TD unknown
Clozapine (Clozaril)	Chronic psychotics who are neuroleptic resistant	1-2 days	300-600	Same as olanzapine	Sedation Sialorrhea (severe) Arrhythmia Orthostatic Dizziness Anticholinergic (most severe)	Agranulocytosis (2%) Cardiac death Delirium in elderly Seizures 5% at high doses 600-900 mg/day) Avoid with benzodiazepine (can produce respiratory arrest)
Quetiapine (Seroquel)	Chronic psychosis	3 hours	200-400	Complicated	Mild sedation Mild constipation Dry mouth	No major adverse effects No prolactinemia

Some Commonly Used Anxiolytics

Class	Primary Indication(s)	Pharmacokinetics Half-life/Dose (mg)	Pharmacodynamics	Side Effects
Anxiolytics				
Buspirone (Buspar)	Generalized anxiety disorder Agitation in TBI and demented patients	1-10 hours 30-60/d	5HT & 5HT2	Dizziness Headache Nausea Nervousness
Benzodiazepines				
Lorazepam (Ativan)	Acute panic attack Agitation in nonpsychotic patients Catatonia Alcohol detoxification	Intermediate 6-20 hrs. 1-6 mg/day	GABA/benzodiazepine receptors	Tolerance Sedation Confusion Dizziness/ataxia Cannot use with clonazepam
Clonazepam (Klonopin)	Panic disorder Short-term treatment of anxiety and agitation in mania	Long >20 hr. 1-4 mg/day	GABA/benzodiazepine receptors	Tolerance Sedation Confusion Dizziness Depression
Diazepam (Valium)	Same as lorazepam	Long >20 hr. 5-40 mg/day	GABA/benzodiazepine receptors	Tolerance Confusion Dizziness/ataxia

Some Commonly Used Anxiolytics

Class	Primary Indication(s)	Pharmacokinetics	Pharmacodynamics	Side Effects
		Half-life/Dose (mg)		
Alprazolam (Xanax)	Panic disorder Short-term management of anxiety	Intermediate 6-20 hrs. 1-10 mg/day	GABA/benzodiazepine receptors	Tolerance Confusion Dizziness Memory Impairment Fatigue

GABA = gamma amino butyric acid

Commonly Used Mood Stabilizers and Anticonvulsants

Class	Primary Indication(s)	Pharmacokinetics Half-life/ Dose (mg)	Pharmacokinetics Other	Pharmacodynamics	Side Effects	Adverse Effects
Lithium	Bipolar disorder Depression enhancer TBI with aggression	24-36 hours	No liver metabolism Not protein bound	Second messenger systems	Weight gain Tremor GI problems Sedation	Rash Diabetes insipidus Hypothyroidism Parathyroidism Toxicity
Carbamazepine	Bipolar disorder Depression enhancer Epilepsy Anticraving TBI Stroke with aggression	24 hours	1st pass Induces hepatic metabolism	GABA turnover is reduced due to inactivation of sodium channels. Antikindling	Orthostatic Headaches Nausea Sedation	Liver failure Agranulocytosis Rash
Valproate	Bipolar disorder Epilepsy	6-16 hours	Protein bound	GABA turnover is reduced due to blockage of sodium channels. GABA transmission is enhanced. Prevents and blocks kindling	Tremor Sedation Weight gain Ataxia	Liver failure High ammonia levels Thrombocytopenia

392

Commonly Used Mood Stabilizers and Anticonvulsants

Class	Primary Indication(s)	Pharmacokinetics		Pharmacodynamics	Side Effects	Adverse Effects
		Half-life/ Dose (mg)	Other			
Lamotrigine	Depressed phase bipolar disorder	25-32 hours	Does not induce hepatic enzyme	Bocks sodium and, to a lesser extent, calcium channel	Headache Nausea Vomiting Dizziness Sedation Ataxia	Rash, significantly worse if co-administered with valproate Steven Johnson's syndrome (serious rash with multisystem failure

Some Commonly Used Antidepressants

CLASS	PRIMARY INDICATION(S)	PHARMACOKINETICS		PHARMACO-DYNAMICS	SIDE EFFECTS	ADVERSE EFFECTS
		Half-life/ Dose (mg)	Other			
Nonselective reuptake inhibitors						
Imipramine (Tofranil) Amitriptyline (Elavil)	Melancholia Chronic pain Enuresis	20-24 hours 100-200	1st pass	NE,5HT	Anticholinergic Quinidine-like Orthostatic Sedation	Fractured hip (in elderly) DeliriuM (in elderly) Paralytic ileus
Partially specific reuptake inhibitors						
Clomipramine (Anafranil)	OCD	1 day 200-300	1st pass can be used IV	5HT > NE	Some anticholinergic Sedation Orthostatic	Fractured hip (in elderly) Delirium (in elderly)
Desipramine (Norpramin)	Depression	1-2 days 100-200	1st pass	NE > 5HT	Some anticholinergic Quinidine-like Sedation	Same as above

NE = norepinephrine
5HT = 5 hydroxytryptamine
DA = dopamine

Some Commonly Used Antidepressants

CLASS	PRIMARY INDICATION(S)	PHARMACOKINETICS Half-life/ Dose (mg)	PHARMACOKINETICS Other	PHARMACO-DYNAMICS	SIDE EFFECTS	ADVERSE EFFECTS
Nortriptyline (Pamelor, Aventyl)	Depression	1 day 75-150	1st pass Rt. U-shaped dose response curve (50-170 ng/ml)	NE > 5HT	Sedation Orthostatic Quinidine-like Some anticholinergic	Same as above
Selective reuptake inhibitors						
Fluoxetine (Prozac) (SSRI)	Nonmelancholic depression Anxiety disorder OCD	7-14 days 20-60	1st pass inhibits liver enzymes	5HT	Decreased libido Anorgasmia Delayed ejaculation Akathisia Weight loss Headache Tremors Agitation	Serotonin reaction Incompatible with MAOI
Paroxetine Paxil) (SSRI)	Nonmelancholic depression OCD Eating disorders	18 hrs 20-50		5HT	Insomnia Sweating Nausea Vomiting Fatigue	Incompatible with MAOI

SSRI = selective serotonin reuptake inhibitor

Some Commonly Used Antidepressants

CLASS	PRIMARY INDICATION(S)	PHARMACOKINETICS Half-life/ Dose (mg)	PHARMACOKINETICS Other	PHARMACO-DYNAMICS	SIDE EFFECTS	ADVERSE EFFECTS
Nefazodone (Serzone) (SSRI)	Depression	3 hours 200-500	1st pass	5HT 5HT auto receptor	Sedation Fatigue Drowsiness Orthostatic Upper respiratory problems	Incompatible with MAOI
Sertraline (Zoloft) (SSRI)	Depression Anxiety disorder	1-2 days 50-200	1st pass	5HT>NE,DA	Diarrhea Tremors Dry mouth	Incompatible with MAOI
Citalopram (Celexa) Escitalopram* (Lexapro) (SSRI)	Depression	35 hours	1st pass	Highly selective for 5HT Minimal NE, DA	Somnolence Insomnia GI upset Fatigue	May cause hyponatremia and SIADH Incompatible with MAOI
Venlafaxine (Effexor) (NSRI)	Depression Anxiety disorder OCD	6-12 hours 225-475	1st pass	5HT, NE Higher doses also DA	Sexual problems Sedation Sweating	Hypertension (higher doses)

NSRI = norepinephrine serotonin reuptake inhibitor

*Escitalopram is an isomer of citalopram and presumably has fewer side effects and better tolerability

Some Commonly Used Antidepressants

CLASS	PRIMARY INDICATION(S)	PHARMACOKINETICS Half-life/ Dose (mg)	PHARMACOKINETICS Other	PHARMACO- DYNAMICS	SIDE EFFECTS	ADVERSE EFFECTS
Bupropion (Wellbutrin) (DA and NE RI)	Nonmelancholic depression Anticraving	12 hours 150-300	1st pass U-shaped dose response curve	DA NE	Restlessness Hyperactivity Tremors Insomnia	Seizures
Mirtazapine (Remeron)	Depression	1-2 days		5 HT, alpha 2 & NE receptor blocker	Sedation Weight gain	Hypertension (higher doses)
MAOI (monoamine oxidase inhibitor)						
Phenelzine (Nardil)	Depression Anxiety disorders Used less often these days	1 day 90-120		All monoamine neuro-transmitters	Orthostatic Weight gain Excitement Muscle twitching	Hypertensive crisis Cannot use with stimulants or opioids Avoid foods with tyramine

References

Abrams R: *Electroconvulsive Therapy, Fourth Edition.* New York, Oxford University Press, 2002.

Abrams R, Taylor MA: The importance of schizophrenic symptoms in the diagnosis of mania. *Am J Psychiatry* 1981;138:658-661.

Agras WS: Treatment of eating disorder. In Schatzberg A, Nemeroff C (eds): *Textbook of Psychopharmacology, 2nd Edition.* Washington DC, American Psychiatric Press, 1998.

Aharanovich E, Liu X, Nunes E, Hasin DS: Suicide attempts in substance abusers: Effects of major depression in relation to substance use disorders. *Am J Psychiatry* 2002;159:1600-1602.

Akiskal HS: Towards a definition of dysthymia: Boundaries with personality and mood disorders. In Burton SW, Akiskal HS (eds), *Dysthymic Disorder.* Gaskell, Royal College of Psychiatrists, 1990, pp. 1-12.

Akiskal HS: The temperamental borders of affective disorders. *Acta Psychiatr Scand* 1994;89:32-37.

Akiskal H, Chen S, Glenn D, Puzantian V, Kashgarian M, Bolinger J: Borderline: An adjective in search of a noun. *J Clin Psychiatry* 1985;46:41-48.

Alden LE: Short-term structured treatment for avoidant personality disorder. *J Consult Clin Psychol* 1989;57:756-764.

Alexander GE, Crutcher MD, De Long MR: Basal ganglia-thalamocortical circuits: Parallel substrates for motor, oculomotor, "prefrontal" and "limbic" functions. In Ulyings HMB, Van Eden CG, De Bruin JPC, Corner MA, Feenstra MA (eds): *The Prefrontal Cortex: Its Structure, Function and Pathology. Progress in Brain Research, Vol. 85.* Amsterdam, Elsevier, 1990, pp. 119-146.

Alexander GE, De Long MR: Strict parallel organization of functionally segregated circuits linking basal ganglia and cortex. *Ann Rev Neurosci* 1986;9:357-381.

Alving J: Serum prolactin levels are elevated also after pseudoepileptic seizures. *Seizure* 1998;7:85-89.

Altshuler LL: Bipolar disorder: Are repeated episodes associated with neuroanatomic and cognitive changes? *Biol Psychiatry* 1993;33:563-565.

Altshuler LL, Cohen L, Szuba MP, Burt VK, Gitlin M, Mintz J: Pharmacologic management of psychiatric illness during pregnancy: Dilemmas and guidelines. *Am J Psychiatry* 1996;153:592-606.

Ambrosini PJ, Bennett DS, Cleland CM, Haslam N: Taxonicity of adolescent melancholia: A categorical or dimensional construct? *J Psychiatr Res* 2002;36:247-256.

American Psychiatric Association: *Practice Guidelines.* Washington DC, American Psychiatric Association, 1996.

American Psychiatric Association Task Force on ECT: *The Practice of Electroconvulsive Therapy: Recommendations for Treatment, Training, and Privileging.* Washington DC, American Psychiatric Association Press, 1990.

American Psychiatric Association Task Force on Laboratory Tests in Psychiatry: The dexamethasone suppression test: An overview of its current status in psychiatry. *Am J Psychiatry* 1987;144:1253-1262.

Andersen K, Balldin J, Gottfries CG, Granerus AK, Modigh K, Svennerholm L, Wallin A: A double-blind evaluation of electroconvulsive therapy in Parkinson's disease with "on-off" phenomenon. *Acta Neurol Scand* 1987;76:191-199.

Atre-Vaidya N, Hussain SM: Borderline personality disorder and bipolar mood disorder: Two distinct disorders or a continuum? *J Nerv Ment Dis* 1999;187:313-315.

Atre-Vaidya N, Jampala VC: Electroconvulsive therapy in Parkinsonism with affective disorder. *Brit J Psychiatry* 1988;152:55-58.

Atre-Vaidya N, Taylor MA: The sensitization hypothesis and importance of psychosensory features in mood disorder: A review. *J Neuropsychiatry Clin Neurosci* 1997;9:525-533 1997.

Atre-Vaidya N, Taylor MA, Seidenberg MS, Reed R, Perrine A, Glick-Oberwise F: Cognitive deficits, psychopathology, and psychosocial functioning in mood disorders. *Neuropsychiatry Neuropsychol Behav Neurol* 1998;11:120-126.

Aylward GP, Brager P: Relations between visual and auditory continuous performance tests in a clinical   population. *Dev Neuropsychol* 2002;21:285-303.

Ballenger JC: Benzodiazpines. In Schatzberg A, Nemeroff C (eds), *Textbook of Psychopharmacology,* Washington DC, American Psychiatric Press, 1998a, pp. 271-286.

Ballenger JC, Davidson JR, Lecrubier Y, Nutt DJ, Baldwin DS, den Boer JA, Kasper S, Shear MK: Consensus statement on panic disorder from the International Consensus Group on Depression and Anxiety. *J Clin Psychiatry* 1998b;59(suppl 8):47-54.

Barker WW, Yoshii F, Loewenstein DA, Chang JY, Apicella A, Pascal S, Boothe TE, Ginsberg MD, Duara R: Cerebrocerebellar relationship during behavioral activation: A PET study. *J Cereb Blood Flow and Metab* 1991;11:48-54.

Battaglia M, Bernardeschi L, Franchini L, Bellodi L, Smeraldi E: A family study of schizotypal disorder. *Schizophr Bull* 1995;21:33-45.

Baum AL, Misri S: Selective serotonin-reuptake inhibitors in pregnancy and lactation. *Harvard Rev Psychiatry* 1996;4:117-125.

Behl C, Rupprecht R, Skutella T, Holsboer F: Haloperidol-induced death—mechanism and protection with vitamin E in vitro. *Neuroreport* 1995;7:360-364.

Beitchman JH, Wilson B, Johnson CJ, Atkinson L, Young A, Adlaf E, Escobar M, Douglas L: Fourteen-year follow-up of speech/language impaired and control children: Psychiatric outcome. *J Am Acad Child Adolesc Psychiatry* 2001;40:75-82.

Benson DF, Ardila A: *Aphasia: A Clinical Approach*. New York, Oxford University Press, 1996, pp. 29-41.

Berner P, Musalek M, Walter H: Psychopathological concepts of dysphoria. *Psychopathology* 1987;20:93-100.

Betts T, Boden S: Pseudoseizures (non-epileptic attack disorder). In Trimble MR (ed): *Women and Epilepsy,* New York, John Wiley & Sons, 1991, pp.243-258.

Binder LM: Persisting symptoms after mild head injury: a review of the post-concussive syndrome. *J Clin Exp Neuropsychol* 1986;8:323-346.

Black B, Uhde TW: Treatment of elective mutism with fluoxetine: a double-blind, placebo controlled study. *J Am Acad Child Adolesc Psychiatry* 1994;33:1000-1006.

Blumer D: Epilepsy and disorders of mood. *Adv Neurol* 1991;55:185-195.

Bodkin JA, Amsterdam JD: Transdermal selegiline in major depression: a double-blind, placebo-controlled, parallel-group study in outpatients. *Am J Psychiatry* 2002;159:1869-1875.

Bolla KI, Cadet JL, London ED: The neuropsychiatry of chronic cocaine abuse. *J Neuropsychiatry Clin Neurosci* 1998;10:289-289.

Boutros NN, Bowers MB: Chronic substance-induced psychotic disorders: state of the literature. *J Neuropsychiatry Clin Neurosci* 1996;3:262-269.

Bowman ES, Coons PM: The differential diagnosis of epilepsy, pseudoseizures, dissociative identity disorder, and dissociative disorder not otherwise specified. *Bull Menninger Clin* 2000;64:164-180.

Bredesen DE: Potential role of gene therapy in the treatment of Parkinson's disease. *Clin Neurosci* 1993;1:45-52.

Bremner JD, Krystal JH, Charney DS, Southwick SM: Neural mechanisms on dissociative amnesia for childhood abuse: Relevance to the current controversy surrounding the "false memory syndrome." *Am J Psychiatry* 1996;153(suppl):71-82.

Brodaty H, Hickie I, Mason C, Prenter L: A prospective follow-up study of ECT outcome in older depressed patients. *J Affect Disord* 2000;60:101-111.

Brown ES, Rush AJ, McEwen BS: Hippocampal remodeling and damage by corticosteroids: implications for mood disorders. *Neuropsychopharmacology* 1999;21:474-484.

Brown RJ, Trimble MR: Dissociative psychopathology, non-epileptic seizures, and neurology. *J Neurol Neurosurg Psychiatry* 2000;69:285-289.

Bush G, Fink M, Petrides G, Dowling F, Francis A: Catatonia. I. Rating scale and standardized examination. *Acta Psychiatr Scand* 1996a ;93:129-136.

Bush G, Fink M, Petrides G, Dowling F, Francis A: Catatonia. II. Treatment with lorazepam and electroconvulsive therapy. *Acta Psychiatr Scand* 1996b;93:137-143.

Butzlaff RL, Hooley JM: Expressed emotion and psychiatric relapse: A meta-analysis. *Arch Gen Psychiatry* 1998;55:547-552.

Caine ED, Grossman H, Lyness JM: Delirium, dementia, and amnestic and other cognitive disorders and mental disorders due to a general medical condition. In Kaplan KI, Sadock NJ (eds): *Comprehensive Textbook of Psychiatry, Volume 1, 6th Edition*. Baltimore; Williams & Wilkins, 1995, pp. 705-754.

Camfield P, Camfield C: How often does routine pediatric EEG have an important unexpected result? *Can J Neurol Sci* 2000;27:321-324.

Campbell JJ III, Duffy JD: Treatment strategies in amotivated patients. *Psychiatr Ann* 1997;27:44-49.

Campbell M, Malone RP: Mental retardation and psychiatric disorders. *Hosp Community Psychiatry* 1991;42:374-479.

Carney RM, Freedland KE, Sheline YI, Weiss ES: Depression and coronary heart disease: A review for cardiologists. *Clin Cardiol* 1997;20:196-200.

Caroff SN, Mann SC, Keck PE: Specific treatment of the neuroleptic malignant syndrome. *Biol Psychiatry* 1998;44:378-381.

Castellanos FX, Sharp WS, Gottesman RF, Greenstein DK, Giedd JN, Rapoport JL: Anatomic brain abnormalities in monozygotic twins discordant for attention deficit hyperactivity disorder. *Am J Psychiatry* 2003;160:1693-1696.

Chanpattana W: Combined ECT and clozapine in treatment-resistant mania. *J ECT* 2000;16:204-207.

Chanpattana W, Chakrabhand ML, Sackeim HA, Kitaroonchai W, Kongsakon R, Techakasem P, Buppanharun W, Tuntirungsee Y, Kirdcharoen N: Continuation ECT in treatment-resistant schizophrenia: A controlled study. *J ECT* 15:178-192, 1999.

Charney DS, Nagy LM, Bremer JD, Goddard AW, Yehuda R, Southwich SM: Neurobiological mechanisms of human anxiety. In Fogel BS, Schiffer RB, Rao SM (eds), *Neuropsychiatry*. Baltimore; Williams & Wilkins, 1996.

Charney DS, Nestler EJ, Bunney BS: *Neurobiology of Mental Illness.* New York; Oxford University Press, 1999.

Christen-Zaech S, Draftsik R, Pillevuit O, Kiraly M, Martins R, Khalili K, Miklossy J: Early olfactory involvement in Alzheimer's disease. *Can J Neurol Sci* 2003;30:20-25.

Chu JW, Matthias DF, Belanoff J, Schatzberg A, Hoffman AR, Feldman D: Successful long-term treatment of refractory Cushing's disease with high-dose mifepristone (RU 486). *J Clin Endocrinol Metab* 2001;86:3568-3573.

Chung TK, Lau TK, Yip AS, Chiu HF, Lee DT: Antepartum depressive symptomatology is associated with adverse obstetric and neonatal outcomes. *Psychosom Med* 2001;63:830-834.

Cloninger CR: Brain networks underlying personality development. In: Carroll BJ, Barrett JE (eds), *Psychopathology and the Brain.* American Psychopathological Association Series. New York; Raven Press, 1991, pp. 183-208.

Cloninger CR, Svrakic DM, Przybeck TR: A psychobiological model of temperament and character. *Arch Gen Psychiatry* 1993;50:975-990.

Combes A, Peytavin G, Theron D: Conduction disturbances associated with venlafaxine. *Ann Int Med* 2001;134:166-167.

Cooper TB, Simpson GM: The 24-hour lithium level as a prognosticator of dosage requirements: A 2-year follow-up study. *Am J Psychiatry* 1976;133:440-443.

Coryell W, Schlesser M: The dexamethasone suppression test and suicide prediction. *Am J Psychiatry* 2001;158:748-753.

Cummings JL: Organic psychoses. Delusional disorders and secondary mania. *Psychiatr Clin North Am* 1986;9:293-311.

Cummings JL: Behavioral complications of drug treatment of Parkinson's disease. *J Am Geriatr Soc* 1991;39:708-716.

Cummings JL: Frontal-subcortical circuits and human behavior. *Arch Neurol* 1993;50:873-880.

Cummings JL: Behavioral and psychiatric symptoms associated with Huntington's disease. *Adv Neurol* 1995;65:179-186.

Cummings JL, Benson DF: *Dementia: A Clinical Approach, 2nd Edition.* Boston; Butterworth-Heinemann, 1992.

Cummings JL, Mega MS: *Neuropsychiatry and Behavioral Neuroscience.* New York; Oxford University Press, 2003, pp. 234-243.

Curyto KJ, Johnson J, TenHave T, Mossey J, Knott K, Katz IR: Survival of hospitalized elderly patients with delirium: a prospective study. *Am J Geriatr Psychiatry* 2001;9:141-147.

Cutting DJ: Body image disturbances in neuropsychiatry. In Reynolds EH, Trimble MR (eds), *The Bridge Between Neurology and Psychiatry.* Edinburgh; Churchill Livingstone, 1989.

Dark FL, McGrath OJ, Ron MA: Pathological laughing and crying. *Aust N Z J Psychiatry* 1996;4:472-479.

Davidson JR: Pharmacotherapy of social phobia. *Acta Psychiatr Scand Suppl* 2003;417:65-71.

de Lignieres B, Vincens M: Differential effects of exogenous oestradiol and progesterone on mood in post-menopausal women: Individual dose/effect relationship. *Maturitas* 1982;4:67-72.

DeLong MR, Wichmann T: Basal ganglia-thalamocortical circuits in Parkinsonian signs. *Clin Neurosci* 1993;1:18-26.

Denicoff KD, Meglathery SB, Post RM, Tandeciarz SI: Efficacy of carbamazepine compared with other agents: a clinical practice survey. *J Clin Psychiatry* 1994;55:70-76.

Devanand DP, Michaels-Marston KS, Liu X, Pelton GH, Padilla M, Marder K, Bell K, Stern Y, Mayeux R: Olfactory deficits in patients with mild cognitive impairment predict Alzheimer disease at follow-up. *Am J Psychiatry* 2000;157:1399-1405.

DeVane CL: Principles of pharmacokinetics and pharmacodynamics. In Schatzberg A, Nemeroff C (eds), *Textbook of Psychopharmacology.* Washington DC; American Psychiatric Press, 1998, pp. 155-170.

Diener HC, Kaube H, Limmroth V: Antimigraine drugs. *J Neurol* 1999;246:515-519.

Dietrich DE, Emrich HM: The use of anticonvulsants to augment antidepressant medication. *J Clin Psychiatry* 1998;59(suppl 5):51-58.

Donovan S, Clayton A, Beeharry M, Jones S, Kirk C, Waters K, Gardner D, Faluding J, Madeley R: Deliberate self-harm and antidepressant drugs: Investigation of a possible link. *Brit J Psychiatry* 2000;177:551-556.

Dulcan MK, Bregman J, Weller EB, Weller R: Treatment of childhood and adolescent disorders. In Schatzberg AF, Nemeroff CB (eds), *The American Psychiatric Press Textbook of Psychopharmacology, 2nd Edition.* Washington DC; American Psychiatric Press, 1998.

Dunn LM, Dunn LM: *Peabody Picture Vocabulary Test-Revised.* Circle Pines, MN; American Guidance Service, 1981.

Dvoredsky AE, Cooley HW: Comparative severity of illness in patients with combined medical and psychiatric diagnoses. *Psychosomatics* 1986;27:625-630.

Dwight MM, Stoudemire A: Effects of depressive disorders on coronary artery disease: A review. *Harv Rev Psychiatry* 5:115-122, 1997.

Eisenberg L: School phobia. *Am J Psychiatry* 1958;114:172-178.

Eisendrath SJ: Psychiatric aspects of chronic pain. *Neurol* 1995;45(suppl 9):S26-S34.

Edwards RH: Pathogenesis of Parkinson's disease. *Clin Neurosci* 1993;1:46-44.

Emslie G, Rush AJ, Weinberg WA, Kowatch RA, Hughes CW, Carmody T, Rintelmann J: Double-blind, randomized placebo-controlled trial of fluoxetine in depressed children and adolescents. *Arch Gen Psychiatry* 1997;54:1031-1037.

Emslie GJ, Weinberg WA, Kowatch RA: Mood disorders. In Coffey CE, Brumback RA: *Textbook of Pediatric Neuropsychiatry.* Washington DC; American Psychiatric Press, 1998, pp. 359-392.

ENRICHD Investigators: Enhancing recovery in coronary heart disease patients (ENRICHD): study design and methods. *Am Heart J* 2000;139:1-9.

ENRICHD Investigators: Enhancing recovery in coronary heart disease (ENRICHD) study intervention: rationale and design. *Psychosom Med* 2001;63:747-755.

Erdemoglu AK, Ozbakir S: Valproic acid in prophylaxis of refractory migraine. *Acta Neurol Scand* 2000;102:354-358.

Evans DL, Staab JP, Petitto JM, Morrison MF, Szuba MP, Ward HE, Wingate B, Luber MP, O'Reardon JP: Depression in the medical setting: Biopsychological interactions and treatment considerations. *J Clin Psychiatry* 1999;60(suppl 4):40-55.

Fall PA, Ekman R, Granerus AK, Thorell LH, Walinder J: ECT in Parkinson's disease. Changes in motor symptoms, monoamine metabolites and neuropeptides. *J Neural Transm Park Dis Dement Sect* 1995;10:129-140.

Fallon BA, Liebowitz MR, Campeas R, Schneier FR, Marshall R, Davies S, Goetz D, Klein DF: Intravenous clomipramine for obsessive-compulsive disorder refractory to oral clomipramine: a placebo-controlled study. *Arch Gen Psychiatry* 1998;55:918-924.

Fals-Stewart W, Lucente S: Effect of neurocognitive status and personality functioning on length of stay in residential substance abuse treatment: an integrative study. *Psychol Addict Behav* 1994;8:179-190.

Fava G, Grandi S, Zielezny M, Canestrari R, Morphy M: Cognitive behavioral treatment of residual symptoms in primary major depressive disorder. *Am J Psychiatry* 1994;151:1295-1299.

Fava GA, Molnar G, Block B, Lee JS, Perini GI: The lithium loading dose method in a clinical setting. *Am J Psychiatry* 1984;141:812-813.

Fava M: Management of nonresponse and intolerance: Switching strategies. *J Clin Psychiatry* 2000;61(suppl 2):10-12.

Fava M, Davidson KG: Definition and epidemiology of treatment resistant depression. *Psychiatr Clin North America* 1996;19:179-200.

Fenwick P: Evocation and inhibition of seizures: behavioral treatment. In Smith DB, Treiman DM, Trimble MR (eds): *Advances in Neurology, Volume 55, Neurobehavioral Problems in Epilepsy.* New York; Raven Press, 1991.

Ferrell MJ, Kehoe WA, Jacisin JJ: ECT during pregnancy: physiologic and pharmacologic considerations. *Convulsive Therapy* 1992;8:186-200.

Fink JS: Neurobiology of basal ganglia receptors: Targets for future therapy in Parkinson's disease. *Clin Neurosci* 1993;1:27-35.

Fink M: Convulsive therapy in delusional disorders. *Psychiatr Clin North Am 18:*393-405, 1995.

Fink M: Toxic serotonin syndrome or neuroleptic malignant syndrome. *Pharmacopsychiatry* 1996;29:159-161.

Fink M, Taylor MA: *Catatonia: A Clinician's Guide to Diagnosis and Treatment.* Cambridge, UK; Cambridge University Press, 2003.

Fishbain DA: The association of chronic pain and suicide. *Semin Clin Neuropsychiatry* 1999;4:221-227.

Folstein MF, Folstein SE, McHugh PR: "Mini-mental state". A practical method for grading the cognitive state of patients for the clinician. *J Psychiatry Res* 1975;12:189-198.

Forssman H: Follow-up study of sixteen children whose mothers were given electric convulsive therapy during gestation. *Acta Psychiatr Neurol Scand* 1955;30:437-441.

Fountoulakis KN, Lacovides A, Nimatoudis I, Kaprinis G, Lerodiakonou C: Comparison of the diagnosis of melancholic and atypical features according to DSM-IV and somatic syndrome according to ICD-10 in patients suffering from major depression. *Eur Psychiatry* 1999;14:426-433.

Frankenburg WK, Dick NP, Carland J: Development of preschool-aged children of different social and ethnic groups: implications for developmental screening. *J Pediatrics* 1975;87:125-132.

Frankenburg WK, Dodds JB, Fandal AW: *Denver Developmental Screening Test – Manual/Workbook for Nursing and Paramedical Personal.* Denver; Ladoca Project and Publishing Foundation, 1973.

Frijda, NH: *The Emotions.* Cambridge; Cambridge University Press, 1986, pp. 379-381.

Fulton M, Winokur G: A comparative study of paranoid and schizoid personality disorders. *Am J Psychiatry* 1993;150:1363-1367.

Gagne Jr GG, Furman MJ, Carpenter LL, Price LH: Efficacy of continuation ECT and antidepressant drugs compared to long-term antidepressants alone in depressed patients. *Am J Psychiatry* 2000;157:1960-1965.

Galer BS: neuropathic pain of peripheral origin: advances in pharmacologic treatment. *Neurology* 1995;45(suppl 9):S17-S25.

Geller B, Fox LW, Clark KA: Rate and predictions of prepubertal bipolarity during follow-up of 6 to 12 year old depressed children. *J Am Acad Child Adolesc Psychiatry* 1994;33:461-468.

Ghaziuddin M, Ghaziuddin N, Greden J: Depression in persons with autism: Implications for research and clinical care. *J Autism Dev Disord* 2002;32:299-306.

Gilmore WS: Anticonvulsants in the treatment of mood disorders: assessing current and future roles. *Expert Opin Pharmacother* 2001;2:1597-1608.

Gitlin MJ: Pharmacotherapy of personality disorders: conceptual framework and clinical strategies. *J Clin Psychopharmacol* 1993;13:343-353.

Gladstone GL, Mitchell PB, Parker G, Wilhem K, Austin MP, Eyers K: Indicators of suicide over 10 years in a specialist mood disorders unit sample. *J Clin Psychiatry* 2001;62:945-951.

Glassman AH, Kanter SJ, Shostak M: Depression, delusions, and drug response. *Am J Psychiatry* 1975;132:716-719.

Glassman AH, O'Connor CM, Califf RM, Swedberg K, Schwartz P, Bigger JT Jr, Krishnan KR, van Zyl LT, Swenson JR, Finkel MS, Landau C, Shapiro PA, Pepine CJ, Mardekian J, Harrison WM, Barton D, McIvor M; Sertraline Antidepressant Heart Attack Randomized Trial (SADHEART Group): Sertraline treatment of major depression in patients with acute MI or unstable angina. *JAMA* 2002;288:701-709.

Glassman AH, Shapiro PA: Depression and the course of coronary artery disease. *Am J Psychiatry* 1998;155:4-11.

Glaxo-SmithKline. Data on file. Study 603, file RM1997/00712/00. Durham, NC, 1997.

Goldberg JF, Frye MA, Dunn RT: Pramipexole in refractory bipolar depression. *Am J Psychiatry* 1999;156:798. (Letter to the Editor)

Goldstein LB: Potential effects of common drugs on stroke recovery. *Arch Neurol* 1998;55:454-456.

Gonzales GR: Central pain: Diagnosis and treatment strategies. *Neurology* 1995;45(suppl 9):S11-S16.

Goodwin DW, Gabrielli WF Jr: Alcohol: Clinical aspects. In Lowinson JH, Ruiz P, Millman RB, Langrod JG (eds), *Substance Abuse: A Comprehensive Textbook, 3rd Edition.* Baltimore; Williams & Wilkins, 1997.

Goodwin FK, Jamison KR: *Manic-Depressive Illness.* New York; Oxford University Press, 1990.

Grafman J, Salazar A: Traumatic brain injury. In Fogel BS, Schiffer RB, Rao SM (eds), *Neuropsychiatry.* Baltimore; Williams & Wilkins, 1996.

Graybiel AM: Functions of the nigrostriatal system. *Clin Neurosci* 1993;1:12-17.

Grigoroiu-Serbanescu M, Wickramaratne PJ, Hodge SE, Milea S, Mihailescu R: Genetic anticipation and imprinting in bipolar I illness. *Br J Psychiatry* 1997;170:162-166.

Grodernberger D: Medical emergencies. In Cary CF, Lee HH, Woeltje KF (eds), *Washington Manual of Therapeutics, 29th Edition.* Philadelphia; Lippincott Raven, 1998.

Gultekin SH, Rosenfeld MR, Voltz R, Eichen J, Posner JB, Dalmau J: Paraneoplastic limbic encephalitis: Neurological symptoms, immunological findings and tumour association in 50 patients. *Brain* 2000;123:1481-1494.

Guze SB (ed), David RB (series ed): *Washington University Adult Psychiatry.* St. Louis; Mosby, 1997.

Guze SB, Woodruff RA Jr, Clayton PJ: The significance of psychotic affective disorders. *Arch Gen Psychiatry* 1975;32:1147-1150.

Hammen C: Generation of stress in the course of unipolar depression. *J Abnorm Psychol* 1199;100:555-561.

Harkness KL, Monroe SM, Simons AD, Thase M: The generation of life events in recurrent and non-recurrent depression. *Psychol Med* 1999;29:135-144.

Hanlon TE, Schoenrich C, Freinek W, Turek I, Kurland AA: Perphenazine-benztropine mesylate treatment of newly admitted psychiatric patients. *Psychopharmacologia* 1966;9:328-339.

Harrison P, Jonas J, Hudson J, Cohen B, Gunderson J: The validity of DSM-III borderline personality disorder. *Arch Gen Psychiatry* 1983;40:23-30.

Hellerstein DJ, Kocsis JH, Chapman D, Steward JW, Harrison W: Double-blind comparison of sertraline, imipramine, and placebo in the treatment of dysthymia effects on personality. *Am J Psychiatry* 2000;157:1436-1444.

Himadi WG, Cerny JA, Barlow DH, Cohen S, O'Brien GT: The relationship of marital adjustment to agoraphobia treatment outcome. *Behav Res Ther* 1986:24:107-115.

Hirschfeld RM, Allen MH, McEvoy JP, Keck PE Jr, Russell JM: Safety and tolerability of oral loading divalproex sodium in acutely manic bipolar patients. *J Clin Psychiatry* 1999;60:815-818.

Hoffman B, Ladwig KH, Schapperer J, Deisenhofer I, Marten-Mittag B, Schmitt C: Psycho-neurogenic factors as a cause of life-threatening arrhythmia. *Nervenarzt* 1999;70:830-835.

Hoffman RS, Koran LM: Detecting physical illness in patients with mental disorders. *Psychosomatics* 198425:654-660.

Hogan DB, Patterson C: Progress in clinical neurosciences: Treatment of Alzheimer's disease and other dementias – review and comparison of the cholinesterase inhibitors. *Can J Neurol Sci* 2002;29:306-314.

Horrigan JP, Barnhill LJ: Guanfacine and secondary mania in children. *J Affect Disord* 1999;54:309-314.

Horst WD, Preskorn SH: Mechanisms of action and clinical characteristics of three atypical antidepressants: Venlafaxine, nefazodone, bupropion. *J Affect Disord* 1998;51:237-254.

Howland RH: Thyroid dysfunction in refractory depression: implications for pathophysiology and treatment. *J Clin Psychiatry* 1993;54:47-54.

Huang HM, Ou HC, Hsieh SJ: Antioxidants prevent amyloid peptide-induced apoptosis and alteration of calcium homeostasis in cultured cortical neurons. *Life Sci* 2000;66:1879-1892.

Hurley SC: Lamotrigine update and its use in mood disorders. *Ann Pharmacother* 2002;36:860-873.

Inoue T, Tsuchiya K, Miura J, Sakakibara S, Denda K, Kasahara T, Koyama T: Bromocriptine treatment of tricyclic and heterocyclic antidepressant-resistant depression. *Biol Psychiatry* 1996;40:151-153.

Irani DN: The neuropsychiatry of the transmissible spongiform encephalopathies (prion diseases). *Psychiatr Ann* 2001;31:207-214.

Izumi T, Inoue T, Kitagawa N, Nishi N, Shimanaka S, Takahashi Y, Kusumi I, Odagaki Y, Denda K, Ohmori T, Koyama T: Open pergolide treatment of tricyclic and heterocyclic antidepressant-resistant depression. *J Affect Disord* 2000;16:127-132,.

Jagust WJ: Functional imaging in dementia: A review. *J Clin Psychiatry* 1994;55(suppl):5-11.

Jagust WJ, Johnson KA, Holman BL: SPECT perfusion imaging in the diagnosis of dementia. *J Neuroimaging* 1995;5 (suppl):S45-52.

Jamison KR: Suicide and bipolar disorder. *J Clin Psychiatry* 2000;61(suppl 9):47-51.

Jampala C, Abrams R, Taylor MA: Mania with emotional blunting. Affective disorder or schizophrenia? *Am J Psychiatry* 1985;145:608-612.

Jampala VC, Atre-Vaidya N, Taylor MA, Schrift MJ, Srinivasraghavan J, Sierles FS. Profile of psychomotor symptoms in psychiatric patients. *Neuropsychiatry Neuropsychol Behav Neurol* 1992;5:15-19.

Jelic V, Nordberg A: Early diagnosis of Alzheimer disease with positron emission tomography. *Alzheimer Dis Assoc Disord* 2000;14 (suppl):S109-S113.

Jones B, Taylor CC, Meehan K: The efficacy of a rapid-acting intramuscular formulation of olanzapine for positive symptoms. *J Clin Psychiatry* 2001;62(suppl 2):22-24.

Joyce PR, Mulder RT, Cloninger CR: Temperament predicts clomipramine and desipramine response in major depression. *J Affect Disord* 1994; 30:35-46.

Kales HC, Dequardo JR, Tandon R: Combined electroconvulsive therapy and clozapine in treatment-resistant schizophrenia. *Prog Neurpsychopharmacol Biol Psychiatry* 1999;23:547-556.

Kantor SJ, Glassman AH: Delusional depressions: Natural history and response to treatment. *Br J Psychiatry* 1977;131:351-360.

Kapfhammer HP, Hippius H: Special feature: Pharmacotherapy in personality disorders. *J Personal Disord* 1998;12:277-288.

Kaplan HI, Saddock BJ: *Pocket Handbook of Emergency Psychiatric Medicine.* Baltimore; Williams & Wilkins, 1993, pp. 115-117.

Kaplan R: Epilepsy syndrome. In Coffey E, Brumback R (eds), *Textbook of Pediatric Neuropsychiatry.* Washington DC; American Psychiatric Press, 1998.

Kauffer D, Cummings JL: Personality alteration in degenerative brain disease. In Ratey J, *Neuropsychiatry of Personality Disorders.* Cambridge, MA; Blackwell Science, 1995.

Keck PE Jr, McElroy SL, Tugrul KC, Bennett JA: Valproate oral loading in the treatment of acute mania. *J Clin Psychiatry*1993; 54:305-308.

Keepers GA, Clappison VJ, Casey DE: Initial anticholinergic prophylaxis for neuroleptic-induced extrapyramidal syndromes. *Arch Gen Psychiatry*1983;40:1113-1117.

Keitner GI, Ryan CE, Miller IW, Kohn R, Epstein NB: 12-month outcome of patients with major depression and comorbid psychiatric or medical illness (compound depression). *Am J Psychiatry* 1991;148:345-350.

Keller MB, Harrison W, Fawcett JA, Gelenberg A, Hirschfeld RM, Klein D, Kocsis JH, McCullough JP, Rush AJ, Schatzberg A, Thase ME: Mood disorders: Treatment of chronic depression with sertraline or imipramine: Preliminary blinded response rates and high rates of undertreatment in the community. *Psychopharmacol Bull* 1995;31:205-212.

Kendler KS, Masterson CC, Davis KL: Psychiatric illness in first-degree relatives of patients with paranoid psychosis, schizophrenia and medical illness. *Br J Psychiatry* 1985;147:524-531.

Ketter TA, Pazzaglia PJ, Post RM: Synergy of carbamazepine and valproic acid in affective illness: case report and review of the literature. *J Clin Psychopharm* 12:276-281, 1992.

Khan A, Warner HA, Brown WA: Symptom reduction and suicide risk inpatients treated with placebo in antidepressant clinical trials: An analysis of the Food and Drug Administration database. *Arch Gen Psychiatry* 2000;57:311-317.

Kobak KA, Greist JH, Jefferson JW, Katzelnick DJ, Henk H: Behavioral versus pharmacological treatments of obsessive compulsive disorder: a meta-analysis. *Psychopharmacology* 1998;136:205-216.

Kogure D, Matsuda H, Ohnishi T, Asada T, Uno M, Kunihiro T, Nakano S, Takasaki M: Longitudinal evaluation of early Alzheimer's disease using brain perfusion SPECT. *J Nucl Med* 2000;41:1155-1162.

Kolb B, Whishaw IQ: *Fundamentals of Human Neuropsychology, 4th Ed.* New York; W.H. Freeman, 1996.

Koller WC, Silver DE, Lieberman A (suppl eds): Algorithm for the management of Parkinson's disease. *Neurology* 1994;44(suppl):S1-S52.

Koran LM: *Obsessive-Compulsive and Related Disorders In Adults. A Comprehensive Clinical Guide.* Cambridge; Cambridge University Press, 1999, pp. 75-76.

Koren G, Pastuszak A, Ito S: Drugs in pregnancy. *N Engl J Med* 1998;338:1128-1137.

Kornstein SG, Schatzberg AF, Thase ME, Yonkers KA, McCullough JP, Keitner GI, Gleenberg AJ, Davis SM, Harrison WM, Keller MB: Gender differences in treatment response to sertraline versus imipramine in chronic depression. *Am J Psychiatry* 2000;157:1445-1452.

Kovacs M: Presentation and course of major depressive disorder during childhood and later years in the life span. *J Am Acad Child Adolesc Psychiatry* 1996;35:705-715.

Kowatch RA, DelBello MP: The use of mood stabilizers and atypical antipsychotics in children and adolescents with bipolar disorders. *CNS Spectrums* 2003;8:273-280.

Kowatch RA, Sethuraman G, Hume JH, Kromelis M, Weinberg WA: Combination pharmacotherapy in children and adolescents with bipolar disorder. *Biol Psychiatry* 2003;53:978-984.

Kowatch RA, Suppes T, Carmody TJ, Bucci JP, Hume JH, Kromelis M, et al: Effect size of lithium, divalprox sodium and carbamazepine in children and adolescents with bipolar disorder. *J Am Acad Child Adolesc Psychiatry* 2000;39:713-720.

Krakauer J, Balmaceda C, Gluck JT, Posner JB, Fetell MR, Dalmau J: Anti-Yo-associated paraneoplastic cerebellar degeneration in a man with adenocarcinoma of unknown origin. *Neurology* 1996;46:1486-1487.

Kroessler D: Relative efficacy rates for therapies of delusional depression. *Convulsive Ther* 1985;1:173-182.

Kraus JF, Sorenson SB: Epidemiology. In Silver JM, Yudofsky SC, Hales RE (eds): *Neuropsychiatry of Traumatic Brain Injury.* Washington DC; American Psychiatric Press, 1994.

Krauthammer C, Klerman GL: Secondary mania: Manic syndromes associated with antecedent physical illness or drugs. *Arch Gen Psychiatry* 1978;35:1333-1339.

Kupchik M, Spivak B, Mester R, Reznik I, Gonen N, Weizman A, Kotler M: Combined electroconvulsive-clozapine therapy. *Clin Neuropharmacol* 2000;23:14-16.

Landau WM, Kleffner FR: Syndrome of acquired aphasia with convulsive disorder in children. *Neurology* 1957;7:523-530.

Landre NA, Taylor MA: Formal thought disorder in schizophrenia: Linguistic, attentional, and intellectual correlates. *J Nerv Ment Dis* 1995;183:673-680.

Lang AE, Lozano AM: Parkinson's disease. First of two parts. *N Engl J Med* 339:1044-1053 1998a.

Lang AE, Lozano AM: Parkinson's disease. Second of two parts. *N Engl J Med* 1998b;339:1130-1143.

Lavoie KL, Fleet RP: The impact of depression on the course and outcome of coronary artery disease: Review for cardiologists. *Can J Cardiol* 2000;16:563-662.

Leckman JF, Cohen DJ (eds): *Tourette's Syndrome. Tics, Obsessions, Compulsions: Developmental Psychopathology and Clinical Care.* New York; John Wiley & Sons, 1999.

Leckman JF, Cohen DJ: Tic disorders. In Lewis M (ed), *Child and Adolescent Psychiatry, 2nd Edition.* Williams & Wilkins; Baltimore, 1996, p. 625.

Leibenluft E, Charney DS, Pine DS: Researching the pathophysiology of pediatric bipolar disorder. *Biol Psychiatry* 2003;53:1009-1020.

Leichnetz GR, Astruc J: Efferent connections of the orbitofrontal cortex in the marmoset (Saguinus oedipus). *Brain Res* 1975a;84:169-180.

Leichnetz GR, Astruc J: Preliminary evidence for a direct projection of the prefrontal cortex to the hippocampus in the squirrel monkey. *Brain Behav Evol* 1975b;11:355-364.

Lezak MD: *Neuropsychological Assessment, 3rd Edition.* New York; Oxford University Press, 1995.

Li G, Silverman JM, Altstiel LD, Haroutunian V, Perl DP, Purohit D, Birstein S, Lantz M, Mohs RC, Davis KL: Apolipoprotein E-epsilon 4 allele and familial risk in Alzheimer's disease. *Genet Epidemiol* 1996;13:285-298.

Liddell MB, Lovestone S, Owne MJ: Genetic risk of Alzheimer's disease: Advising relatives. *Br J Psychiatry* 2001;178:7-11.

Litman RE, Curphy T, Shneidman ES, Farberow NL, Tabachnik N: Investigations of equivocal suicides. *JAMA* 1963;184;924-929.

Litvan I, MacIntyre A, Goetz CG, Wenning GK, Jellinger K, Verny M, Bartko JJ, Jankovic J, McKee A, Brandel JP, Cahudhuri KR, Lai EC, D'olhaberriague L, Pearce RKB, Agid Y: Accuracy of the clinical diagnoses of Lewy body disease, Parkinson disease, and dementia with Lewy bodies. *Arch Neurol* 1998;55:969-978.

Livingston R: Anxiety disorders. In Lewis M (ed), *Child and Adolescent Psychiatry, 2nd Edition.* Baltimore; Williams & Wilkins, 1996.

Loftis JM, Hauser P: Co-management of depression and HCV treatment. *Psychiatr Ann* 2003;33:385-391.

Lucchinetti CF, Kimmel DW, Lennon VA: Paraneoplastic and oncologic profiles of patients seropositive for type 1 antineuronal nuclear autoantibodies. *Neurology* 1998;50:652-657.

Maes M, Cosyns P, Maes L, D'Hondt P, Schotte C: Clinical subtypes of unipolar depression: Part I. A validation of the vital and nonvital clusters. *Psychiatry Res* 1990;34:29-41.

Maes M, Maes L, Schotte C, Vandewoude M, Martin M, D'Hondt P, Blockx P, Scharpe S, Cosyns P: Clinical subtypes of unipolar depression: Part III. Quantitative differences in various biological markers between the cluster analytically generated nonvital and vital depression classes. *Psychiatry Res* 1990;34:59-75.

Maes M, Schotte C, Maes L, Cosyns P: Clinical subtypes of unipolar depression: Part II. Quantitative and qualitative clinical differences between the vital and nonvital depressive groups. *Psychiatry Res* 31990;4:43-57.

Magee WJ, Eaton WW, Wittchen H-U, McGonagle KA, Kessler RC: Agoraphobia, simple phobia, and social phobia in the National Comorbidity Survey. *Arch Gen Psychiatry* 1996;53:159-168.

Mamelak M: The Motor vehicle collision injury syndrome. *Neuropsychiatry Neuropsychol Behav Neurol* 2000;13:125-135.

Markham CH, Diamond SG: Clinical overview of Parkinson's disease. *Clin Neurosci* 1993;1:5-11.

Marneros A, Tsuang MT(eds): *Schizoaffective Psychoses.* Berlin-Heidelberg; Springer-Verlag, 1986.

Marra C, Silveri MC, Gainotti G: Predictors of cognitive decline in the early stage of probable Alzheimer's disease. *Dement Geriatr Cogn Disord* 2000;11:212-218.

Masi G, Mucci M, Millepiedi S: Separation anxiety disorder in children and adolescents: epidemiology, diagnosis and management. *CNS Drugs* 2001;15:93-104.

McAllister TW: Mild traumatic brain injury and the postconcussive syndrome. In Silver JM, Yudofsky SC, Hales RE: *Neuropsychiatry of Traumatic Brain Injury.* Washington DC; American Psychiatric Press, 1994.

McCombs JS, Stimmel GL, Hui RL, White TJ: The economic impact of treatment non-response in major depressive disorders. In Amsterdam JD, Hornio M, Nierenberg AA (eds), *Treatment-Resistant Mood Disorders.* Cambridge UK; Cambridge University Press, 2001, pp. 491-516.

McCracken JT: Attention-deficit/hyperactivity disorder II: Neuropsychiatric aspects. In Coffey CE, Brumback RA (eds): *Textbook of Pediatric Neuropsychiatry*, Washington DC; American Psychiatric Press, 1998.

Mesulam MM: *Principles of Behavioral and Cognitive Neurology, 2nd Edition.* New York; Oxford University Press, 2000.

Miller JR: Multiple sclerosis. In Rowland LP (ed), *Merritt's Neurology, 10th Edition,* Philadelphia; Lippincott Williams & Wilkins, 2000, pp. 773-791.

Miller LJ: Use of electroconvulsive therapy during pregnancy. *Hosp Community Psychiatry* 1994;45:444-450.

Miller R, Chouinard G: Loss of striatal cholinergic neurons as a basis for tardive and L-dopa-induced and neuroleptic-induced supersensitivity psychosis and refractory schizophrenia. *Biol Psychiatry* 1993;34:713-738.

Moellentine C, Rummans T, Ahlskog E, Harmsen WS, Suman VJ, O'Connor MK, Black JL, Pileggi T: Effectiveness of ECT in patients with Parkinsonism. *J Neuropsychiatry Clin Neurosci* 1998;10:187-193.

Moldavsky M, Lev D, Lerman-Sagie T: Behavioral phenotypes of genetic syndromes: a reference Guide for psychiatrists. *J Am Acad Child Adolesc Psychiatry* 2001;40:749-761.

Molho ES, Factor SA: Worsening of motor features of parkinsonism with olanzapine. *Mov Disord* 1999;14:1014-1016.

Monk C: Stress and mood disorders during pregnancy: implications for child development. *Psychiatr Q* 2001;72:347-357.

Motto J: Liability issues and liability prevention in suicide. In Jacobs DG (ed): *Suicide Assessment and Intervention.* San Francisco; Jossy Bass, 1999.

Mukherjee AB, Svoronos S, Ghazanfari A, Martin PR, Fisher A, Roecklein B, Rodbard D, Staton R, Behar D, Berg CJ, et al: Transketolase abnormality in cultured fibroblasts from familial chronic alcoholic men and their male offspring. *J Clin Invest* 1987;79:1039-1043.

Mukherjee S, Sackeim HA, Schnur DB: Electroconvulsive therapy of acute manic episodes: a review of 50 years' experience. *Am J Psychiatry* 1994;151:169-176.

Murphy BEP: Antiglucocortoid therapies in major depression: A review. *Psychoneuroendocrinology* 1997;22:S125-132.

Musselman DL, Marzec UM, Manatunga A, Penna S, Reemsnyder A, Knight BT, Baron A, Hanson SR, Nemeroff CB: Platelet reactivity in depressed patients treated with paroxetine: preliminary findings. *Arch Gen Psychiatry* 2000;57:875-882.

Nagaratnam N, Pathma-Nathan N: Behavioural and psychiatric aspects of silent cerebral infarction. *Br J Clin Pract* 1997;51:160-163.

Nathan PE, Gorman JM (eds): *A Guide to Treatments That Work*. New York; Oxford University Press, 1998.

National Pharmaceutical Council, Inc: *Pain: Current Understanding of Assessment, Management, and Treatments* (monograph), 2001.

Nazoe S, Naruo T, Yonekura R, Nakabeppu YU, Soejima Y, Nagai N, Nakajo M, Tanaka H: Comparison of regional cerebral blood flow in patients with eating disorders. *Brain Res Bull* 1995;36:251-255.

Nelson EC, Cloninger CR: The tridimensional personality questionnaire as a predictor of response to nefazodone treatment of depression. *J Affect Disord* 1995;35:51-57.

Neufeld MY, Chistik V, Vishne TH, Korczyn AD: The diagnostic aid of routine EEG findings in patients presenting with a presumed first-ever unprovoked seizure. *Epilepsy Res* 2000;42:197-202.

Neuman JK, Peeples B, East J, Ellis AR: Nicotine reduction: Effectiveness of bupropion. *Br J Psychiatry* 2000;177:87-88.

Nicoll JA, Roberts GW, Graham DI: Apolipoprotein E epsilon 4 allele is associated with deposition of amyloid beta-protein following head injury. *Nat Med* 1995;1:135-137.

Nigl AJ, Jackson B: Electromyograph biofeedback as an adjunct to standard psychiatric treatment. *J Clin Psychiatry* 1979;40:433-436,

Nutt JG: Pharmacotherapy of Parkinson's disease. *Clin Neurosci* 1993;1:64-68.

O'Donohue NV: *Epilepsies of Childhood I, 3rd Edition*. Oxford, UK; Butterworth-Heinemann, 1994.

O'Hara K, Suzuki Y, Ochiai M, Yoshida K, Ohara K: Age of onset anticipation in anxiety disorders. *Psychiatry Res* 89:215-221, 1999.

O'Hara MW, Zekoski EM, Philipps LH, Wright EJ: Controlled prospective study of postpartum mood disorders: comparison of childbearing and nonchildbearing women. *Abnorm Psychol* 1990;99:3-15.

Olson RP: A long-term, single-group follow-up study of biofeedback therapy with chronic medical and psychiatric patients. *Biofeedback Self Regul* 1988;13:331-346.

Oquendo MA, Ellis SP, Greenwald S, Malone KM, Weissman MM, Mann JJ: Ethnic and sex differences in suicide rates relative to major depression in the United States. *Am J Psychiatry* 2001;158:1652-1658.

Oribe E, Amini R, Nissenbaum E, Boal B: Serum prolactin levels are elevated after syncope. *Neurology* 1996;47:60-62.

Oshima A, Higuchi T: Treatment guidelines for geriatric mood disorders. *Psychiatry Clin Neurosci* 1999;53 Suppl:S55-59.

Pandurangi AK, Devi V, Channabasavanna SM: Caudate atrophy in irreversible tardive dyskinesia - a pneumoencephalographic study. *J Clin Psychiatry* 1980;41:229-231.

Papka M, Rubio A, Schiffer RB: A review of Lewy body disease, an emerging concept of cortical dementia. *J Neuropsychiatry Clin Neurosci* 1998;10:267-279.

Parker G: Classifying depression: Should paradigms lost be regained? *Am J Psychiatry* 2000;157:1195-1203.

Parker G, Roy K, Hadzi-Pavlovic D: Psychotic (delusional) depression: a meta-analysis of physical treatments. *J Affect Disord* 24:17-24, 1992.

Patel SP, Gaw AC: Suicide among immigrants from the Indian subcontinent: a review. *Psychiatr Serv* 1996;47:517-521.

Paul R: Disorders of communication. In Lewis M (ed): *Child and Adolescent Psychiatry, 2nd Edition.* Baltimore; Williams & Wilkins, 1996.

Paykel ES: Epidemiology of refractory depression. In Nolen WA, Zohar J, Roose JP, Amsterdam JD (eds), *Refractory Depression: Current Strategies and Future Directions.* Chichester, UK; John Wiley, 1994, pp. 3-17.

Pechard A, Besson AS, Mialon A, Berny C, Manchon M: Critical analysis of different methods used for toxicology screening in emergency laboratory. *Ann Biol Clin* 1999;57:525-537.

Pelham WE, Bender ME, Caddell J, Booth S, Moorer SH: Methylphenidate and children with attention deficit disorder. *Arch Gen Psychiatry* 1985;42:948-952.

Perry PJ, Alexander B, Liskow BI: *Psychotropic Drug Handbook, 7th Edition.* Washington DC; American Psychiatric Press, 1997.

Peskind ER: Pharmacologic approaches to cognitive deficits in Alzheimer's disease. *J Clin Psychiatry* 1998;59 (suppl):22-27.

Petersen RC: Mild cognitive impairment: Transition between aging and Alzheimer's disease. *Neurologia* 2000;15:93-101.

Petrides G, Dhossche D, Fink M, Francis A: Continuation ECT: Relapse prevention in affective disorders. *Convuls Ther* 1994;10:189-194.

Petrides G, Fink M, Husain MM, Knapp RG, Rush AJ, Mueller M, Rumm TA, O'Connor KM, Rasmussen KG Jr, Bernstein HJ, Biggs M, Bailine SH, Kellner CH: ECT remission rates in psychotic versus nonpsychotic depressed patients: A report from CORE. *J ECT* 2001;17:244-253.

Petrides G, Divadeenam KM, Bush G, Francis A: Synergism of lorazepam and electroconvulsive therapy in the treatment of catatonia. *Biol Psychiatry* 1997;42:375-381.

Petronis A, Kennedy JL: Unstable genes-unstable mind? *Am J Psychiatry* 1995;152:164-172.

Pies R: Adverse neuropsychiatric reactions to herbal and over-the-counter "antidepressants." *J Clin Psychiatry* 2000;61:815-820.

Pliszka SR: Non-stimulant treatment of attention-deficit/hyperactivity disorder. *CNS Spectrums* 2003;8;253-258.

Pomerleau CS, Pomerleau OF, Flessland KA, Basson SM: Relationship of tridimensional Personality Questionnaire scores and smoking variables in female and male smokers. *J Subst Abuse* 1992; 4:143-154.

Popper CW: Psychopharmacologic treatment of anxiety disorders in adolescents and children. *J Clin Psychiatry* 1993;54(suppl):52-63.

Posner JB, Dalmau JO: Paraneoplastic syndromes of the nervous system. *Clin Chem Lab Med* 2000;38:117-122.

Post RM, Kopanda RT: Cocaine, kindling, and psychosis. *Am J Psychiatry 133*:627-634, 1976.

Post RM, Rubinow DR, Ballenger JC: Conditioning sensitization and kindling: implications for course of affective illness. In Post RM, Ballenger JC (eds), *Neurobiology of Mood Disorders.* Baltimore; Williams & Wilkins, 1984, pp. 432-466.

Post RM, Weiss S: Kindling and manic depressive illness. In Bolwig TG, Trimble MR (eds), *The Clinical Relevance of Kindling.* New York; John Wiley and Sons, 1989, pp. 209-230.

Preskorn SH: *Clinical Pharmacology of Selective Serotonin Reuptake Inhibitors, 1st Edition.* Caddo, OK; Professional Communications, 1996.

Preskorn SH, Burke M: Somatic therapy for major depressive disorder: selection of an antidepressant. *J Clin Psychiatry* 1992;53(suppl):5-18.

Pridmore S, Yeo PT, Pasha MI: Electroconvulsive therapy for the physical signs of Parkinson's disease without depressive disorder (letter). *J Neurol Neurosurg Psychiatry* 1995;58:641-642.

Prudic J, Sackeim HA: Electroconvulsive therapy and suicide risk. *J Clin Psychiatry* 1999;60 (suppl 2):104-110.

Pullicino PM, Pordell R: Computed tomography and magnetic resonance of subcortical ischemic lesions. In Pullicino PM, Caplan, Hommel M (eds), *Advances in Neurology, Vol. 62.* New York; Raven Press, 1993.

Rabins PV, Folstein MF: Delirium and dementia: Diagnostic criteria and fatality rates. *Br J Psychiatry* 1982;140:149-153.

Rao V, Lyketsos C: Neuropsychiatric sequelae of traumatic brain injury. *Psychosomatics* 2000;41:95-103.

Rasmussen KG, Abrams R: Treatment of Parkinson's disease with electroconvulsive therapy. *Psychiatr Clin North Am* 1991;14:925-933.

Rauh SL, Renshaw P: Clinical neuroimaging in psychiatry. *Harvard Rev Psychiatry* 1995;2:297-312.

Remick RA, Maurice WL: ECT in pregnancy (letter). *Am J Psychiatry* 1978;135:761-762.

Renneberg B, Goldstein AJ, Phillips D, Chambless DL: Intensive behavioral group treatment of avoidant personality disorder. *Behavior Therapy* 1990;21:363-377.

Reznik I, Rosen Y, Rosen B: An acute ischaemic event associated with the use of venlafaxine: a case report and proposed pathophysiological mechanisms. *J Psychopharmacol* 1999;13:193-195.

Richelson E: Pharmacology of antidepressants – characteristics of the ideal drug. *Mayo Clin Proc* 1994;69:1069-1081.

Robinson R, Starkstein S: Neuropsychiatric aspects of cerebrovascular disorders. In Yudofsky SC, Hales RE, *The American Psychiatric Press Textbook of Neuropsychiatry, 3rd Edition.* Washington DC; American Psychiatric Press, 1997.

Rojas I, Graus F, Keime-Guibert F, Rene R, Delattre JY, Ramon JM: Long-term clinical outcome of paraneoplastic cerebellar degeneration and anti-Yo antibodies. *Neurology* 2000;55:713-715.

Roose SP, Dalack GW, Glassman AH, Woodring S, Walsh BT, Giardina EG: Cardiovascular effects of bupropion in depressed patients with heart disease. *Am J Psychiatry* 1991;148:512-516.

Roose SP, Glassman AH, Attia E, Woodring S: Comparative efficacy of selective serotonin reuptake inhibitors and tricyclics in the treatment of melancholia. *Am J Psychiatry* 1994;151:1735-1739.

Rosenblatt A, Leroi I: Neuropsychiatry of Huntington's disease and other basal ganglia disorders. *Psychosom* 2000;41:24-30.

Rowbotham MC: Chronic pain: From theory to practical management. *Neurol* 1995;45(suppl 9):S5-S10.

Rubia K, Overmeyer S, Taylor E, Brammer M, Williams SC, Simmons A, Bullmore ET: Hypofrontality in attention deficit hyperactivity disorder during higher order motor control: a study with functional MRI. *Am J Psychiatry* 1999;156:891-896.

Rucci P, Frank E, Kostelnik B, Fagiolini A, Mallinger AG, Swartz HA, Thase ME, Siegel L, Wilson D, Kupfer DJ: Suicide attempts in patients with bipolar I disorder during acute and maintenance phases of intensive treatment with pharmacotherapy and adjunctive psychotherapy. *Am J Psychiatry* 2002;159:1160-1164.

Ryan ND: Medication treatment for depression in children and adolescents. *CNS Spectrums* 2003;8:283-287.

Salloway S, White J: Paroxysmal limbic disorders in neuropsychiatry. *J Neuropsychiatry Clin Neurosci* 1997;9:403-419.

Sapolsky RM, Krey LC, McEwen BS: The neuroendocrinology of stress and aging: The glucocorticoid cascade hypothesis. *Endocr Rev* 7:284-301, 1986.

Sapolsky RM: Glucocorticoids and hippocampal atrophy in neuropsychiatric disorders. *Arch Gen Psychiatry* 2000;57:925-935.

Sato T, Hirano S, Narita T, Kusunoki K, Kato J, Goto M, Sakado K, Uehara T: Temperament and character inventory dimensions as a predictor of response to antidepressant treatment in major depression. *J Affect Disord* 1999;56:153-161.

Saxena A: Issues in newborn screening. *Genet Test* 2003;7:131-134.

Schatzberg AF, Cole JO: *Manual of Clinical Psychopharmacology, 2nd Edition.* Washington DC; American Psychiatric Press, 1991.

Scheibel AB: The thalamus and neuropsychiatric disease. *J Neuropsychiatry Clin Neurosci* 1997;9:342-353.

Schmahmann JD (ed): *The Cerebellum and Cognition.* San Diego, CA; Academic Press, 1997.

Schneider K: *Clinical Psychopathology.* New York; Grune and Stratton, 1959 (Hamilton MW, translator).

Schneider B, Philipp M, Muller MJ: Psychopathological predictors of suicide in patients with major depression during a 5-year follow-up. *Eur Psychiatry* 2001;16:283-288.

Schneier FR: Treatment of social phobia with antidepressants. *J Clin Psychiatry* 2001;(suppl 1):43-48.

Schneier FR, Johnson J, Hornig CD, et al: Social phobia. Comorbidity and morbidity in an epidemiologic sample. *Arch Gen Psychiatry* 1992;49:282-288.

Selkoe DJ: Alzheimer's disease: Genotypes, phenotype, and treatments. *Science* 1997;275:630-631.

Seltzer EG, Gerber MA, Cartter ML, Freudigman K, Shapiro ED: Long-term outcomes of persons with Lyme disease. *JAMA* 2000;283:609-616.

Sergent J, Signoret JL: Implicit access to knowledge derived from unrecognized faces in prosopagnosia. *Cereb Cortex* 1992a;2:389-400.

Sergent J, Signoret JL: Varieties of functional deficits in prosopagnosia. *Cereb Cortex* 1992b;2:375-388.

Serretti A, Lattuada E, Cusin C, Macciardi F, Smeraldi E: Analysis of depressive symptomatology in mood disorders. *Depress Anxiety* 1998;8:80-85.

Sharma V, Yatham LN, Haslam DR, Silverstone PH, Parikh SV, Matte R, Kutcher SP, Kusumakar V: Continuation and prophylactic treatment of bipolar disorder. *Can J Psychiatry* 1997;42(Suppl 2):92S-100S.

Shay KA, Roth DL: Association between aerobic fitness and visuospatial performance in healthy older adults. *Psychol Aging* 1992;1:15-24.

Sheline YI: Neuroimaging studies of mood disorder effects on the brain. *Biol Psychiatry* 2003;54:338-352.

Shprintzen RJ, Goldberg RB, Lewin ML, Sidoti EJ, Berkman MD, Argamaso RV, Young D: A new syndrome involving cleft palate, cardiac anomalies, typical facies, and learning disabilities. Velo-cardio-facial syndromes. *Cleft Palate J* 1978;15:56-62.

Siegel BV Jr, Asarnow R, Tanguay P, Call JD, Abel L, Ho A, Lott I, Buchsbaum MS: Regional cerebral glucose metabolism and attention in adults with a history of childhood autism. *J Neuropsychiatry Clin Neurosci* 1992;4:406-414.

Sierles FS, Chen JJ, McFarland RE, Taylor MA: Posttraumatic stress disorder and concurrent psychiatric illness: a preliminary report. *Am J Psychiatry* 1983;140:1177-1179.

Silberman EK, Post RM, Nurnberger J, Theodore W, Boulenger JP: Transient sensory, cognitive and affective phenomena in affective illness. A comparison with complex partial epilepsy. *Br J Psychiatry* 1985;146:81-89.

Silver JM, Yudofsky SC, Hales RE (eds): *Neuropsychiatry of Traumatic Brain Injury.* Washington DC; American Psychiatric Press, 1994.

Silverman JM, Li G, Zaccario ML, Smith CJ, Schmeidler J, Mohs RC, Davis KL: Pattern of risk in first-degree relatives of patients with Alzheimer's disease. *Arch Gen Psychiatry* 1994;51:577-586.

Simard M, van Reekum R, Cohen T: A review of the cognitive and behavioral symptoms in dementia with Lewy bodies. *J Neuropsychiatry Clin Neurosci* 2000;12:425-450.

Simon, GE: Management of somatoform and factitious disorders. In Nathan PE, Gorman JM (eds), *Treatments That Work.* New York, Oxford University Press, 1998.

Simon RI: *Clinical Psychiatry and the Law, 2nd Edition.* Washington DC; American Psychiatric Press, 1992.

Simon RI: Psychiatry and law. In Talbott J, Hales RE, Yudofsky (eds), *Textbook of Psychiatry, 2nd Edition.* Washington DC; American Psychiatric Press, 1994.

Slater E: Diagnosis of hysteria. *Br Med J* 1965;1:1395-1399.

Slater E, Glithero E: A follow-up of patients diagnosed as suffering from "hysteria." *J Psychosom Res* 1965;9:9-13.

Slaughter JR, Slaughter KA, Nichols D, Holmes SE, Martens MP: Prevalence, clinical manifestations, etiology, and treatment of depression in Parkinson's disease. *J Neuropsychiatry Clin Neurosci* 2001a;13:187-196.

Slaughter JR, Martens MP, Slaughter KA: Depression and Huntington's disease: prevalence, clinical manifestations, etiology, and treatment. *CNS Spectrums* 2001b;6:306-326.

Small GW: Treatment of Alzheimer's disease: current approaches and promising developments. *Am J Med* 1998;104:32S-38S.

Small JG, Klapper MH, Milstein V, Marhenke JD, Small IF: Comparison of therapeutic modalities for mania. *Psychopharmacol Bull* 1996;32:623-627.

Sohn YH, Jeong Y, Kim HS, Im JH, Kim JS: The brain lesion responsible for Parkinsonism after carbon monoxide poisoning. *Arch Neurol* 2000;57:1214-1218.

Spiker DG, Dealy RS, Hanin I, Weiss, JC, Kupfer DJ: Treating delusional depression with amitriptyline. *J Clin Psychiatry* 1986;47:243-245.

Squire LR: *Memory and Brain.* New York; Oxford University Press, 1987.

Sramek JJ, Simpson GM, Morrison RL, Heiser JF: Anticholinergic agents for prophylaxis of neuroleptic-induced dystonic reactions: A prospective study. *J Clin Psychiatry* 1986;47:305-309.

Stahl SM: *Essential Psychopharmacology, Neuroscientific Basis and Clinical Applications.* Cambridge; Cambridge University Press, 1996.

Stahl SM: Mental illness may be damaging to your brain. *J Clin Psychiatry* 1997;58:289-290.

Stahl SM: Neurotransmission of cognition, Part 1. Dopamine is a hitchhiker in frontal cortex: norepinephrine transporters regulate dopamine. *J Clin Psychiatry* 2003;64:4-5.

Starkstein SE, Manes F: Apathy and depression following stroke. *CNS Spectrums* 2000;5:43-50.

Statham DJ, Heath AC, Madden PA, Bucholz KK, Bierut L, Dinwiddie SH, Slutske WS, Dunne MP, Martin NG: Suicidal behaviour: An epidemiological and genetic study. *Psychol Med* 1998;28:839-855.

Stewart SE, Geller D, Spencer T, Gianini L: Tics and Tourette's disorder: Which therapies, and when to use them. *Current Psychiatry* 2003;2:45-56.

Stompe T, Ortwein-Swoboda G, Strobl R, Friedmann A: The age of onset of schizophrenia and the theory of anticipation. *Psychiatry Res* 2000;93:125-134.

Strakowski SM, MCElroy SL, Keck PE: Clinical efficacy of valproate in bipolar illness: Comparisons and contrasts with lithium. In Halbreich U, Montgomery SA (eds), *Pharmacotherapy for Mood, Anxiety, and Cognitive Disorders.* Washington DC; American Psychiatric Press, 2000, pp.143-157.

Sulllivan PF, Kessler RC, Kendler KS: Latent class analysis of lifetime depressive symptoms in the national comorbidity survey. *Am J Psychiatry* 1998;155:1398-1406.

Sullivan M, LaCroix A, Russo J, Swords E, Sornson M, Katon W: Depression in coronary heart disease. What is the appropriate diagnostic threshold? *Psychosomatics* 1999;40:286-292.

Suominen K, Isometsa E, Heila H, Lonnqvist J, Henriksson M: General hospital suicides--a psychological study in Finland. *Gen Hosp Psychiatry* 2002;24:412-416.

Suominen KH, Isometsa ET, Henriksson MM, Ostamo AI, Lonnqvist JK: Inadequate treatment for major depression both before and after attempted suicide. *Am J Psychiatry* 1998;155:1778-1780.

Sussman N: The role of antidepressants in sexual dysfunction. *J Clin Psychiatry Monograph* 1999;17:9-14.

Sutton I, Winer J, Rowlands D, Dalmau J: Limbic encephalitis and antibodies to Ma2: A paraneoplastic presentation of breast cancer. *J Neurol Neurosurg Psychiatry* 2000;69:266-268.

Swedo SE, Leonhard HL, Mittleman BB, Allen AJ, Rapoport JL, Dow SP,Kanter ME, Chapman F, Zabriskie J: Identification of children with pediatric autoimmune neuropsychiatric disorders are with a streptococcal infection by a marker associated with rheumatic fever. *Am J Psychiatry* 1997;154:110-112.

Swoboda E, Conca A, Konig P, Waanders R, Hansen M: Maintenance electroconvulsive therapy in affective and schizoaffective disorder. *Neuropsychobiology* 2001;43:23-28.

Tagami M, Yamagata K, Ikeda K, Nara Y, Fujino H, Kubota A, Numano F, Yamori Y: Vitamin E prevents apoptosis in cortical neurons during hypoxia and oxygen reperfusion. *Lab Invest* 1998;78:1415-1429.

421

Taylor CA, Price TRP: Neuropsychiatric assessment. In Silver JM, Yudofsky SC, Hales RE (eds): *Neuropsychiatry of Traumatic Brain Injury.* Washington DC; American Psychiatric Press, 1994.

Taylor MA: *The Fundamentals of Clinical Neuropsychiatry.* New York; Oxford University Press, 1999.

Tew JD Jr, Mulsant BH, Haskett RF, Prudic J, Thase ME, Crowe RR, Dolata D, Begley AE, Reynolds CF 3rd, Sackeim HA: Acute efficacy of ECT in the treatment of major depression in the old-old. *Am J Psychiatry* 1999;156:1865-1870.

Thase ME, Carpenter L, Kupfer DJ, Frank E: Clinical significance of reversed vegetative subtypes of recurrent major depression. *Psychopharmacol Bull* 1991;27:17-22.

Thase ME, Greenhouse JB, Frank E, Reynolds CF 3rd, Pilkonis PA, Hurley K, Grochocinski V, Kupfer DJ: Treatment of major depression with psychotherapy or psychotherapy-pharmacotherapy combinations. *Arch Gen Psychiatry* 1997;54:1009-1015.

Thompson AJ, McDonald WI: Multiple sclerosis and its pathophysiology. In Asbury AK, McKhann GM, McDonald WI: *Diseases of the Nervous System Clinical Neurobiology, Volume II, 2nd Edition.* Philadelphia; WB Saunders Company,1992, pp. 1209-1228.

Thompson TL II: Psychosomatic disorders. In Talbott JA, Hales RE, Yudofsky SC (eds), *The American Psychiatric Press Textbook of Psychiatry.* Washington DC; American Psychiatric Press, 1988.

Tomb DA: Other organic treatments. In Lewis M (ed), *Child and Adolescent Psychiatry. A Comprehensive Textbook.* Baltimore; Williams & Wilkins, 1996, pp. 912-914.

Tondo L, Baldessarini RJ: Reduced suicide risk during lithium maintenance treatment. *J Clin Psychiatry* 2000;61:97-104.

Tondo L, Baldessarini RJ, Hennen J, Floris G, Silvetti F, Tohen M: Lithium treatment and risk of suicidal behavior in bipolar disorder patients. *J Clin Psychiatry* 1998;59:405-414.

Trimble MR, Bolwig TG (eds): *Aspects of Epilepsy and Psychiatry.* New York; John Wiley & Sons, 1986.

Trimble MR: *The Psychoses of Epilepsy.* New York; Raven Press, 1991.

Tsuang MT, Woolson RF, Fleming JA: Long-term outcome of major psychoses. Schizophrenia and affective disorders compared with psychiatrically symptom-free surgical conditions. *Arch Gen Psychiatry* 1979;39:1295-1301.

Tyrer P, Casey P, Ferguson B: Personality disorder in perspective. *Br J Psychiatry* 1991;159:463-471.

Tyrer P, Seivewright N: Pharmacological treatment of personality disorders. *Clin Neuropharmacol* 1988;11:493-499.

van der Kolk BA, Fisler R: Dissociation and the fragmentary nature of traumatic memories: overview and exploratory study. *Journal of Traumatic Stress, 8:*505-525, 1995.

Vanelle JM, Loo H, Galinowski A, de Carvalho W, Bourdel MC, Brochier P, Bouvet O, Brochier T, Olie JP: Maintenance ECT in intractable manic-depressive disorders. *Convulsive Therapy* 1994;10:195-205.

van Reekum R, Black SE, Conn D, Clarke D: Cognition-enhancing drugs in dementia: A guide to the near future. *Can J Psychiatry* 42(suppl 1):35S-50S, 1997.

van Waarde J, Stolker JJ, van der Mast RC: ECT in mental retardation: A review. *J ECT* 2001;17:236-243.

Varma SL, Sharma I, Chugh S: Psychiatric morbidity in the families of paranoid and non-paranoid schizophrenia patients. *Singapore Med J* 1992;33:67-69.

Verkes RJ, Van der Mast RC, Hengeveld MW, Tuyl JP, Zwinderman AH, Van Kempen GM: Reduction by paroxetine of suicidal behavior in patients with repeated suicide attempts but not major depression. *Am J Psychiatry* 1998;155:543-547.

Volavka J*: Neurobiology of Violence*. Washington, DC; American Psychiatric Press, 1995.

Wade AG: Antidepressants in panic disorder. *Int Clin Psychopharmacol* 1999;14(suppl 2):S13-17.

Wade JB, Taylor MA, Kasprisin A, Rosenberg S, Fiducia D: Tardive dyskinesia and cognitive impairment. *Biol Psychiatry* 1987;22:393-395.

Wade TD, Bulik CM, Neale M, Kendler KS: Anorexia nervosa and major depression: Shared genetic and environmental risk factors. *Am J Psychiatry* 2000;157:469-471.

Walker R, Swartz CM: Electroconvulsive therapy during high-risk pregnancy. *Gen Hosp Psychiatry* 1994;16:348-353.

Weddington WW: The mortality of delirium: An underappreciated problem? *Psychosomatics* 1982;23:1232-1235.

Weinrieb RM, O'Brien CP: Persistent cognitive deficits attributed to substance abuse. *Neurol Clinics* 1993;11:663-691.

Weiss G: Attention deficit hyperactivity disorder. In Lewis M (ed), *Child and Adolescent Psychiatry, 2nd Edition*. Baltimore; Williams & Wilkins, 1996.

Weller EB, Weller RA, Svadjian H: Mood disorders. In Lewis M (ed), *Child and Adolescent Psychiatry. A Comprehensive Textbook, 2nd Edition*. Baltimore; William & Wilkins, 1996.

Winokur G, Coryell W, Keller M, Endicott J, Akiskal H: A prospective follow-up of patients with bipolar and primary unipolar affective disorder. *Arch Gen Psychiatry* 1993;50:457-465.

Wisner KL, Zarin DA, Holmboe ES, Appelbaum PS, Gelenberg AJ, Leonard HL, Frank E: risk-benefit decision making for treatment of depression during pregnancy. *Am J Psychiatry* 2000;157:1933-1940.

Wittling W, Block A, Genzel S, Schweiger E: Hemisphere asymmetry in parasympathetic control of the heart. *Neuropsychologia* 1998;36:461-468.

Woodside DB, Field LL, Garfinkel PE, Heinmas M: Specificity of eating disorders diagnoses in families of probands with anorexia nervosa and bulimia nervosa. *Compr Psychiatry* 1998;39:261-264.

Yatham LN, Kusumakar V, Calabrese JR, Rao R, Scarrow G, Kroeker G: Third generation anticonvulsants in bipolar disorder: A review of efficacy and summary of clinical recommendations. *J Clin Psychiatry* 2002;63:275-283.

Yeragani VK, Pesce V, Jayaraman A, Roose S: Major depression with ischemic heart disease: effects of paroxetine and nortriptyline on long-term heart rate variability measures. *Biol Psychiatry* 2002;52:418-429.

Yerby M: Pregnancy and teratogenesis. In Trimble M (ed), *Women and Epilepsy*. Chichester, UK; John Wiley & Sons, 1991, pp. 167-185.

Yonkers KA, Dyck IR, Keller MB: An eight-year longitudinal comparison of clinical course and characteristics of social phobias among men and women. *Psychiatr Serv* 2001;52:637-643.

Yudofsky SC, Hales RE: *The American Psychiatric Press Textbook of Neuropsychiatry, 2nd Edition.* Washington DC; American Psychiatric Press, 2003.

Zisook S, Schuchter SR: Uncomplicated bereavement. *J Clin Psychiatry* 1993;54:365-372.

Zisook S, Schuchter SR, Sledge PA, Paulus M, Judd LL: The spectrum of depressive phenomena after spousal bereavement. *J Clin Psychiatry* 1994;55(suppl):29-36.

GLOSSARY

Affect. Global emotional tone. The capacity to experience and convey feelings. Components include relatedness, intensity, stability, tone of voice, modulation, facial expressivity and gestures. Loss of affect, or emotional expression, is called *emotional blunting*.

Agitation. Increased frequency of motor behavior (e.g., pacing, fidgeting) usually associated with an intense mood.

Agnosia. Literally, not knowing. The inability to "recognize" or make sense of perceptions. Examples are inability to identify objects by sight, while being able to do so by touch.

Agoraphobia. Fear of losing control and panicking in a public place and not be helped promptly. Agoraphobics' fears include leaving home, leaving the neighborhood, being in traffic, being on a bridge, or being in a shopping mall.

Akathisia. Inner restlessness that causes rocking and pacing. ("I feel like I'm jumping out of my skin.") Different from agitation which is associated with anxiety. Antipsychotic drugs and pure SSRIs can cause severe akathisia.

Akinetic mutism. A state of immobility, mutism and unresponsiveness during which the patient may follow the examiner's movements with his eyes. Commonly associated with other catatonic features, and frontal circuitry lesions. Differs from the "locked-in" syndrome which is associated with cranial nerve signs and full alertness during which the patient communicates with eye blinks.

Altered sensorium. A state of reduced arousal

Alzheimer's disease. The most common type of dementia that early-on attacks the perceptual-integrating brain. Prevalence increases with age, from <2% of the population at age 65 to 25-35% by age 90.

Amnesia Loss of memory. A qualifier is always added to indicate the type of amnesia, e.g. retrograde, anterograde, global, etc

Anhedonia. Inability to experience pleasure

Anorexia nervosa. Most often diagnosed in teenage girls and young women. The obsession that one is overweight and must diet even after losing huge amounts of weight. Despite the term anorexia, appetite is usually normal, and despite the weight loss, energy is often normal. Is fatal in about 9% of sufferers.

Anosognosia. The nonrecognition of one's illness, seen in non-dominant parietal lobe and frontal lobe disease.

Anterograde amnesia. Inability to acquire new information.

Antisocial personality disorder. A Cluster B personality disorder. More common in men than women. Decreases in prevalence with age, due to premature death or "mellowing out." Disregards and violates the rights of others. Doesn't conform to legal norms. Deceitful, impulsive, aggressive, reckless, irresponsible, remorseless.

Apathy. A state of low energy and disinterest

APOE. A lipoprotein allele in the human genome associated with risk for Alzheimer's disease and other neurologic conditions. The 2/2 version carries no risk while the 4/4 the most for Alzheimer's disease.

Apraxia (dyspraxia). Severe difficulty performing a simple action despite normal strength and sensory function, and understanding the instruction.

Apraxia, constructional. See constructional dyspraxia.

Apraxia, gait. See gait apraxia.

Asperger disease. A pervasive developmental disorder in which patients have poor social skills with relatively preserved language skills.

Ataxia. Unsteady movement that can involve the head, limbs and trunk.

"A" test. A sensitive test of arousal and sustained attention. A helpful test in identifying delirium. Consists of reading a standardized set of 60 letters to the patient and asking him to tap the table with a pen when you speak the letter A. Five or more errors (or <90% of answers correct) suggests poor sustained attention.

Atypical psychotic disorder. A psychotic patient who does not meet criteria for another DSM psychotic condition. Atypical presentations (e.g., different age or type of onset, symptom pattern) strongly suggests the condition is secondary.

Automatic obedience. A catatonic feature in which the patient responds to touch despite verbal instructions to the contrary. For example, the examiner says, "Don't shake my hand," and then extends his hand to shake the patient's hand, and then the patient shakes the examiner's hand."

Avoidant personality disorder. A Cluster C personality disorder. Socially inhibited; hypersensitive to criticism; feels inadequate; avoids interpersonal contact and risks; views self as inept, inferior and unappealing. Comorbid with anxiety disorders and nonmelancholic depressions.

Avolition. Reduced motivation, concern, drive and planning. Common in schizophrenia and other dysfunctions of the dorsolateral prefrontal cortex. Ways of eliciting avolition include asking the patient how he or she spends a typical day, what he or she plans to do after discharge from the hospital, and what he or she would do if he or she won the state lottery. Along with reduced emotional expressivity, avolition is a component of emotional blunting.

Binswanger's disease. Vascular dementia, most often a frontal lobe dementia, associated with disease of hemispheric white matter, due most often to sustained hypertension.

Bipolar disorder. A mood disorder in which the patient exhibits both manic and depressive episodes.

Bipolar I disorder. The patient has recurrent episodes of mania, or manic episodes alternating with depressive episodes.

Bipolar II disorder. Episodes of major depressive disorder requiring treatment, interspersed with hypomanic episodes (or having an abnormal temperament) not requiring hospitalization. Fifty percent will make suicide attempts.

Bipolar III disorder. Childhood or early teen onset of abnormal temperament (lability, moodiness, emotionality, intense interpersonal interactions and stormy relationships), but no clear-cut episodes. Associated with drug abuse and strong family history of mood disorder. Can be mistaken for borderline personality disorder.

Bipolar spectrum disorder. Disorders that may be variants of bipolar disorder. Includes borderline personality disorder (50% meet criteria for mood disorder, cyclothymia, soft bipolar temperament; creativity; alcohol and drug abuse, alone or co-occurring with the bipolar disorder; migraine;

and irritable bowel syndrome. Bipolar II patients are more likely to be creative, and creative persons are more likely to have bipolar II disorder, than population rates predict.

Borderline personality disorder. A Cluster B personality disorder. A substantial number of such patients are bipolar and 25-50% meet criteria for bipolar II disorder or cyclothymia. Characterized by unstable relationships and self-image; outbursts of anger; impulsiveness; fearfulness about abandonment; suicidal; self-mutilating; intense, reactive and having unstable moods.

Bradyphrenia. Slowing of cognition seen in depression, frontal lobe and white matter disease, and during sedation.

Bradykinesia. Reduced motor behavior. Can reflect depression, reduced level of consciousness, Parkinson's disease and other action brain conditions.

Brief psychotic disorder with marked stressor. A psychosis with acute onset following a stressful event, with the content of hallucinations and delusions relating to the event. Also characterized by intense moods like crying, screaming or cursing; no emotional blunting; a duration of 1-2 weeks; an increased suicide risk; often initially responsive to sedation; may be a mood disorder variant and can be treated like one. Parents get this a lot. Clerkship supervisors, too.

Bulimia nervosa. Most common in young women. Characterized by binges in which the patient ingests excessive quantities of high-calorie, sweet fattening foods followed by purging behavior, which typically consists of self-induced vomiting or using emetics or laxatives. Weight is usually normal or slightly overweight.

Cachectic. Gaunt associated with weight loss and wasting.

Capgras' syndrome. The delusion that one's friends, relatives and associates are impostors. Most often associated with dysfunction of the nondominant temporoparietal cortex.

Catalepsy. A catatonic feature characterized by maintaining a position for a prolonged time.

Cataplexy. Associated with narcolepsy. Abrupt decrease or loss of muscle tone (except for eye movement and respiration) following strong emotion or, sometimes, spontaneously (in which case the cataplexy is mild). Like sleep paralysis, may be terminated by another's touch.

Catatonia. A motor regulation disturbance characterized by one (possible catatonia), two (definite catatonia) or more of these: catalepsy, waxy flexibility, stereotypy, verbigeration, Gegenhalten, echolalia, echopraxia, mitgehen, mitmachen, automatic obedience and stupor with mutism. Most often seen in major mood disorder (mania, melancholia), but also occurs in other disorders with brainstem, thalamus, basal ganglia or frontal dysfunction and schizophrenia. Observed in about 10% of acutely ill psychiatric admissions.

Circumstantiality. Responding relevantly and accurately but providing far too many details. Seen in mania, alcoholism, stimulant abuse, and epilepsy, and sometimes with normal aging. An example: "How long have I been working in Chicago? Let me tell you, it hasn't been easy. All that political stuff, then the recessions. My own health problems added to that, you know, but after all the time things have finally turned out okay. It took 15 years, however."

Cluster A personality disorders. Odd, eccentric personality disorders. Includes paranoid, schizoid and schizotypal personality disorders.

Cluster B personality disorders. Dramatic, emotional personality disorders (PDs). Includes antisocial, histrionic, narcissistic, and borderline PDs. Persons with Cluster B PDs have increased risk for somatization or conversion disorder, substance abuse, criminality, STD and conduct disorder. The cluster's diagnostic validity is limited, with 25% of persons with one Cluster B PD meeting criteria for another PD, but people can have one personality.

Cluster C personality disorders. Anxious-fearful personality disorders PDs. Includes avoidant, dependent and obsessive compulsive PD. Persons with a Cluster C PD have increased risk for anxiety disorder, non-melancholic depression, eating disorders, adjustment disorders and benzodiazepine abuse, and increased likelihood of family members having a Cluster C PD.

Cognition. General term to describe mental activities associated with think, learning and memory.

Comorbidity. The co-occurrence of two or more conditions that are presumed related in their expression in some way, e.g. bipolar disorder and alcohol abuse. When two or more conditions are present, but not directly related that is co-occurrence, e.g. sleep apnea and male pattern baldness.

Complete auditory hallucinations. Clear voices that are sustained and experienced as coming from an external source. Often the voices comment on the patient's actions or converse about the patient. Most common in schizophrenia, but can occur in other conditions like major depression with melancholic features, and mania.

Complex partial seizure. A type of seizure during which there is some alteration in arousal and responsiveness, but not full unconsciousness. The seizure is typically less than a minute and associated with complex behaviors (e.g. taking clothes off) and experiences (e.g. visual distortions).

Compulsion. Repetitive behavior performed stereotypically in response to obsessions to reduce distress or prevent a dreaded event. Examples include special prayers repeated in a set manner, hand-washing, checking, mental counting, mental list-making and mental reviewing. A key feature of obsessive compulsive disorder. Occasionally, compulsions occur without obsessions, or vice versa.

Computed axial tomography (CT). A method of brain imaging developed in the 1970s, for which its creators won the Nobel Prize. Uses ionizing radiation, so not used in pregnant women. Better than MRI for visualizing acute bleeding and bony lesions, and is the diagnostic modality of choice for acute head trauma.

Constructional apraxia. The complete inability to copy simple geometric shapes.

Constructional dyspraxia. Difficulty in copying the outline of a simple geometric shape. Associated with dysfunction of the non-dominant parietal lobe or the corpus callosum.

Constructional praxis. The ability to copy the outline of a simple geometric shape. Primarily a function of the non-dominant parietal lobe, but also requires normal functioning of other structures like the corpus callosum.

Conversion disorder. The patient has one or more medically unexplained symptoms related to sensory or voluntary motor function (i.e., pseudoneurologic symptoms). Common in somatization disorder. Twenty to 30% of patients have a general medical or neurologic disorder that explains the symptoms.

Cortical dementia. The most common cortical dementia is Alzheimer's disease. A mnemonic for cortical dementia is "four A's": amnesia (that doesn't respond to cuing); apraxia (e.g., constructional apraxia); aphasia (typically posterior aphasia, with normal fluency); and agnosia (such as anosognosia, the non-recognition of one's illness).

Cueing. Giving hints to help "jog" memory.

Cyclothymia. A mild variant of bipolar disorder. Characterized by gradual mood swings, lasting weeks or months, varying from extroverted, outgoing, optimistic, high energy, cheerful and impulsive to moody, irritable, low energy and pessimism. Each phase often causes social and job problems.

Declarative memory. Being able to state what you know, like the information in this excellent book.

Déjà vu. Been there, done that…but wasn't and didn't. When intense and frequent a psychosensory feature of limbic system dysfunction.

Delirium. Seen in 10-15% of hospitalized acutely ill general medical patients. When severe, can cause psychosis and other behavioral disturbances. Characterized by diffuse cognitive impairment with impaired alertness, attention and concentration.

Delusional perception. Giving a delusional meaning to a real perception, with no apparent connection between the perception and the interpreted meaning. For example, a person sees a robin, and believes this is a sign that the FBI is following him. Most common in schizophrenia, but can occur in other severe conditions such as melancholia and mania.

Delusion. A fixed (the patient cannot be persuaded that the belief is false) false belief that is not commonly shared by persons of similar background. A sign of psychosis, but not diagnostically specific.

Delusion, primary. A primary delusion develops de novo, from arbitrary thinking. For example, "The funny sound of the telephone and my cable TV going out means I'm being spied upon."

Delusion, secondary. A delusion that arises from other psychopathology such as a hallucination or an abnormal mood state. Two examples: 1) A person hears a hallucinated voice and concludes that what the voice says is correct; 2) A melancholic person concludes that she has done sinful things and deserves punishment.

Delusion, systematized. A delusion is that is detailed and structured like a movie plot. A central feature of delusional disorder, but sometimes occurs in other conditions such as psychosis due to a general medical condition.

Delusional mood. A nonspecific feeling of unease and suspiciousness. Not precise enough to be labeled as a delusion, and not specific for any disorder.

Delusion, mood-congruent. A delusion that occurs during a depressive or manic episode and the content of which fits the mood state, e.g., "I'm manic and the King of Bavaria."

Delusion, mood-incongruent. A delusion in a depressed or manic patient, the content of which differs from the mood state, e.g., I'm manic and the King of Bavaria, and oh, by the way, Martians have taken over Club Med."

Delusion (idea) of reference. A delusion in which others' actions, or events, are directly related to oneself, e.g., strangers in the street are looking at me and somehow know about what's been happening to me.

Delusional disorder. An uncommon disorder, with typical age of onset of 30-50. The most prominent finding is a systematized delusional story on a mundane topic like work, love, sex or trust; where the mood is normal except when the patient is responding to the delusion. If hallucinations occur, they are exclusively on the subject of the delusion. Can be subtyped as erotomanic, grandiose, jealous or somatic. May be due to a general medical condition.

Dementia. A group of conditions characterized by substantial cognitive dysfunction with poor memory, initially in the presence of normal alertness and consciousness. Although many dementias are irreversible, some are reversible (e.g., due to medications, depression in late life). The prevalence of dementia increases with age.

Dementia, cortical pattern. See cortical dementia.

Dementia due to Huntington's disease. Typically begins between 30-50 years of age, is progressive, and usually leads to death within 15-20 years of the first symptoms. Due to autosomal dominant transmission of a trinucleotide repeat (>35 CAG) on the short arm of chromosome 4, with the larger number of repeats associated with the most severe disease. A subcortical dementia. In later stages bilateral caudate atrophy presents a CT "butterfly" pattern.

Dementia due to Parkinson's disease. The most common basal ganglia disorder associated with dementia. Presents as a frontal lobe dementia, with memory impairment early on helped by cuing, motor slowing, and dorsolateral prefrontal syndrome. Classic features include motor disturbances (bradykinesia, rigidity, pill-rolling resting tremor, often in the preferred limb) and mood disturbances (non-melancholic depression in 50% of patients, mania in 5%). Associated with Lewy bodies.

Dementia, subcortical. See subcortical dementia.

Dependent personality disorder. A Cluster C personality disorder. Submissive; fears separation; indecisive; unassertive; low self-confident.

Depersonalization disorder. Persistent or recurrent experiences of feeling detached from one's body, as if one were an outside observer. Does not have established validity. Transient depersonalization is experienced by at least a third of persons exposed to danger. Depersonalization is common during panic attacks, and can be a feature of psychomotor/psychosensory epilepsy.

Derailment. The sudden, disrupted switch from one line of thought to a new, parallel line of thought. An example: "I started in the lumber business what the environmentalists don't understand trees mean jobs." An example of aphasic speech or formal thought disorder.

Derealization. The experience that the surrounding environment seems unreal, like a dream or cartoon. Can be seen in patients with anxiety disorder, drug intoxications, seizure related conditions, and mood disorder.

Desmopressin. An analog of vasopressin that can be prescribed as a nasal spray. Can effective in treating enuresis.

Digit Span. The distance from thumb to pinky OR the number of digits that can be recalled, either forward or in reverse. It is a test of working memory.

Dissociative amnesia. One or more episodes of inability to recall important personal information, usually of a traumatic or stressful nature. Common features include disorientation to person but not to time and place; indifference to memory loss; and onset under 40. Does not have established validity. Check for traumatic brain injury, high blood pressure, substance abuse or history of seizures.

Dissociative disorders. Poorly understood, of unclear diagnostic validity. Dissociation has a neurologic basis. Some of the phenomena can be explained by temporal lobe epilepsy, anxiety disorders with panic attacks, head trauma, substance abuse, and cluster B personality disorders. Should not be diagnosed until neurologic disorders known to cause dissociative symptoms have been ruled out.

Dissociative fugue. Sudden unexpected travel away from home or one's customary workplace or work, with inability to recall one's past, associated with uncertainty about one's memory. Does not have established validity. Check for drug and alcohol consumption, head trauma, history of seizures, and personality disorder.

Dissociative identity disorder (multiple personality disorder). Two or more distinct personality states co-exist, and each may suddenly take over the patient's behavior. Does not have established validity. When the patient has two identities, think of epilepsy; when he or she has many personalities, think of Cluster B personality disorders.

Dissociative (disorders) symptoms. A category in DSM that diagnostically gets you nowhere. They include depersonalization, derealization, conversion and ???

Dominant hemisphere. The hemisphere that handles language. In 99% of right handers, the left hemisphere is dominant. In 60% of left handers, the left hemisphere is dominant. The dominant hemisphere handles details, not Gestalts; processes information sequentially; uses reasoning and logic; and handles sensation and movement on the opposite side of the body.

Dorsolateral avolitional syndrome. The avolitional syndrome associated with dysfunction in the dorsolateral prefrontal cortical circuit.

Dorsolateral prefrontal circuit. Brodmann areas 9 and 10 project to the caudate head which projects to the globus pallidus and substantia nigra which, in turn, send information to the thalamus, which sends feedback to the dorsolateral prefrontal cortex. Lesions cause executive function deficits: Patients cannot generate new ideas or shift sets; lack fluency or flexibility of thought; and have problems organizing information. In presenting their history, their details may be accurate, but the history's organization is poor. Lesions in the circuit produce avolition and emotional blunting.

Dressing apraxia. The loss of the ability to dress oneself. It is endemic in second year medical students.

Driveling (jargon) speech. Fluent double-talk with good balance of large and small words seeming to form a sentence (i.e., seemingly normal syntax), but having no meaning. **Word salad** is its most severe form. An example: "I'm not rejected by the mechanistic frame, but back-hoe or not, who needs that done if he couldn't."

Dysmegalopsia. Perceived changes in an object's size. A distortion that is typically seen in drug-induced states, epilepsy and mood disorder, particularly bipolar disorder.

Dysmorphopsia. Perceived changes in an object's shape. A distortion that is typically seen in drug-induced states, epilepsy and mood disorder, particularly bipolar disorder.

Dysphoria. Anxious irritability, often but not exclusively associated with major depressive disorder with melancholic features.

Dysprosodia. Impairment of the emotional, melodic, intonation and rhythmic component of speech. Associated with non-dominant hemisphere dysfunction.

Dysprosodia, expressive. Impaired spontaneous expression of emotion and gesturing, associated with dysfunction of the homologue of Broca's area in the non-dominant hemisphere.

Dysprosodia, receptive. Impaired comprehension of the prosody of others, associated with non-dominant temporoparietal dysfunction.

Dysthymia. A silly DSM depression category that requires the patient to be chronically but only moderately depressed. Often associated with severe depressive episodes, and with poor treatment.

Dystonia. A sudden abnormal and usually painful increase in muscle tension. It can be localized to the tongue and neck or involving the whole body as in oculogyric crisis. Seen in some patients given antipsychotic drugs and some SSRIs.

Echolalia. When the patient repeats what the examiner says, when this repetition is not called for. Most often seen in catatonia and extra-sylvian global aphasia.

Echopraxia. A catatonic phenomenon in which the patient mimics the examiner's action.

Electroconvulsive therapy (ECT). Developed in the 1930s in Italy. A highly effective treatment for moderate or severe major depressive disorder, particularly melancholia; major depressive disorder with psychotic features; catatonia; mania (12-15 treatments may be necessary for manics); mixed mood states; psychoses due to general medical disorders; psychoses without emotional blunting; neuroleptic malignant syndrome; and delirium. It is most often prescribed in university medical centers and for private patients. It is neuroconversion, analogous to cardioversion. In both, electricity is used to stop an organ's abnormal rhythm, so it can naturally reboot. In cardioversion, 200-400 joules are delivered in a split second, sometimes 2-3 times. In neuroconversion (ECT), 20-100 joules are used over 4-6 seconds several times weekly for 3-4 weeks.

Electroconvulsive therapy procedure. Following informed consent, a procedure done 2-3 times weekly for 3-4 weeks under general anesthesia, full muscle relaxation, anesthesia, ventilation with 100% oxygen and vital sign monitoring. A grand mal brain seizure (no motor convulsion) is induced with electricity. Seizure usually lasts 30-60 seconds. Procedure takes about 10-15 minutes. Remission rates for patients with mood disorders who are treated in a timely fashion are 80-95%. In depressed patients treated unsuccessfully for years with medications the remission rate is about 50%.

Electroconvulsive therapy side effects. Most common immediately post-treatment, side effects include amnesia for events immediately surrounding the treatment (majority of patients, frequency reduced with unilateral ECT), headache (30% of treatments), emergence delirium (5-10% of patients), prolonged apnea (rare, treated with continued anesthesia and assisted respiration) and prolonged seizures (rare, treated with IV lorazepam).

Elliptical speech. Tightly linked associations that "orbit" the point and are on the same topic as the question or conversation, but never reach the point or answer the question. An example: Doctor: What type of work do you do? Patient: I work in Chicago. Doctor: Yes, but what do you do in Chicago? Patient: I've been there a year." Seen in schizophrenia and some dementias. Is a better term than **tangential speech**, which is often used synonymously.

Emotional blunting. The combination of loss of emotional expression and volition.

EPS. See *extrapyramidal symptoms.*

Euthymia. Normal mood range

Extrapyramidal symptoms. Symptoms associated with basal ganglia dysfunction as in Parkinson's disease or from some antipsychotic drugs.

Factitious disorder. Intentional production or feigning of general medical or psychiatric signs or symptoms without an external incentive (e.g., to receive disability payment, to avoid a difficult assignment). The patient purposely fabricates signs and symptoms and other historical data to become a patient and assume a "sick role." Epidemiology, genetics, family history, natural course and pathophysiology are unknown. **Munchausen syndrome** is an extreme example.

Flight of ideas. Jumping from topic to topic, in which the first topic is mildly related to the second, and the second topic mildly related to the third, and so forth. Common in mania. An example: "The examiner says to the patient, "What type of work do you do?" and the patient responds, "I've been working in Chicago for 15 years. The city is too crowded and what is Planned Parenthood doing about it. Being a parent is easy and college is expensive. How do we live within our means? I have the answer and the budget deficit will be solved."

Formal thought disorder. A language disorder that resembles a thalamic or basal ganglia aphasia. Speech is paraphasic and fluent. Examples include private word usage, word approximations, neologisms, nonsequiturs, driveling, phonemic paraphasia, elliptical speech, verbigeration and perseveration. Most often seen in schizophrenia or chronic drug-induced psychosis.

Fregoli syndrome. The delusion that someone in one's environment is a famous person. Most often associated with non-dominant parietal dysfunction.

Frontal lobe (action brain) dementias. Frontal lobe dementias as a group are the second most common dementia syndrome, next to Alzheimer's disease. Characterized by disruption in action (too little in avolition, too much in disinhibition). Often includes apathy and emotional blunting. Memory is usually better than behavior would predict. Cuing helps memory, and details are usually retained, but sequences are impaired. Includes primary frontal lobe cortical dementia, basal ganglia dementias (e.g., Pick's, Parkinson's, Huntington's, Wilson's diseases) and white matter dementias (e.g., vascular dementia, traumatic brain injury, alcoholism, multiple sclerosis, vitamin deficiency) dementias.

Gait apraxia. Severe difficulty in walking despite normal strength and sensory function. Most often associated with frontal lobe disease.

Gegenhalten. A catatonic phenomenon characterized by the patient exerting equal and opposite resistance to the examiner moving the patient's limb.

Generalized anxiety disorder. A low-grade, chronic form of anxiety. Persistent unrealistic worry about life circumstances associated with mild to moderate motor tension, autonomic hyperactivity, increased vigilance and scanning, fatigue and easy fatigability.

Gilles de la Tourette's. See Tourette's disorder.

Grandiose delusion. A delusion characterized by the false belief that one is famous, extraordinarily gifted, powerful or like a deity. Relatively common in mania, but can be seen in other psychoses.

Habituation. a process by which the neuron system reduces or inhibits responsiveness to a stimulus.

Hallucination. A perception in any sensory modality, for which there is no external stimulus. Not diagnostically specific, and can occur in non-pathologic conditions, such as fatigue, distractibility, and when falling asleep or awakening. A huge variety of disorders can produce hallucinations, including melancholia; bipolar disorder, manic or depressed episode; schizophrenia; schizoaffective disorder; drug-induced psychosis; and virtually any general medical or neurologic disorder (e.g., delirium, stroke, head trauma) that impairs brain structure or function. When hallucinations interfere with a person's ability to perform his or her ordinary tasks, the person is said to be psychotic.

Hallucination, command. An hallucination in which the voice directs the patient to do something.

Hallucination, complete auditory. See complete auditory hallucinations.

Histrionic personality disorder. A Cluster B personality disorder. Excessively emotional and attention seeking; seductive, dramatic and suggestible; emotionally unstable and shallow; vague in speech.

Hypergraphia. Excessive, perseverative, overly detailed and pedantic writing seen in patients with chronic temporolimbic disease or in 19th century Russian novelists.

Hypoactivity. Paucity of actions. Often seen along with slow speech in persons with melancholia, and in frontal lobe dementias.

Hypomania. A low-grade abnormal elevation in mood and energy.

Ideomotor apraxia. The inability to demonstrate the use of simple objects, despite adequate motor and sensory function and understanding of the task. Associated with dominant hemisphere disease.

Illusion. A misinterpretation of real stimuli. Can result from an intense mood, distractibility, fatigue or impaired information processing. When not the result of an intense mood, consider a hallucinogen drug-induced state, epilepsy or schizotypal personality disorder.

Jamais vu. False unfamiliarity. A psychosensory feature.

Kinesthetic apraxia. Loss of the ability to do simple movements by command.

Kleptomania. A DSM impulse disorder which is really a variation of OCD. It is the compulsion to steal, typically inexpensive and unneeded objects.

Language disorders in schizophrenia. The speech and language problems observed in schizophrenics. Sometimes referred to as Formal Thought Disorder and characterized by disorganized associations, elements of aphasia and reduced speech production.

Magnetic resonance imaging (MRI). A method of brain imaging using the magnetic properties of the human body, mainly composed of water, rather than ionizing radiation. Produces images with excellent soft-tissue contrast and spatial resolution. Especially useful for white matter lesions and visualizing the posterior fossa. More expensive, but of higher resolution than computed tomography. Can be combined with biochemical and metabolic technologies to give functional MRI.

Major depressive disorder (recurrent depressive illness, unipolar mood disorder). Episodes of substantial depression but no hypomania or mania. Commonly called "unipolar" disorder.

Major depressive disorder with melancholic features (melancholia). A subtype of major depression characterized by unremitting, intensive and dysfunction, apprehension and pessimism, psychomotor disturbance (slowing and agitation), sleep disturbance and other ultradian (90-minute) cycle disturbances and circadian rhythm disturbances (often called vegetative signs) in appetite (anorexia) and libido (loss), and hypothalamic-pituitary axis hyperactivity.

Malingering. Purposeful faking of signs and symptoms and historical information to gain external incentives (e.g., money, avoiding legal problems or difficult assignments). More common in persons with antisocial personality disorder or substance abusers. Psychiatric malingering typically involves complaints about hearing voices or being suicidal. Direct confrontation of malingerers is risky and rarely effective. Let the patient "save face," but discharge him quickly from medical care.

Melancholia. See major depressive disorder with melancholic features.

Mania. An abnormal mood state with excessive intensity, variability and responsivity associated with rapid and pressured speech, flight of ideas, abnormally high energy and inappropriate social behaviors. The necessary and sufficient condition to be classified as having bipolar mood disorder.

Mood disorder. A DSM category of conditions affecting emotions.

Morbid risk. The likelihood that a given relative or a proband has, or will develop, the disorder that the proband has.

Narcissistic personality disorder. A Cluster B personality disorder. Grandiose sense of self importance; sense of entitlement and need for excessive admiration; interpersonally exploitative, lacks empathy.

Narcolepsy. Characteristics include sleep attacks, cataplexy, sleep paralysis, hypnogogic and hypnopompic hallucinations. Sleep begins with REM instead of NREM. Highly familial, with 30-50% of offspring having narcolepsy or excessive daytime sleepiness. An autoimmune process causes dysfunction of the hypothalamic hypocretin (orexin) system.

Neologism. An example of paraphasic or aphasic speech or formal thought disorder in which the patient utters a non-word. An example: "There goes the *silverstarmer*." It is an out-of-class paraphasia.

Neomammalian brain. Part of the triune brain. Consists of the association cortices of the cerebral hemispheres, the cerebellar cortices and the corpus callosum. Functions include action (frontal loops, cerebellum), environmental interpretation (posterior-integrating system), high- (dominant hemisphere) and low-frequency (non-dominant) information processing.

Nonmelancholic depression. An episode of depression without melancholic features.

Obsessions. Intrusive, unwanted thoughts, impulses, images or sensations that cause marked anxiety and are not simply excessive worries about real life problems. A key feature of obsessive compulsive disorder and related syndromes (e.g., kleptomania, Giles de la Tourette's syndrome).

Obsessive compulsive disorder (OCD). Characterized by recurrent intrusive thoughts (obsessions) perceived by the patient (early in the illness, at least) as illogical, and which limit the patient's functioning. Common obsessions include daily decisions, outlandish behaviors, order and symmetry, dirt and contamination, and religion and philosophy. In most OCD patients, obsessions are accompanied by compulsions, which are usually (not always) driven by obsessions. May be associated with frontal-caudate pathway is dysfunction.

Obsessive compulsive personality disorder. A Cluster C personality disorder. Preoccupied with orderliness, perfectionistic, controlling, inflexible; stubborn, lacking in openness, miserly, hoarding, cannot delegate, overly conscientious, scrupulous; workaholic. In dimensional terms, low novelty seeking, high harm avoidance, low reward dependence.

Orbitomedial dysinhibited syndrome. A frontal circuitry syndrome associated with disease in the orbitomedial circuit.

Overvalued idea. A thought that occupies much of one's energies, for which the importance is exaggerated or the accuracy is doubtful, and social and employment dysfunction ensues. Not diagnostically specific. However, if after 20 years of the overvalued idea, you invent the light bulb and you're a genius.

Paleomammalian brain. Part of the triune brain. Consists of the limbic system (cingulate gyrus, septal nuclei, mammillary bodies, fornix, hippocampus, parahippocampus, amygdala, entorhinal area, perirhinal area and hypothalamus). Handles appetitive drives, fight/flight mechanisms, emotions, new learning and memory. Human paleomammalian brain dysfunctions include mania, depression, anxiety disorders, experiential hallucinations and psychosensory symptoms.

Panic disorder. Characterized by spontaneous panic attacks lasting many minutes, occurring from several times yearly to several times weekly, and not linked to specific situations. During a panic attack, several of these are present: dyspnea, paresthesias from respiratory alkalosis, light-headedness, chest discomfort, tachycardia with palpitations, slight blood pressure rise, tremor, sweating, depersonalization, and fear of dying. The typical patient has multiple medical visits and laboratory tests before it is diagnosed. IV lactate induces panic attacks in patients with panic disorder or agoraphobia.

Paranoid personality disorder. A Cluster A personality disorder. Mistrustful, suspicious, unforgiving, and grudge-bearing. Rare. May have a familial relationship with delusional disorder, as relatives of patients with delusional disorder have a higher than expected rate of paranoid personality disorder.

Paraphasia. An aphasic element of speech, e.g. misusing words such as calling a pen a "writer."

Paraphilias. A DSM category of sexual disturbances.

Passive aggressive personality disorder. Tends to express anger indirectly by procrastinating, forgetting, coming late and screwing up tasks. In dimensional terms, low novelty seeking, high harm avoidance, high reward dependence. Not included in newer DSM versions.

Persecutory delusion. A delusion characterized by the false belief that others are plotting against oneself. Can be seen in many psychotic disorders.

Perseveration. Repeating things, repeating things, repeating things.

Personality. One's lifelong, characteristic patterns of behavior, termed traits. Personality traits are highly heritable and interact with the environment.

Personality disorder. Lifelong maladaptive behavior patterns that cause functional impairment—particularly in personal relationships—or distress. Personality disorders are often co-morbid with non-psychotic disorders. For example, 40-60% of persons with anxiety disorders, non-melancholic depressions, eating disorders, and adjustment disorders have a pre-existing personality disorder.

Pharmacodynamics. A drug's effects on the body (e.g., inhibiting neurotransmitter transporters, ion channels, etc.).

Pharmacokinetics. The body's effects on the drug from absorption to excretion.

Phobia, social. See social phobia.

Phobia, specific. See specific phobia.

Pick's disease (a frontotemporal dementia). Accounts for 5% of dementias. Most are misdiagnosed as Alzheimer's disease, in part because symptoms sometimes overlap. Age of onset usually 40-60. Begins frontotemporally, progresses posteriorly. Personality change occurs early with executive function problems, with relative sparing of new learning. Patients can become avolitional or disinhibited. The dorsolateral prefrontal cortex syndrome occasionally leads to a misdiagnosis of schizophrenia.

Pill-rolling tremor. Characterized by involuntary rhythmic apposition of the thumb and forefinger, often—but not necessarily—bilateral and symmetrical. Most often seen in Parkinson's disease or parkinsonism due to antipsychotics, and most prominent when the limb is at rest (i.e., not defying gravity)

Positive symptom, nonaffective psychosis. Not an official DSM term. These patients have hallucinations and delusions, but no mood symptoms and negative symptoms. According to DSM, these patients will satisfy criteria for paranoid schizophrenia.

Positron emission tomography (PET). A method of functional brain imaging based on a) injecting F-fluoro-deoxy-glucose (FDG), which is taken up by neurons using the same active transport system as does glucose. Glucose—and, hence, FDG—metabolism is tightly coupled with neuronal activity (although FDG cannot travel beyond a certain point and becomes stranded within the neutrophil). This is a marker of gross neuronal activation. Much more expensive than computed tomography.

Post-partum psychosis. Postpartum psychosis is not a specific disorder. Rather, the numerous changes of childbirth trigger illness in women vulnerable to psychiatric disorder. Mood disorder is the most common post-partum syndrome, and depression is the most common mood disorder. This is different from "post-partum blues," which is experienced by 50% of women during the first week after delivery, and is related to changes in hormone levels.

Post-traumatic stress disorder (PTSD). An anxiety disorder following a severe traumatic event in which there was actual or threatened death, serious injury, or personal violation. Following the event, the patient emotionally detached, re-experiences the event, and is hyperaroused. If symptoms last less than a month, it is acute stress disorder. High frequency of co-morbid conditions, including OCD, panic disorder, major depressive disorder, alcohol dependence, substance abuse, cluster B personality disorders.

Posturing. What catatonics and politicians do. The difference is that catatonics maintain the posture (the position they are in) for hours, while politicians constantly change their position.

Prefrontal cortex. Brodmann's areas 9-12. Anterior portion of the frontal lobe associated with attention and concentration, working memory, logical reasoning, problem-solving, planning, abstracting ability, generating new ideas, shifting sets, spontaneous generation of language, sticking to a topic and presenting one's history in an organized fashion. Initiates fronto-striato-thalamic circuits.

Premorbid. Preceding the occurrence of disease, e.g., premorbid personality is the personality before the onset of illness.

Premotor cortex. Brodmann's area 6, the motor component of the unimodal association cortex. It contains motor programs, analogous to computer software, that direct actions by way of the corticospinal and corticobulbar tracts. Broca's area is part of the premotor cortex.

Private word usage. An example of paraphasic speech or formal thought disorder in which the patient uses a word that appears irrelevant to the sentence or topic. For example, the patient says "The *green* is going to happen next week." It is an out-of-class paraphasia.

Procedural memory. Memory that is implied in what you do but cannot be declared. If your shoe laces are tied, the implication is that you did it, but you can't relate the movements (the procedures) to prove it, you must show them.

Prosody. The emotional, melodic, intonation and rhythmic component of speech. A non-dominant hemisphere function.

Prosopagnosia. Not recognizing familiar faces or being unable to match faces in a test.

Pseudodementia. Some elderly persons with melancholia develop substantial cognitive dysfunction with normal alertness. Their dysfunction falls into the dementia range, but resolves with successful treatment of their depression. This finding has alternatively been labeled pseudodementia, treatable dementia, and pseudopseudodementia.

Pseudoprofundity. What all professors do some of the time and some patients with chronic temporolimbic disease do all of the time. It is the superficial, often perseverative, opining on an important topic such as philosophy, theology, and cosmology.

Psychosis. A disorder characterized by delusions or hallucinations that severely impair the person's ability to perform the ordinary tasks of life. Psychosis can occur in many disorders, including mood disorder, drug induced states, epilepsy, traumatic brain injury, dementia, delirium, schizophrenia, schizophreniform disorder, delusional disorder, brief psychotic disorder, postpartum psychosis, shared psychotic disorder, and atypical psychosis.

Rapid cycling. A subtype of bipolar mood disorder where the patient experiences four or more episodes in a year.

Relatedness. An ability of an individual to express warmth, to interact emotionally and empathically, and to establish rapport.

REM density. The amount of total REM time related to total sleep time.

Reptilian brain. Part of the triune brain that consists of the brainstem, vestibular system, thalamus, hypothalamus, basal ganglia, primitive amygdala and hippocampus. Handles arousal, activation, balance, information input and output, homeostatic and procreative drives, and fight/fight mechanisms. In humans, reptilian brain dysfunctions include stuporous states, catatonia and anxiety disorders.

Retrograde amnesia. Amnesia for past events that occurred before some brain function change.

RIND. Reversible Ischemic Neurologic Deficit. It lasts more than 24 hours and less than two week.

Schizoaffective disorder. A DSM psychotic disorder category condition for those who can't make up their minds whether the patient is schizophrenic, has a psychotic mood disorder, or a little of both. The patient has mood episodes but prominent psychotic features at other times.

Schizoid personality disorder. A Cluster A personality disorder characterized by a detached and restricted range of emotional expression with a paucity of interests, activities and friendships. Aggregates in the families of patients with schizophrenia. Like schizotypal personality disorder, it is probably a mild illness related to psychoses.

Schizophrenia. A syndrome that results from a complex interaction of genetic vulnerability and prenatal adverse events. As children, they are emotionally odd, motorically and socially awkward and cognitively mildly impaired. The first psychotic episode typically follows puberty. Common findings include avolition; paucity of speech; formal thought disorder; hallucinations, most often auditory; delusions (most often, non-affective primary delusions of persecution); motor disturbances and attention and cognition problems. Tends to have a chronic, deteriorating course.

Schizophreniform disorder. Symptoms and signs are the same as in schizophrenia, but the duration of the acute illness is less than the six months required for diagnosing schizophrenia. Impaired social or job functioning during some part of the illness is not required for the diagnosis. There is no validation for this category, and clinicians rarely use it.

Schizotypal personality disorder. A Cluster A personality disorder. Has schizoid personality disorder traits, plus problems with speech (it's vague); perception (illusions); and having odd beliefs and experiences (e.g., ESP, sensing spirits, and other paranormal phenomena). Like schizoid personality disorder, it is probably a mild illness related to psychoses.

Single photon emission computed tomography (SPECT). SPECT is a functional imaging technique similar to PET, but it exploits a single photon emitting nuclide. It is a less sensitive and has poorer spatial resolution, but it is reasonably priced and easily accessible.

Social phobia. The most common anxiety disorder of males, and equally frequent in males and females. Defining feature is anxiety in anticipation of and during social situations in which the patient fears—almost always inaccurately—scrutiny by others who will detect the patient's anxiety and then disparage the patient. Feared situations include public speaking, interviews, dating, parties, weddings, dances, eating or writing in public, or using public lavatories.

Somatic delusion. A delusion characterized by concerns about having a disease. Relatively common in melancholia, but can be seen in other psychoses.

Somatization disorder. A chronic condition with medically unexplained symptoms in 4 or more organ systems, including 4 or more pain symptoms, 2 or more GI symptoms; 1 or more sexual symptoms; and 1 or more pseudoneurologic symptoms. Symptoms are often presented vaguely. Increased likelihood of unnecessary tests and unnecessary surgery. Tends to run in families, with men having antisocial personality disorder and women having somatization disorder.

Specific phobia. Most common phobic disorder with typical onset in childhood. Unlike social phobia or agoraphobia, specific phobias are fears of a single object or situation. The most Common specific phobias are of animals like insects or cats; situations such as heights (acrophobia), flying or storms; and blood and injury. Persons with specific phobias usually seek treatment only if they are likely to be exposed to the feared object or situation.

Stereotypy. A catatonic phenomenon characterized by repeated automatic complex movement. For example, a patient repeatedly twirls his hands over his head.

Subcortical dementia. A dementia associated with frontal white matter or basal ganglia disease. A mnemonic for subcortical dementia due to basal ganglia disease is the "three M company": **M**ood problems, **M**otor problems, and **M**emory problems that respond to cuing.

Substance abuse. Continued use of a psychoactive substance despite knowledge of having a persistent or recurrent social, occupational, psychological or general medical problem caused or exacerbated by use of that substance, or recurrent use in situations in which use is dangerous. Problems are recurrent but not always present.

Sundown syndrome. Either the hackneyed last scene in a romance where the happy couple ride off into the sunset, OR the emergence of the delirium at night when darkness adds to the ambiguity of perceptions.

Synesthesia. Stimuli in one sensory modality trigger a perception in a different sensory modality (e.g., seeing sound). Typically seen in drug-induced states (classic for LSD), epilepsy and mood disorder, particularly bipolar mood disorder.

Thalamus. The thalamus sits at the center of the brain. It integrates frontal lobe circuits and those circuits with the cerebellar-pontine part of the action brain. The reticular activating system ends in the thalamus, so the thalamus provides arousing "tone" to the frontal circuits. The thalamus helps organize and integrate all sensory input. It also integrates perception with action. It is the "pentium chip" of the brain.

Thought broadcasting. The experience that one's thoughts are leaking out of one's head so that others can hear them. Sometimes associated with thought echo, when the thought is spoken back to the person (as if an echo) by the hallucinated voice. Most common in schizophrenia, but can occur in other severe conditions such as major depression with melancholic features, and mania. A first rank symptom.

Thought echo. See thought broadcasting.

Tics. Sudden, recurrent, involuntary muscle movements or sounds.

Tourette's disorder (Gilles de la Tourette's syndrome). Repetitive, complex tics difficult to distinguish from compulsions. Many patients have obsessions or compulsions. Thought to be related to OCD. Probably an autosomal dominant condition with high penetrance. The sensorimotor-putamen pathway is implicated.

Tremor. Relatively rhythmic involuntary movements. Pill-rolling tremor occurs in Parkinson's disease and parkinsonism due to antipsychotic drugs. Postural tremor occurs with anxiety, hyperthyroidism and multiple medications, including lithium. Intention tremor occurs with cerebellar disease. Flapping tremor occurs with hepatic, pulmonary or renal failure, and delirium.

Trichotillomania. In the DSM impulse control disorder category, but really an OCD variant of compulsive hair pulling sometimes to the point of producing large bald spots.

Triune brain. Described by Paul MacLean to provide an evolutionary framework for understanding brain and behavior relationship. It includes the reptilian, paleomammalian and neomammalian structures. The reptilian brain is characteristic of non-mammals. The paleomammalian brain is an "add on" seen in social mammals. The neomammalian brain is seen in primates and is most developed in Harvard professors.

Unipolar. The widely used unofficial term for the awkward DSM category recurrent major depression.

Vascular dementia. Even though frontal lobe dementias are the second most common group of dementias, vascular brain changes are the second most common cause of dementia. Many vascular dementias have a frontal lobe pattern. Hemispheric white matter is most often affected (called Binswanger's disease). The thalamus, basal ganglia and internal capsule may also be involved. Bradykinesia and psychosis, depression (when dominant frontal circuits are involved) or anxiety are commonly observed. SPECT shows focal hypoperfusion, and MRI shows multiple white matter hyperintensities.

Verbigeration (palilalia). A catatonic phenomenon characterized by a verbal stereotypy in which the patient automatically repeats associations, particularly at the end of a thought. For example, a patient says, "I've been working in Chicago for 15 years, 15 years, years, years."

Viscous/adhesive personality. Personality characterize by perseveration, stubbornness, narrow field of interest, loss of humor and circumstantial speech and pedantic dry manner.

Volition. Aspects of personality and cognition related to ambition, planning and desires.

Waxy flexibility. A catatonic phenomenon in which the examiner manipulates the patient's limbs and feels the initial resistance gradually abating, as if bending a candle.

Wernicke's encephalopathy. Presents as delirium or dementia plus eye signs, typically sixth nerve palsy or nystagmus. Associated with a heritable disturbance in the ability to handle thiamine, precipitated by malnutrition, such as from alcoholism or starvation. May be fatal if untreated. Associated with small hemorrhages in periaqueductal gray matter.

Witzelsucht. Silly shallowness. Associated with lateral orbito-frontal circuit dysfunction.

Word approximations. An example of aphasic speech or formal thought disorder in which the patient uses words that modestly miss the true meaning of what is said. For example, a patient refers to a pen as an "ink writer," or a clock as a "wall time taker." It is an in-class paraphasia.

Word salad. See driveling speech.

Endnotes

Chapter 1

[1] In the real world, this picture is incomplete because we would want to add some statement about her general medical and neurologic health beyond what is apparent. Concerns such as fever, pain, abnormal gait, etc., come to mind. However, for our purposes what we describe is it! It is like the USMLE (United States Medical Licensure Examination) and specialty board exams. If the question does not mention a clinical finding or lab result, the ground rule is that you assume the finding is absent and the lab test, if done, will be normal.

[2] If you have to apply the Rule of Parsimony, by definition, you are dealing with a complicated, not typical, situation. Thus, the rule of parsimony sometimes leads to zebras, but that is okay, because zebras (uncommon conditions) do exist and need to be recognized. Acanthocytosis, although rare, does occur and if you only applied the Duck Principle, you would never think of it. To read more about movement disorders, refer to Berman, 1992.

[3] See Berman, 1992

[4] Dopamine blockers are used to suppress the choreiform movements seen in Huntington's disease (Fahn, 2000). We chose risperidone because it is also used to enhance the effects of SSRIs in OCD, and in low doses it is less likely to cause extrapyramidal symptoms (Owens, 1994). Olanzapine, which also may have some mood stabilizing properties might also be an option.

[5] One way of estimating pre-illness IQ is assessing the patient's vocabulary. The better the vocabulary, the higher the IQ.

[6] See Gorman, 1999. These are behavioral techniques that patients learn and practice with the aim of stress reduction. In systematic desensitization, patients are asked to visualize anxiety provoking scenes followed by a series of relaxation, whereas in autogenic relaxation, they learn to visualize a relaxing scene and relax their muscles.

[7] There is no one article or source that we can refer to that would compile all this information. The factors listed in *Table 1.4* are a summary of the articles we have reviewed over the years. However, the following can be used for additional information: Altshuler 1993; Atre-Vaidya et al, 1998; Harrow et al, 1990; Silverstone and Romans-Clarkson, 1989; Tohen et al, 1990; 1992; Tsuang et al, 1979; Winokur et al, 1993; Jampala et al, 1985; Guze, 1975.

[8] See Chapter 7

[9] Antipsychotics are classified as high potency (e.g., haloperidol) vs. low potency (e.g., thorazine), and typical vs. atypical. Typical antipsychotics are older and primarily work through blockade of D2 receptor (e.g., haloperidol, fluphenazine); atypical antipsychotics exert their action by serotonin dopamine antagonism and have a higher 5HT2/D2 blockade ratio. These have fewer extrapyramidal effects.

[10] Barbiturates, such as sodium amytal, were routinely used in the past for control of agitation. However, the concerns of respiratory depression associated with barbiturates have led to the decrease in its use. In our experience, if given very slowly, sodium amytal is relatively safe. Lorazepam and oxazepam are metabolized by conjugation and, therefore, compared to long-acting benzodiazepines, such as diazepam, are safer in patients with liver disease. Additionally, unlike diazepam they are also absorbed completely when given intramuscularly (Schatzberg, 1991; Perry et al, 1997).

[11] Tardive dyskinesia is an irreversible debilitating side effect of typical neuroleptics as a result of dopaminergic supersensitivity of the neurons. It is associated with basal ganglia abnormality and cognitive deficits (Pandurangi et al, 1980; Wade and Taylor, 1987). Antipsychotics can induce cell death by necrosis and apoptosis through anticholinergic

and dopaminergic blocking effects. They can cause cognitive deficits as well as various extrapyramidal symptoms (Behl, 1997; Miller and Chouinard, 1993; Stahl, 1996). In their manual of clinical psychopharmacology, Schatzberg and Cole provide a concise yet informational overview of the treatment.

[12] Most studies show that prophylaxis is useful for high risk patients (e.g., younger, male, on high dose of high potency neuroleptic with history of acute dystonic reaction), but not for routine use (Hanlon, 1966; Sramek, 1986). Doctors who favor the use claim that compliance is better due to less EPS (Schatzberg and Cole, 1991). However, those who show better compliance with prophylactic antiparkinsonians, use very high doses of antipsychotics (Keepers et al, 1983).

[13] One of us was covering an inpatient service for a colleague and had to discuss several potentially unpleasant disposition plan alternatives with a patient who was known to be assaultive toward staff members. The patient had alternatively received diagnoses of borderline personality (a stormy emotionally labile pattern of behaviors) or bipolar mood disorder. She was physically tough, verbally often abusive to the staff, and no one wanted to confront her for fear of injury. The covering physician met the patient in her room, opened the discussion with "Here's the deal," laid out the alternatives matter-of-factly, using language from the patient's perspective, and left the choices to her. She picked what was considered her best choice. Six months later, she was back on the unit, more manic than before. Seeing the covering physician she said to the staff near her, "Oh, he's tough. He doesn't BS me. I like him."

[14] "NOS in DSM-ese means "not otherwise specified." Can you imagine a patient coming home from the doctor and a spouse asking "Well, what did the doctor say?" and the response "The doctor said I was not otherwise specified."

[15] See Grodernberger D, 1998. Physostigmine crosses the blood-brain barrier, whereas neostigmine does not.

[16] Beware of little old ladies. One of us (NAV) was humbled by ignoring the evidence from Volavka, 1995, when during teaching rounds a partially treated manic woman threw her cup, hurting NAV's lip, but more so her pride.

[17] See Landre and Taylor, 1995. Formal thought disorder refers to abnormal speech and language that is aphasic-like.

[18] Perry et al, 1997

[19] See Fink and Taylor, 2003

[20] We will discuss depression in Chapter 3. Our position is that the DSM major depression category includes two broad subtypes: melancholia (what used to be called "endogenous" depression) and several other forms we refer to as nonmelancholic depressions. Throughout the book we use the term *melancholia* to differentiate between major depression without melancholic features from that with melancholic features. As we discuss in Chapter 2, we make this distinction because we believe that melancholic depression is a more severe form of depression and responds primarily to biologic treatments, such as antidepressants and ECT. Major depression without melancholic features or nonmelancholic depression often involves a combination of interpersonal, social, psychological and biologic factors, and each of these may need to be addressed individually. For a recent review of this, see Parker, 2000.

[21] See Ballenger, 1998

[22] Of course, we do not mean to single out ECT for the "or else" treatment. Anytime a patient or family asks you to do or not do something that you think is bad for the patient, you must refuse to comply. However, if it comes to a referral, make sure you refer to a specific person, and the family and patient are clear (in writing) whom they are to see and why.

[23] ENRICHD investigators 2000, 2001; also see Thase, 1991

[24] Fava et al, 1994; Thase et al, 1997

[25] This model assumes that these patients have personalities, experiences, learning, brain injuries that can not be reversed by analyzing the original events, and that the therapy should focus on trying to help these individuals adapt to the environment. Some people may argue that the only difference between this and what we call *supportive therapy* is the name. Even if this is true, the name, rehabilitative psychotherapy, helps us understand the focus better. For further discussion, refer to Guze, 1997, and Taylor, 1999.

[26] See Fenwick, 1991

[27] See Devane, 1998

[28] With the overabundance of herbal remedies, it is essential that you are aware of neuropsychiatric effects of herbal supplements. A review by Pies (2000) will be of significant help.

Chapter 2

[1] See Mesulam, 2000

[2] Schizophrenia typically begins before age 30, 75% of the first psychosis between ages 15-25.

[3] See Sergent and Signoret, 1992a; Sergent and Signoret, 1992b; Cutting DJ, 1989

[4] See Benson and Ardila, 1996

[5] See Rauh and Renshaw, 1995; Pullicino et al, 1993

[6] See Goldstein, 1998

[7] For more details, read the chapter by Cutting listed in footnote 3. Critchley's monograph is *The Parietal Lobes*, New York, Hafner Press, 1953.

[8] See Devanand et al, 2000; Kogure et al, 2000; Jelic and Nordberg, 2000

[9] See Christen-Zaech et al, 2003

[10] See Kauffer and Cummings, 1995; Frijda, 1986

[11] See footnote 2

[12] The syndromes associated with frontosubcortical circuits can occur due to disruption anywhere in the circuit. A small lesion in the cortex can produce a syndrome from one circuit. The same sized lesion in the basal ganglia or thalamus might affect several circuits because they are jammed into the smaller space of these structures (Cummings, 1993).

[13] If you recognized Patient 2-4's behaviors as manic-like, you are correct. The dysinhibited syndrome and primary mania substantially overlap. We distinguish primary from secondary mania in Chapter 4.

[14] See Kauffer and Cummings, 1995.

[15] See Kauffer and Cummings, 1995. Frontal lobe dementias often exhibit early personality changes. Vascular dementia may not show early personality changes if the ischemic strokes primarily occur in posterior circuits.

[16] *Motor sequencing* is tested by asking patients to make a fist and bring it down onto the table, then the edge of their open hand down onto the table, and then their palm down onto the table in the sequence: fist-edge-palm. Five sequences as rapidly as possible with each hand is a good test of contralateral dorsolateral prefrontal cortex and circuit functioning. Asking the patient to maintain 3 or 4 postures (closing eyes, holding arms out with palms downward, making a fist, sticking out one's tongue) for about 20 seconds each is a test for *motor persistence*.

[17] See Schmahmann, 1997

[18] See Barker et al, 1991

[19] See McLean, 1990

[20] To understand the brain functioning and to make a clinical diagnosis in a neuropsychiatric patient, a basic understanding of normal cognitive function and typical findings in a patient are necessary. Kolb and Whishaw (1996) provide a good overview. A simple clinical test that can be used to determine if cueing helps is to give the patient three unrelated words. If he is not able to remember them, give him the category; and if he still cannot remember, then give him the first letter of each word. Patients who have learned the information but have retrieval problems are able to recall learned information with cueing (Mesulam, 2000).

[21] Working memory is short-term. It is the memory you use to briefly hold a bit of information while you actively use it to do something. If you do not try to remember the information in working memory, it will decay and be discarded, clearing the "desktop" for the next job. An example of working memory is looking up a phone number and then "holding" it in working memory while you go to the phone to punch in the number. Without the working memory of their customers, pizza delivery and other take-out businesses would be in trouble.

[22] In recent years, we have learned a lot about the role of the thalamus in human brain and behavior. An excellent summary of findings can be found in an article by Scheibel, 1997, whereas Cummings and Benson's (1992) book on dementia gives clinical findings in specific dementias.

[23] See Scheibel, 1997. The *ventral basal complex* of the thalamus receives somatosensory information and transfers this to the primary somatosensory cortices. The *nucleus reticularis* of the thalamus receives input from the RAS. It is an inhibitory nucleus acting as a sensory gate so that the cortex is not flooded with too many irrelevant stimuli (noise). The *lateral geniculate nucleus* receives visual information and transfers it to the primary visual cortex. The *medial geniculate nucleus* receives auditory information and transfers it to the primary auditory cortex. The *ventral pulvinar* is involved in associational visual and auditory processing. The *medial pulvinar* relates to the amygdala and temporal and paralimbic cortices, and the parietal lobe heteromodal cortex. The *ventral posterior-lateral nucleus* is involved with motor associational processes (skilled motor tasks) and with the parietal lobes associational cortices; it integrates movement in three-dimensional space. The *anterior tubercle* relates to the posterior cingulate cortex and the mammilothalamic tract (it is compromised in Wernicke's encephalopathy). The *medial dorsal nucleus* relates to the prefrontal heteromodal cortex, orbitofrontal and paralimbic cortex, the amygdala and septal region. Wow!

[24] See Sohn et al, 2000

[25] The basal ganglia are part of the brain circuits that modulate cognitive as well as motor behaviors. Five frontosubcortical circuits are identified. Three (dorsolateral, lateral, orbito frontal and anterior cingulate) are relevant to many behaviors observed in psychiatric patients. These cortical areas connect to the thalamus through the basal ganglia. The dysfunction of dorsolateral circuits causes executive system problems and avolition. Dysfunction of the lateral orbitofrontal circuit causes disinhibition, and lesions of anterior cingulate circuit cause apathy and poor self-monitoring. A lesion anywhere in the circuitry can lead to these behavior changes. For more detail refer to Alexander et al, 1990; Alexander and DeLong, 1986; Cummings, 1993.

[26] Procedural memory is information and skills we learn automatically and unconsciously from repeated exposure to a task or problem, such as riding a bike. Procedural memory is a function of the basal ganglia and cerebellum (Squire, 1987).

[27] See Cummings, 1993

[28] There are several reports of use of dopaminergic agents in avolitional syndromes (Campbell and Duffy, 1997). However, none of the reports specifically give us an algorithm of which one to choose first. We used the agent that will also help the co-morbidity. D_2 stimulation plays an essential role in mediating neuropsychiatric effects of Parkinsonian patients treated with these agents. Of the patients receiving D_2 agonists,

about 30% develop visual hallucinations, 10% have delusions, 10% report euphoria, and about 1% actually have mania (Cummings, 1991). We need to be concerned about these side effects.

Chapter 3

[1] Akiskal (1990) in his monograph about dysthymic disorder categorizes early onset chronic low-grade depression as a) subaffective dysthymia, and b) characterological depression due to personality disorder. According to Akiskal, the first group is similar to major mood disorder and responds to medications in similar fashion. In DSM, chronic low grade depression secondary to chronic medical or other axis I illness is considered secondary dysthymia.

[2] There are many studies since the 1960s that repeatedly demonstrate the existence of melancholia (used to be called endogenous depression). These studies use powerful statistical approaches that establish the syndrome. What is unclear, is whether melancholia stands by itself as a distinct disease, or is a severe pathophysiologic phase of depression. Whether a distinct subtype or phase of illness, identifying melancholia is important for treatment. Think of cancer as an analogy. Knowing the stage of the cancer can change the treatment options. So, too, for depression. See Maes et al (1990), Part I, II, III; Sullivan et al, 1998; Serretti et al, 1998; Fountoulakis et al, 1999; Ambrosini, 2002.

[3] In our experience, patients who exhibit recurrent adjustment disorder with depressive or anxious features often have mild to moderate mood disorder and may respond to antidepressants. Adjustment disorders in the teens predicts major depression later in life.

[4] In DSM-IV, bereavement is not considered a psychiatric illness unless the duration is more than 2 months or features listed above are present. Patients with a previous history of depressive episodes should be treated earlier if they meet the criteria for depression. For more information, see articles by Zisook et al, 1993, 1994.

[5] High doses of estrogen can cause irritability and aggression, although estrogen itself has antidepressant properties when given in moderate doses. See de Lignieres and Vincens, 1982.

[6] Several studies of cardiac patients have shown the relationship between emotions, tachyarrhythmia and sudden cardiac death. (Hoffman et al, 1999; Wittling et al, 1998.)

[7] For a thorough discussion of liability issues, see Motto, 1999

[8] Oquendo et al, 2001; Gladstone et al, 2001; Schneider et al, 2001; Statham et al, 1998; Fishbain, 1999; Aharonovich et al, 2002; Jamison, 2000

[9] The DSM category of major depression uses "melancholia" as a modifier. The criteria essentially reflect Patient 3-3's symptoms for major depression with melancholic features. Although there is some controversy about the separation of depression into melancholic and nonmelancholic types, we like the dichotomy because it helps us clinically. Melancholics are more likely to become psychotic, catatonic, or stuporous. They are more likely to respond to ECT or to broad pharmacodynamic spectrum antidepressant drugs such as nortriptyline or venlafaxine. Nonmelancholics are more likely to have an associated personality disorder and be dysthymic as well as having episodes of depression. When treating nonmelancholic patients, we chose an antidepressant drug in part based on the patient's personality, whereas for melancholic patients, personality does not seem to affect medication choice. See the following documenting some of the above points: Abrams, 1997; Parker, 2000.

[10] The overall response rates of each disorder vary depending on the study and patient selection criteria. A comprehensive review of treatment response can be found in Nathan and Gorman (1998); Petrides et al (2001).

[11] Environmental stressors (like those of Patient 3-3) or internally generated stress (e.g., an anxious-fearful person who makes stressful mountains out of inconvenient molehills)

affect the immune system primarily through endocrine and neurologic pathways. Alterations in the immune system increase an individual's susceptibility to various disorders. For further discussion of this, see the chapter on psychosomatic disorders by Thompson R, 1988.

[12] The lethal dose of SSRI drugs is higher than the lethal dose of the older tricyclic antidepressants (TCAs) and patients are more likely to die from a TCA overdose than from an SSRI overdose. Nevertheless, lethal doses can be calculated and the prescription limited. Also, why give a month's supply of a drug before knowing if it will work.

[13] All SSRIs cause anxiety and agitation, but fluoxetine has the highest incidence of nervousness and anxiety. A recent study by Donovan et al (2000) found that the incidence of deliberate self-harm is higher in SSRIs than with TCAs. Amitriptyline had the lowest incidence, whereas fluoxetine had the most. There are several articles by Preskorn S, 1992, 1995, that compare and contrast the SSRIs. When fluoxetine was first introduced, clinicians routinely used either a benzodiazepine or trazodone to reduce initial anxiety and drop-out rates.

[14] The causes of antidepressant-induced sexual dysfunction are not well understood. Several mechanisms are postulated. These include increased serotonin activity, anticholinergic effect, D_2 blockade, $5HT_2$ blockade and nitrous oxide inhibition. When choosing an antidepressant, first we need to determine what specific type of antidepressant is needed for a given patient. Then, in that category, we need to pick the drug that has the least effect on the above-mentioned receptors. For further reading, see Sussman, 1999; Richelson, 1994. Recently, one of us (NAV) had an influx of a large number of elderly male patients in her clinic. Almost all of these patients were receiving an SSRI for late onset depression. Ninety percent requested a change in medication because of sexual side effects. This was an important lesson for us. We have to think about the sexual side effects of antidepressants even in the elderly. This also confirms an old saying, "Just because there is snow on the roof, it does not mean there is no fire in the fireplace."

[15] Borderline personality disorder defines a person with long-standing mood instability that results in a stormy life with unstable relationships and other uproars. These patients are famous for making suicide attempts, cutting and burning themselves, and threatening these actions if not appeased. This diagnosis is listed among the personality disorders (axis II) because persons with "it" appear to have abnormal traits rather than illness states.

[16] Based on the available data and our experience, we prefer never to diagnose a patient "borderline." Too many times we have seen depressed and bipolar patients labeled "borderline" because the therapist did not get along with the patient or the patient appeared dependent. See Atre-Vaidya, 1999; Akiskal, 1994, 1985; Harrison et al, 1983.

[17] Litman et al, 1963; Suominen et al, 2002

[18] Suominen et al, 1998

[19] Goodwin and Jamison, 1990, chapter 7; Keller et al, 1995

[20] Schizophrenia is rare (about .05% lifetime risk in the general population when modern criteria are used) and, therefore, the percentage of psychotic inpatients who have schizophrenia will be small compared to other disorders. Fewer than 4% of admissions to an acute psychiatric unit meet the criteria for schizophrenia (Taylor, 1999).

[21] For further understanding, refer to Chapters 6 and 15 in Goodwin and Jamison, 1990. Genetic anticipation, an increase in severity or a decrease in age of onset inherent in the transmission of a disease gene from a parent to a child is being described in several psychiatric disorders including schizophrenia, bipolar disorder, and anxiety disorder. You can read more about genetic anticipation and psychiatric illness in articles by Grigoroiu-Serbanescu et al, 1997; O'Hara et al, 1999; Petronis and Kennedy, 1995; Stompe et al, 2000.

[22] See Patel and Gaw, 1996, and also Note 15.

[23] Several studies (Kantor and Glassman, 1977; Kroessler, 1986; Spiker et al, 1985; Parker, 1992; APA Practice Guidelines, 1996) have demonstrated the ineffectiveness of antidepressant medication alone in psychotic depression.

[24] Donovan et al, 2000; Khan et al, 2000; Verkes et al, 1998; Tondo et al, 1998; Tonds and Baldessarini, 2000; Prudic and Sackeim, 1999

[25] Treatment resistance has never been well defined. The implication, however, is that the patient has not responded to at least two adequate trials with different antidepressant drugs. Some 30-60% of depressed patients are still symptomatic after their first course of antidepressant treatment (Preskorn et al, 1992) and 20% are substantially ill after two years of treatment (Paykel et al, 1994).

[26] See Fava and Davidson, 1996; McCombs et al, 2001.

[27] "Adequate response" is also not clearly defined. In modern drug studies, a 50% or more drop in symptom severity is considered adequate. We are not happy unless the patient gets all better.

[28] See Goodwin and Gabrielli, 1997.

[29] See Starkstein and Manes, 2000

[30] Taylor, 1999

[31] Keitner et al, 1991; Howland, 1993; Musselman et al, 2000

[32] See Fava , 2000

[33] Continuation electroconvulsive therapy is shown to be an effective treatment for those patients who either do not respond to continuation antidepressant treatment or who have frequent relapses or who do not tolerate antidepressant side effects. For more discussion of continuation or maintenance ECT, see Gagne et al, 2000; and Petrides et al, 1994. Maintenance ECT is also helpful in schizoaffective and bipolar disorder, and schizophrenia . Maintenance ECT can be used alone or in combination with medication (Sharma et al, 1997; Swoboda et al, 2001).

[34] See Hammen, 1991; Harkness et al, 1999.

[35] As discussed in Note 5, although both of us prefer a broad spectrum antidepressant for melancholia, one of us (NAV) prefers to start with venlafaxine, whereas the other (MAT) prefers nortriptyline, if the patient is a young healthy adult without cardiac history.

[36] It is our practice to routinely offer ECT when available as a choice for all patients with melancholic depression. APA guidelines of treating depression (APA ECT Task Force, 1990). The safety of ECT is well established, and morbidity and mortality less than that of drugs. For detailed information about ECT, see Abrams R, 2002.

[37] Post-partum depression refers to a depression within 4-6 weeks of childbirth. Most such depressions begin within 1-2 weeks of childbirth. The quip, "mental illness is inherited, you get it from your children," refers to the stresses of parenthood not the massive hormonal changes at parturition.

[38] See Glassman et al, 1975; Kroessler, 1985; Parker et al, 1992

[39] One of us (MAT) recently saw an 80-year-old woman who was depressed and given 0.5 mg risperidone as part of her outpatient treatment. Despite three months of venlafaxine and risperidone, her depression became worse and she was hospitalized and the risperidone abruptly stopped. Dyskinetic movements of her mouth appeared within a few days. So, how much antipsychotic is "too much?" If it were our "granny," the answer would be "a single molecule." Don't give what you don't have to give. Don't do what you don't have to do. Do no harm.

To beat this horse one more time, MAT also saw a patient labeled treatment resistant who did not respond to any antidepressant drug and was then given olanzapine along with her sertraline. She developed an oculogyric crisis, could not breathe and was hospitalized for this. She recovered. She had an atypical depression and had never received an MAOI. An MAOI was prescribed and she did well for the first time in years. The new drugs are marketed better than the old ones, but the *oldies are still the goodies*.

[40] Monk, 2001; O'Hara et al, 1990; Chung et al, 2001

[41] For a detailed description of ECT in pregnancy, refer to Miller, 1994; and Walker and Swartz, 1994

[42] To read more, refer to the following articles: Wisner et al, 2000, Miller, 1994, Ferrill et al, 1992, Remick and Maurice, 1978, Forssman, 1955, Koren et al, 1998, Altshuler et al, 1996.

[43] Every drug that is found to be teratogenic in humans has caused teratogenesis in nonhumans. However, there are drugs that have teratogenic effects in high doses in nonhumans that are not teratogenic in humans in clinical doses (Koren, 1998). For example, antipsychotics cause behavioral abnormalities in laboratory animals, but not in humans, and benzodiazepines cause oral clefts in laboratory animals but not in humans. Although tricyclic antidepressants do not cause organ dysgenesis in humans, in laboratory animal studies they cause low density of serotonin receptors, high agonist affinity for brain dopamine receptor and low adrenergic binding (Altshuler, 1996). SSRIs are generally safe but, again, laboratory animal studies show abnormalities in serotonin brain receptor binding and craniofacial malformations, birth related hematoma, and inhibition of milk ejection reflux (Baum and Misri, 1996).

[44] In cardioconversion, 200-400 joules is delivered to the chest in a split-second. In ECT, the average joules delivered is about 40-50 joules, and the maximum about 100 joules, but delivered over 4-8 seconds. Cardioconversion shuts down the dysrhythmic heart in hope that it will convert to normal rhythm naturally. ECT shuts down the brain in hope that it will reboot naturally. The goal is not the seizure, but producing temporary brain electrical quiet. In cardioconversion, 2-3 or more stimulations may be needed to convert. In ECT, 8-15 stimulations may be needed to convert. The brain is clearly more complicated than the heart.

[45] ECT works somewhat better in the elderly than in the young. No one knows why. The side effects of ECT are independent of age. Medication side effects, however, are age-dependent, and drug choice is often matched by the patient's age requirements. Refer to Brodaty et al, 2000, Tew et al, 1999, Oshima and Higuchi, 1999.

[46] See Berner et al, 1987

[47] Bodkin and Amsterdam, 2002

[48] See notes 18-21 in chapter 7 for further discussion of treating depression in Parkinson' disease.

[49] The only other diagnosis that is equally controversial as PTSD is borderline personality disorder. Starting from its validity to etiology to treatment response, PTSD has been hotly debated. We do not claim to be experts in dealing with PTSD. When we encounter a patient with chronic PTSD symptoms, our main focus remains in identifying a treatable mood disorder, treating pre-existing anxiety and personality disorders, and/or ruling out a seizure disorder. Other conditions that can result in a chronic PTSD picture are traumatic brain injury and substance abuse. Articles by Charney et al, 1996 and Fichtner et al, 1997 and Sierles et al, 1983 are helpful in understanding this disorder.

[50] See Sheline YI, 2003

[51] About 60-70% of melancholics will be nonsuppressors of cortisol to dexamethasone challenge (1-2 mg given at 11:00 pm, cortisol levels taken prior to administration and then at 8:00 and 4:00 am the next day with cortisol levels above 5 mcg/dl indicating nonsuppression). The dexamethasone suppression test is a test that assesses the functioning of the pituitary hypothalamic adrenal axis. In normal patients, exogenous cortisol suppresses the body's cortisol through the pituitary hypothalamic feed back loop. Melancholic depression increases cortisol through its effect on the pituitary adrenal axis. It is no longer considered useful in identifying melancholia from other syndromes, but it is still helpful in predicting relapse in high risk patients. A depressed patient with a pretreatment abnormal DST should convert to a normal DST after clinical improvement. Failure to convert predicts relapse. See APA Task Force on Laboratory Tests in

Psychiatry, 1987 for an excellent review of DST in psychiatry. For a more recent evaluation of the merits of the test, see Coryell and Schlesser, 2001.

[52] Lyme disease is associated with long-term neuropsychiatric symptoms (see Seltzer et al, 2000).

Chapter 4

[1] A review of the studies comparing bipolar and unipolar depression can be found in Chapter 3 of the textbook, *Manic-Depressive Illness*, by Goodwin and Jamison (1990).

[2] See the following for discussions of lithium and other mood stabilizers in the treatment of bipolar depressions: Strakowski et al, 2000; Pies, 2002; Rucci et al, 2002; Gilmer, 2001; Dietrich and Emrich,1998; Yatham et al, 2002; Hurley, 2002.

[3] Although most clinicians are not aware of it, studies demonstrate the efficacy of ECT in mania. See the textbook by Abrams (2002), the APA Task Force. The articles by Mukherjee et al, 1994, and Vanelle et al, 1994 provide a good overview of the topic.

[4] In some states, other than emergency management, informed written consent is needed to give psychotropics. In Michigan, for example, valproic acid prescribed for epilepsy does not require consent. If it is prescribed by a psychiatrist for epilepsy, consent is required. If it is prescribed for bipolar disorder by a generalist, consent is not required; but if it is prescribed by a psychiatrist for bipolar disorder, consent is required. If you are not now outraged on reading this, you are not a psychiatrist or mental health professional.

[5] To diagnose mania accurately, one must be familiar with all the features and presentations of mania. A detailed clinical description of mania can be found in Goodwin and Jamison (1990), Chapter 2.

[6] Catatonic excitement is most likely an outburst of mania during a catatonic episode. Today, mania remains the leading underlying process inducing a catatonia (see Fink and Taylor, 2003).

[7] See Marneros and Tsuang, 1986

[8] *Table 3.4* approximates the guidelines recommended by the APA (APA Practice Guidelines Supplement, 1994). Because lorazepam is easily absorbed by IM injections (unlike other benzodiazepines), it is particularly useful for agitated patients and is the drug of choice for controlling agitation in nonpsychotic mania. It also is a powerful GABA-a agonist so it may offer some protection for the excited manic not becoming catatonic. In choosing an antipsychotic for an excited psychotic manic, the most important factor we consider is the avoidance of NMS. Atypical antipsychotics, such as olanzapine and risperidone, can be used if you do not anticipate the need for parental administration. Olanzapine has been approved recently for treatment in mania, but in our experience, we have had only modest success with it for highly excited patients. Risperidone may be a more potent choice. The disadvantage of risperidone is that a parental form is not yet available, and in younger men we have had to use doses greater than 8 mg, exposing the patient to EPS risks similar to that of the typical antipsychotics. For a more detailed discussion of our rationale, see Taylor (1999), Chapter 8; *Journal of Clinical Psychiatry,* Supplement 8, vol. 61, 2000; Abrams, 2002.

[9] Krauthammer and Klerman (1978) were first to systematically describe secondary mania. Patients with secondary mania tend to be more irritable and assaultive. They are older and without a family history of bipolar mood disorder. The presentation is more atypical. For example, silly instead of euphoric affect, presence of thought disorder or absent vegetative symptoms. More systematic descriptions can be found in Yudofsky and Hales, *APA Textbook of Neuropsychiatry, 2nd Edition* (2003), and in Goodwin and Jamison, 1990.

[10] Of the three loading strategies, valproate loading is done most frequently. Although Abrams (2002), in his book, states that routine ECT works as well as what we refer to as

loading ECT, in our practice, we have been able to obtain a quicker control with "ECT loading." We have had similar experience with lithium. We do not routinely obtain lithium levels the next day as suggested by Fava et al (1984). However, if the anticipated dose is greater than 1800 mg/day, then we would recommend a 24-hour blood level and using the method described by Cooper and Simpson (1976). Given the narrow therapeutic index and possibility of toxicity, we do not load lithium if the anticipated dose (based on age and medical status) is greater than 1800 mg/day. For further information about loading, see the following references: Fava et al, 1984, Keck et al 1993, Hirschfeld et al, 1999, Perry, et al, 1997.

[11] Many clinicians are surprised by the large doses of lorazepam needed to resolve a catatonia, but these doses work and are well tolerated. Begin at 1-2 mg TID, increasing every day or so, if needed (Fink and Taylor, 2003).

[12] Most experts agree that catatonia responds both to lorazepam and ECT equally well. The choice often depends on immediate availability of ECT and patient preference; sometimes these two treatments are used together. For further discussion see Bush et al, 1996a,b; Petrides et al, 1997; and Fink and Taylor, 2003.

[13] See Fink and Taylor, 2003

[14] Although medications are the mainstay of the treatment for bipolar disorder, psychosocial treatment has been shown to improve overall outcome (Nathan and Gorman, 1998). Biofeedback, as well as relaxation training, is helpful for the psychiatric patient in reducing symptom severity, although some patients find relaxation training to be more helpful (Olson, 1988, Nigl and Jackson, 1979).

[15] As always, drug/drug interactions are important elements when we use combined pharmacotherapy. Combinations can lead to a synergist therapeutic effect, or increase side effects and toxicity. Ketter et al (1992) provides a good overview of using carbamazepine and valproic acid together. We do not use this combination any more. Carbamazepine metabolism is increased by valproic acid's induction of liver enzymes so carbamazepine levels drop when valproic is added. The combination may also lead to an epoxy carbamazepine metabolite which is a neurotoxin. Lithium and valproic acid both produce tremors, and when they are combined, severe tremors are more likely.

[16] See footnote 8, chapter 1.

[17] Post and colleagues (1984, 1989) introduced the sensitization model to explain the cause of chronic bipolar mood disorder. Psychosensory features are clinical phenomena that reflect temporolimbic sensitization, and there is some evidence their presence may indicate a better response to anticonvulsants (Atre-Vaidya and Taylor, 1997).

[18] See Brown et al, 1999; Sapolsky et al, 1986; Sapolsky, 2000

[19] See Charney et al, 1999. The data about familial risk are clinically helpful in educating patients about individual risk. The percentages often vary from study to study, but do not worry, the exact numbers do not make a substantial difference in clinical practice. For that purpose, a rough estimate is okay. First-degree relatives include parents, siblings, and children.

[20] Flight of ideas is the classic speech of mania. Associations move rapidly from topic to topic, often further and further from the point. Distracting stimuli and the patient's own thoughts seem to enter the speech unfiltered. Formal thought disorder is the classic speech of schizophrenia. It is fluent and sometimes makes sense, but also includes made-up words (neologisms – literally new words, like "bunderfunder") paraphasic speech (word approximations, like "graphite stick" for pencil, and jargon speech (unintelligible strings of words) like "the red wire touched the paper floor light switch").

[21] See Boutros and Bowers, 1996

[22] Molho and Factor, 1999

[23] Chronic substance use results in neurocognitive deficits that you have to consider in planning treatment for these patients (Fals-Stewart, 1994). For a detailed discussion of the management of traumatic brain injury, see Silver et al, 1994.

[24] Arterial border zones termed watershed areas surround Broca's and Wernicke's areas and are involved in language. Strokes in these areas produce various language difficulties.

[25] Diener et al, 1999; Erdemoglu and Ozbakir, 2000

Chapter 5

[1] See Wade, 1999; Ballenger et al, 1998

[2] Another Greek tragedy. The "agora" was the main market and meeting place in ancient Athens. Thus, agoraphobia is a fear of public places.

[3] Social phobia involves the build-up of various fears associated with social situations and include fears of public speaking, talking on the phone, meeting new people, urinating in a public toilet. If the number and severity of social phobias become overwhelming, the patient may not leave home, anticipating encounters with the social phobia situations. Thus, social phobia, like panic disorder, can end up producing agoraphobia.

[4] Psychologists are usually better trained than physicians to use CBT.

[5] See Himadi et al, 1986

[6] See Chapter 7, Patient 2 for discussion of procedural memory. Procedural memory is a function of basal ganglia pons and cerebellum. Abnormality of frontal-striatal circuitry is demonstrated in patients with obsessive compulsive features. Brain regions that are most consistently involved are anterior cingulate cortex, orbitofrontal cortex and head of the caudate nuclei. Functional imaging studies have shown these areas to be hypermetabolic. Similarly, subcortical diseases such as Huntington's and Parkinson's exhibit obsessive compulsive features. See Cummings and Mega, 2003.

[1] Gradual exposure to feared stimuli evokes less tension and is easier for the patient and is as effective as flooding (sudden exposure). Both exposure and response prevention are essential. See Koran, 1999; Kobak et al, 1998.

[2] These disorders often meet the criteria for OCD and can be treated with selective serotonin reuptake inhibitors. See Taylor, 1999.

[9] See Swedo et al, 1997

[10] See Fallon et al, 1998

[11] The term epilepsy spectrum disorder was introduced by Roberts (91) to describe a group of patients who have a history of head injury, and several psychomotor/psychosensory features in absence of clinical or EEG evidence of seizures.

[12] See Charney, 1996

[13] See Magee et al, 1996

[14] See Maggee et al, 1996; Schneier et al, 1992

[15] See Yonkers et al, 2001

[16] See Schneier, et al 2001

Chapter 6

[1] Recently there have been several case and open trial studies suggesting that a combination of ECT and an antipsychotic are effective in treatment resistant patients (Chanpattana et al, 1999; Kupchik et al, 2000; Kales et al, 1999). Most of these reports describe using clozapine as the antipsychotic. Patients were treated repeatedly with various antipsychotics without success. Clozapine was tried with some improvement.

Then ECT was added and fuller improvement occurred. The question is whether it was the ECT alone that did it or the combination. The combination point of view rests on the idea that ECT alters the blood-brain barrier permitting more drug to get in. At present, there is a large multicenter collaborative study being conducted that is evaluating the ECT/clozapine combination.

[2] See Denicoff et al, 1994

[3] There are several subtypes of delusional disorder described in DSM-IV. These include erotomanic, persecutory, jealous, grandiose, somatic, mixed and unspecified type. It is a rare disorder with a population prevalence of .03% (DSM-IV).

[4] Because delusional disorder is a late occurring condition, secondary causes must be ruled out. Cummings in 1986 provided an extensive review of secondary delusion, its phenomenology and anatomical correlations. We highly recommend this article and a chapter on secondary psychosis, delusions, and schizophrenia, also by Cummings (1986).

[5] See Volavka, 1995.

[6] Clozapine has been hailed as a miracle drug, but pharmaceutic hype usually covers up blemishes. When thinking about prescribing clozapine, keep the following in mind: 1) It is expensive and requires blood tests weekly; 2) It has very strong anticholinergic properties making it more dangerous for use in the elderly than the older antidepressants; 3) Copious salivation is an intolerable side effect for many patients; 4) 3% of patients at 300 mg daily and 6% at 600 mg daily have seizures (Do not use if you suspect epilepsy or an epilepsy spectrum disorder.); and 5) it works for some patients who have not responded to other drugs, but not to the degree the manufacturer would have you believe.

[7] Chanpattana et al, 2000b

[8] Expressed emotion is a measure of family environment that is demonstrated to be a reliable predictor of relapse in schizophrenia. It has been shown that those patients who have overly critical family members have frequent relapse. Butzlaff and Hooley (1998) did a meta-analysis of all the published studies and found that not only the relapse rate was higher not only in schizophrenic patients, but also for patients with mood disorders and eating disorders.

[9] Kurt Schneider describes signs that he thought as pathognomic of schizophrenia. These are 1) audible thoughts, 2) voices arguing, 3) voices commenting on patient's actions, 4) the experience of influences "playing on body" (somatic passivity), 5) thought withdrawal (experience of thoughts being taken out of the brain), 6) diffusion of thought (thoughts leaking out of the brain), 7) delusional perception of all feelings, and 8) impulses and volitional acts that are experienced by the patient as work or influence of others (Kurt Schneider, 1959). Investigators have demonstrated these features and their presence in other disorders, especially in acute mania (Abrams and Taylor, 1981).

[10] Kendler, 1985

[11] Soft neurologic signs are less localizing than other features such as an aphasic syndrome or limb paralysis. Soft signs reflect motor dysregulation. Examples are: motor overflow (choreiform movements and other extraneous movement [sticking your tongue out while writing]), motor impersistence (unable to maintain a posture – fist, eyes closed, mouth open – for 20 seconds).

[12] Illusions are misperceptions of real stimuli, whereas hallucinations are perceptions without the stimulus.

[13] There is ample research to back our statement (Kendler et al, 1985; Battaglia, 1995; Varma et al, 1992; Fulton, 1993). Treatments should mainly focus on etiological factors (Table 6.12) responsible for schizotypal symptoms. The treatment of primary schizotypal disorder is similar to schizophrenia (Gitlin, 1993; Kapfhammer and Hippius, 1998).

[14] It is not all about medication. Many pharmacologists or pharmacists know a lot more about drugs than we do. Prescription involves more than just writing a script. You can choose the best medication for the patient, but if you do not pay attention to the costs,

convenience of use, side effects and drug-drug interactions, the toilet bowl is more likely to receive medication than your patient.

[15] See Stanilla and Simpson, 1998

[16] This dose is excessive by most ER standards. Many use 5 mg haloperidol plus 1 or 2 mg lorazepam together, but problems can still arise from giving a powerful antipsychotic broad D_2 blocker to a patient you have not fully evaluated.

[17] A *synesthesia* is when a person experiences a stimulus in a different sensory domain, e.g., seeing sound

[18] See Post and Kopanda (1976)

[19] Electroconvulsive therapy is more effective in treating acute than chronic drug-induced psychosis (Abrams, 1997). Although there are no organized studies, case literature suggests that ECT is effective in drug-induced psychosis (Fink, 1995). In our experience we have been able to achieve clinically significant symptom reduction for many patients with chronic drug induced conditions whey they are having acute exacerbations.

[20] See Bolla et al, 1998; Weinrieb and O'Brien, 1994

[21] See Fals-Stewart, 1992; Fals-Stewart and Lucente, 1993

Chapter 7

[1] Hint: The clue in the vignette has to do with risperidone.

[2] Dementia with Lewy body is a relatively common cause of dementia. Controversy exists if Parkinson's disease with dementia, Lewy body disease and Lewy body variant of Alzheimer's are distinct entities or represent a spectrum of a single entity. We recommend three articles for further reading: 1) Simard, 2000; 2) Litvan et al, 1998; and 3) Papka, 1998.

[3] We did not mention schizophreniform disorder in the psychotic disorder chapter, because, frankly, we do not think much of the idea of it. By definition it looks like schizophrenia, but it either resolves within 6 months or it last longer and the patient is now called schizophrenic. Most studies show that the patient initially labeled as schizophreniform is eventually diagnosed schizophrenic.

[4] The limbic system generates primary emotions such as fear, anger, sadness, happiness. However, social emotions, such as gratitude, social smile, and pride are processed through the neocortex (see Frijda, 1986). Patients who are mild to moderately depressed may be able to continue to have appropriate social encounters. However, they reveal their mood by their distractibility, smiling without an engaging quality, reduced eye contact, and decreased animation.

[5] Human memory consists of several independent systems. An injury or disease can selectively affect the memory system. One can have profound deficits in one memory system with relatively intact other systems. A simple clinical test can help assess different memory systems. There are several classifications of the human memory system, however, most experts agree that human memory systems can be divided into a cognitive system and a procedural system.

The cognitive representation system. The cognitive representation system involves the cortex and consists of working (primary) memory, one-trial perceptual memory, and declarative memory.

a. *Working memory* is a prefrontal cortical function in which a sensory perception (transmitted via the thalamus or the parahippocampal gyrus) or thought is held for about 30 seconds while the prefrontal cortex decides what to do with that information. Working memory requires attention, a function of the reticular activating system, thalamus, and prefrontal cortex. One test of working memory is to ask the patient to repeat a series of words or digits.

b. *One-trial perceptual memory* allows you to remember information arriving in your sensory cortex without having paid conscious attention to it. It is also called priming. Even densely amnestic people have intact priming.

c. *Declarative memory* is information that you learn consciously, and consists of semantic and episodic memory.

1. *Semantic memory* consists of information known to others in your culture or in the world, such as who is the President or what major events happened in the world from 1935-1945. Semantic memory is associated with functioning of the hippocampus, parahippocampus, entorhinal cortex and perirhinal cortex.

2. *Episodic (autobiographical) memory* is memory for information known only to you and "others who were there at the time." Examples include a 16th birthday party and your first date. Episodic memory is associated with functioning of the hippocampus.

d. *Meta-memory* is knowledge about one's own memory capabilities and knowledge about strategies that can improve memory. It is your self-rating of your performance and can be greatly influenced by mood. Depressed patients typically think they did worse than, in fact, they did cognitive tests, Alzheimer's patients often minimize errors of their performance.

P*rocedural memory (action) system* is information and skill that is learned by practicing the sequence of actions, such as riding a bicycle, performing a physical examination, or solving a computer problem without knowing how you solved it. Procedural memory is a function of the basal ganglia, pons, and cerebellum.

For a more detailed discussion, see Lezak, 1983; Squire, 1987.

[6] Identifying Alzheimer's disease early enables you to start antidementia treatment before extensive brain deterioration occurs. Small (1996) discusses the neuroimaging and genetic techniques of early detection of Alzheimer's in detail. For further clinical description, refer to Taylor, 1999; Cummings, 1992.

[7] See Selkoe, 1997

[8] Cholinesterase inhibitors increase the concentration of available ACh by inhibiting enzymes responsible for hydrolysis. There is some evidence that glutamate is also central to pathology. The degree of glutaminic loss corresponds to the degree of dementia. There is also some evidence that oxidative stress also plays a role. Antioxidants such as vitamin E may help prevent the progression of the disease. See Simard et al, 2000.

[9] van Reekam et al (1997) and Hogan and Patterson (2002) review all cognition enhancing drugs in dementia and treatment strategies based on the pathophysiologic process. These reviews are a good starting point. As new research and papers are being published, MEDLINE should help you with the latest. Another reference is the *APA Guidelines for Treatment of Dementia* (2000). We have two additional drugs, rivastigmine and galantamine. Rivastigmine is an acetyl- and butyrylcholinesterase inhibitor, whereas galantamine is an acetylcholinesterase and nicotinic receptor modulator. All three cholinesterases are equivalent in efficacy. However, patients who do not respond or tolerate one, may respond to another. The usual starting dose for rivastigmine is 1.5 mg PO BID, increased up to 6-12 mg/day. The starting dose for galantamine is 4 mg BID up to 16-24 mg/day. If needed, either can be used as alternatives to donepezil. When switching, one must be careful about cholinergic toxicity. Often you must taper one before starting another.

[10] See Shay and Roth, 1992

[11] Liddell et al (2001) discuss the current status and ways a psychiatrist could advise a first-degree relative. Other articles of interest include Li et al, 1996 and Silverman et al, 1994. In these articles, authors discuss the patterns of risk in first-degree relatives. According to these authors, risk of dementia is higher in relatives. Also, the risk goes down with the increase in age; that is if you do not get the disease by the eighth decade, the risk is lower.

[12] See Marra et al, 2000; Peterson, 2000

[13] See Jagust, 1994; 1995

[14] See Small, 1998; Peskind, 1998

[15] The Mini-Mental State Examination (see Folstein et al, 1975) is a 10-item screening cognitive examination. Use of the MMSE is taught in most US medical schools. Although not comprehensive, it still is widely used for screening for cognitive deficits.

[16] See Cummings, 1995; Slaughter et al, 2001b

[17] Rosenblatt and Leroi, 2000

[18] Although Parkinson's disease was originally considered as a neurologic disorder marked by rigidity, tremor at rest, and mask-like facies, the clinical symptoms include much more. Mood disorders, especially depression, are an integral part of Parkinson's with over half of the patients complaining of depression. The journal, *Clinical Neuroscience* (vol. 1, #1, 1993), has an entire section devoted to Parkinson's disease. We recommend this issue which includes articles by Markham and Diamond, 1993; Graybiel, 1993; DeLong and Wichmann, 1993; Edwards, 1993; for treatment of Parkinson's disease and depression, see Nutt, 1993; Bredesen, 1993; Fink, 1993. Also see Taylor 1999, pp. 362-363; Slaughter et al, 2001.

[19] See Markham and Diamond, 1993; Slaughter et al, 2001

[20] Bromocriptine, a D_2 agonist, pramipexole, a D_3 agonist, and pergolide, a D_2 and D_3 agonist, are all used for treatment of early Parkinson's (Nutt, 1993; Lange and Lozano, 1998). All three have mood elevating properties that have been demonstrated as well in patients without Parkinson's disease (Inoue et al, 1996; Goldberg et al, 1999; Izumi et al, 2000).

[21] ECT is an established treatment for depression and is recommended in Parkinson's patients with depression (Koller et al, 1994). However, it has been demonstrated that Parkinsonian symptoms improve with ECT even in the absence of depression (Atre-Vaidya and Jampala, 1988; Rasmussen and Abrams, 1991). There is also a double-blind study using "sham" ECT to treat nondepressed Parkinsonian patients that also demonstrate its efficacy (Andersen et al, 1987). Also see Pridmore et al, 1995; Fall et al, 1995; Moellentine et al, 1998.

[22] See Mukherjee et al, 1987; Kraus et al, 1994

[23] A number of years ago, there was a public health initiative to add the colorless, tasteless, odorless thiamine to booze the way we add vitamin D to milk. The initiative was blocked because some persons thought once thiamine was in booze, more people would drink! Have you ever turned down a cold beer on a hot day because you were concerned about your thiamine levels?!

[24] See Silver and Yudofsky, 1994. There is a vast and ever-growing literature in traumatic brain injury and its neuropsychiatric consequences. For a trainee interested in this subject, the most comprehensive, yet comprehensible source is the textbook, *Neuropsychiatry of Traumatic Brain Injury* by the authors listed above. Although we cite other literature, for a beginner, we would recommend this book.

[25] The World Health Organization's official listing of all medical diagnoses: *International Classification of Disease*, now in its 10th version, thus ICD-10

[26] Rao and Lyketsos, 2000; Kraus et al, 1994; Taylor and Price, 1994

[27] Several general principles should be used in treating patients with brain injury. Although there is little actual data, most clinicians, including us, have observed an increased tendency towards developing side effects. It is recommended that the starting doses should be much lower (starting at about 25% of the usual dose) and gradually increased to maximum recommended dose as tolerated. More information about pharmacotherapy of TBI can be found in Chapter 6 of McAllister, 1994; Silver and Yudofsky, 1994.

[28] See McAllister, 1994

[29] Povlishock JT: Presented at the 12th Annual Meeting of American Neuropsychiatric Association, Fort Myers, Florida, 2001. See Grafman and Salazer, 1996

[30] See Nicoll et al, 1995

[31] See Binder, 1986; Mamelak, 2000

[32] See Huang et al, 2000; Tagami et al, 1998

[33] Copying geometric shapes: □ △ ○ ⟠ 𝕋 ⌖ and reproducing them immediately afterwards and again 5-10 minutes later is a reasonable test of visuomotor coordination, construction ability and visual memory.

[34] Dissociative symptoms are frequent in neurologic patients. One of the most common differentials is epilepsy. Dissociation is a poorly understood phenomenon. The validity of dissociative disorders remains unclear. Published literature on dissociation suffers from lack of adequate control populations, selection of self-reported cases leading to selection bias and unwarranted conclusions. A recent increase in the prevalence of these disorders is probably due to increased publicity and enthusiastic therapists eager to give these diagnoses. The "official" distinction between so-called "neurological" and "psychological" dissociation only reflects the presence or absence of a precipitating event. The subsequent pathophysiology is similar regardless of etiology. All dissociation has a neurologic basis. Limbic and paralimbic areas in the brain play an important role in integrating and balancing experience, thought, behavior, and affect. Disruption of these relationships results in dissociation. There are several explanatory hypotheses about the neurology of dissociation: 1) Dissociation is a result of an acute trauma resulting in a shutdown of nonemotional or declarative memory pathways and utilization of emotional, episodic, or nondeclarative memory pathways. 2) Dissociation is due to lowering of the firing threshold of limbic neuronal circuits. Early trauma (e.g., severe physical abuse) resulting in premature stimulation of the limbic system alters limbic system development. And 3) dissociation is associated with differential hemispheric activation. For further discussion, see van der Kolk and Fisler, 1995; Bremner, et al, 1996; Bowman and Coons, 2000; Brown and Trimble, 2000.

[35] The EEG has been arbitrarily divided into frequency bands (cycles/sectors or Hertz): 0.5-4.0 delta, 4.5-7.0 theta, 7.5-12.0 alpha, 12.5-18 beta. When alert at rest with eyes closed, normal persons show predominantly alpha rhythm. When doing cognitive tasks, such as mental arithmetic, beta predominates. Drowsiness also diminishes alpha but leads to slowing into the theta range. Localized slowing in the theta or delta range usually indicates a localized pathologic process; localized slowing is a nonspecific finding. SPECT (single positron emission computerized tomography) measures brain metabolism. During a seizure the seizure focus is in a state of hypermetabolism and if a patient is measured in such a state (a rare lucky occurrence), localized hyperperfusion (of the radioactive material) will be the finding. After years of seizures, the area in and around the seizure focus is often dysfunctional and hypometabolic unless a seizure is occurring. So between seizures, it is an area of hypoperfusion.

[36] Epilepsy remains a clinical diagnosis. It is difficult to identify a seizure focus on a routine EEG in all patients with clinical seizures (Camfield and Camfield, 2000; Neufeld et al, 2000). Therefore, for an experienced clinician, the EEG diagnosis of seizure offers very little new information over a careful history. Neurologists may be uncomfortable with the above statement because they frequently rely on EEG, and some have access to sophisticated laboratories. Seventy-two hours of continuous recording and videotaping, perhaps on several occasions, will identify most patients with seizure disorder. The trouble is most clinicians do not have access to these facilities. Keep the following in mind. Hans Berger, a psychiatrist, invented the EEG. Clinicians then wanted to know what the EEG of different types of epileptics looked like. So they recruited epileptic patients (diagnosed, of course, without the aid of EEG) and hooked them up to Berger's machine. The clinical diagnosis came first, and it classified the EEG findings, not the other way around. If the old time clinicians could do it, we can too.

[37] Most epileptologists prefer the term *nonepileptic seizures* to describe the convulsions that are not associated with EEG changes and may have some psychological factors associated with them. The term *pseudoseizure* is outdated. These patients do have convulsions, but some do not have epilepsy (Betts and Boden, 1991). Similarly, there are true seizures that are precipitated by certain psychological states and thoughts (Fenwick, 1991). Elevated prolactin levels are also sometimes seen in nonepileptic seizures. However, these elevations are minimal (Alving, 1998). Similarly, you may find increased prolactin levels after a syncopal attack (Oribe et al, 1996).

[38] See pathophysiology of traumatic brain injury in Silver JM, Yudofsky SC, Hales RE (eds): *Neuropsychiatry of Traumatic Brain Injury*, 1994. Also see discussion of patient 7.

[39] One of our past residents was assigned to a new affiliated hospital inpatient service. A young woman was admitted who periodically did "bad things" that somehow disrupted the unit and gained attention. She was labeled "hysterical" – in DSM: conversion/ dissociative disorder. Our resident thought otherwise, but could not convince her new attending. Rather than slinking away defeated, she waited, armed with knowledge and a set-up to draw blood for prolactin. The patient had another episode. Our resident drew the blood 18 or so minutes afterward. Prolactin levels were markedly elevated. Confronted with the evidence and references, the attending agreed. The patient was placed on an anticonvulsant, and the hysteria resolved.

[40] See Taylor, 1999; Trimble, 1986; Blumer, 1991

[41] See Leichnetz and Astruc, 1975a, 1975b

[42] See Atre-Vaidya and Taylor, 1997

[43] See Jampala et al, 1992; Silberman et al, 1985

[44] See footnote 34. For additional references, read Salloway and White, 1997.

[45] There is no diagnosis more frequently misapplied than borderline personality disorder. In our clinical experience and from the literature, it is clear that borderline disorder is a heterogeneous condition and that more than 50% have a mood disorder, especially bipolar mood disorder. Some have temporal lobe epilepsy and drug abuse, and the rest have a dramatic-emotional personality disorder characterized by impulsivity, excitability and high novelty seeking. The error in not looking for etiology occurs for several reasons: 1) The patient's behaviors are long-standing and not episodic, suggesting a trait disorder rather than a state of illness. 2) Borderline is often applied because of the consequences of signs and symptoms rather than the specific clinical features themselves, thus a stormy life and bad relationships becomes borderline despite the dysphoric moods that explain these problems. 3) Splitting (i.e., a phenomenon in which one person is seen by the patient as all good and others are seen as all bad), a human frailty, is assumed pathognomonic of borderline, despite no evidence to suggest this is so, and so any patient who does this is at risk for the diagnosis. 4) Without a diagnosis treatment is always difficult, and a patient with a fluctuating mood always exasperating. Treaters get upset, disappointed, and then angry, and respond with the pejorative diagnosis, borderline.

[46] Behavioral alterations secondary to epilepsy are frequent. These can be ictal, pre-ictal, or post-ictal or interictal. They consist of disturbances in mood, cognition, and perception. Because of this, epilepsy, especially temporal and frontal lobe epilepsies, are frequently misdiagnosed as schizophrenia or psychosis NOS. Both of us have evaluated dozens of patient with such diagnoses who ultimately had either complex partial seizures or epilepsy related disorders. Almost all of these patients benefited from anticonvulsants. There are several good articles and books that provide an excellent overview of epilepsy and psychosis. For starters, we recommend *Psychosis of Epilepsy* (1991) and *Aspects of Epilepsy (1986) and Psychiatry*, both by Michael Trimble.

[47] SeeYerby, 1991

Chapter 8

[1] See Dvoredsky and Cooley, 1986; Hoffman and Koran, 1984

[2] See Boutros and Bowers, 1996

[3] See Volavka, 1995

[4] See Volavka, 1995

[5] This is a landmark case in psychiatry. By this ruling the court essentially established the "end of confidentiality as it existed before." In this case, a California college student, Prosenjit Poddar, had expressed to his therapist his desire to kill his girlfriend, Tatitiana Tarasoff. The therapist did tell this to campus police, but did not inform Tatiana or her family. After Poddar murdered Tarasoff, her family successfully sued the University of California for failure to inform and protect. The judge in this ruling said "confidentiality ends when public peril begins." (Simon, 1992, 1994)

[6] See Pechard et al, 1999

[7] See Perry et al, 1997

[8] Gastrointestinal, gastrourinary, musculo-skeletal and neurologic are the four biggies.

[9] Patients who have chronic pain are often helped by multimodal treatments. Labeling patient as having psychogenic pain often excludes them from receiving adequate pharmacologic treatment and labeling a patient as having neurologic pain delays their receiving adequate behavioral intervention. Several articles that discuss the management of pathophysiology of chronic pain are Rowbotham, 1995; Gonzales, 1995; Galer, 1995; Eisendrath, 1995; National Pharmaceutical Council, 2001.

[10] Thompson and McDonald, 1992

[11] See Simon, 1998

[12] See Slater 1965; Slater and Glithero, 1965

[13] For a detailed discussion of clinical and pathological diagnosis and management, refer to Miller J, 2000.

[14] See Irani DN, 2001

[15] One of us has seen in consultation several patients labeled "conversion disorder" by both neurologists and psychiatrists. The definitive diagnoses in these patients were: several with partial complex epilepsy, familial cerebellar-pontine degeneration, traumatic brain injury, ophthalmic migraine, and several with psychotic depression.

[16] See Loftis and Hauser, 2003

[17] See Thompson and McDonald, 1992

[18] Chu et al 2001; Murphy, 1997

[19] Fragmented without any obvious goal

[20] See Weddington, 1982; Curyto et al, 2001

[21] See Rabins and Folstein, 1982; Caine et al, 1995

[22] See Kaplan and Saddock, 1993

[23] See Harrison's Principle of Medicine, pp. 2082-2083

[24] See Lucchinetti, 1998; Sutton, 2000; Gultekin et al, 2000

[25] See Posner and Dalmau, 2000; Lucchinetti et al, 1998; Rojas et al, 2000

[26] See Krakauer et al, 1996

[27] See Nazoe et al, 1995. Many practitioners tend to rely heavily on laboratory tests and diagnose patients prematurely. Functional brain studies are extremely sensitive to changes in blood flow. Many psychiatric illnesses exhibit abnormal SPECT findings. We believe that relying on these tests (for diagnosis) without careful consideration of clinical presentation is a gross injustice to patients and their families.

[28] See Perry et al, 1997

[29] See Lavoie and Fleet, 2000, Dwight and Stoudemire, 1997; Glassman and Shapiro, 1998

[30] Roose et al, 1994

[31] Resnik et al, 1999; Combes et al, 2001

[32] Roose et al, 1991

[33] Glassman et al, 2002; ENRICHD, 2000, 2001; Yeragani et al, 2002; Musselman et al, 2000

[34] See Sullivan et al, 1999; Evans et al, 1999; Carney et al, 1997

[35] Personality traits are conceptualized as tendencies to act in a certain way under certain circumstances, and the tendency is characteristic in quality and quantity for each person. For personality trait A, you can have a low dose, a high dose, or be (like most persons) somewhere in the middle. The distribution of doses is a normal bell-shaped curve. Persons on the extremes are likely to have a personality disorder. Any extreme behavior or body trait can get you into difficulties. If you are 6-foot 7 inches, you need to watch your body mechanics when bending down or lifting or you will get lower back pathology. A nonpathologic trait of being very tall (statistically abnormal height) can make you prone to real pathology. Deviant or abnormal personality traits can also make persons prone to real pathology. The way this happens is unclear. For further discussion, see Cloninger et al, 1993.

[36] See Tyrer and Seivewright, 1988; Tyrer et al, 1991

[37] See Kornstein et al, 2000

[38] See Tyrer and Seivewright, 1988, Tyrer et al, 1991

[39] Patients who have avoidant personality disorder respond positively to behavior treatments such as social skills training, graded exposure, group treatment focusing on systematic desensitization, self-image improvement, and behavioral rehearsals (Alden, 1989; Renneberg et al, 1990).

[40] Differential diagnoses are dramatically influenced by the patient's age. In a person over 50, cancer and depression become important considerations. In a person over 70 dementia must be considered.

[41] See Woodside et al, 1998; Wade et al 2000

[42] See Tamai et al, 1993

[43] See Agras, 1998

[44] Cerebrovascular accidents, especially lacunar infarct, frequently result in behavioral change. It is necessary for a neuropsychiatrist to be aware of major stroke syndromes. Any standard book of clinical neurology will provide a good overview. For quick reference, we have often used *Clinical Neurology, 3rd Edition*, by Aminoff, Greenberg, Simon. *The APA Textbook of Neuropsychiatry,* by Yudofsky and Hales provides a detailed account of psychiatric disorders secondary to stroke. However, in individual patients, when we have suspected behavior changes were due to a lacunar infarct, we have found MEDLINE to be most helpful in locating articles that documented the brain behavior correlations.

[45] You would think his undressing would be of more concern than his failure to follow hospital administrative procedures, but the administrative mind is unfathomable.

[46] See Robinson and Starkstein, 1997; Nagaratnam and Pathma-Nathan, 1997

Chapter 9

[1] Parrot-like, senseless repetition of a word or phrase spoken by another person.

[2] See Landau and Kleffner, 1957

[3] See O'Donohue, 1994

[4] See Kaplan, 1998

[5] DDST is a brief screening instrument covering the following areas for years one to six: gross motor, language, fine motor – adaptive and personal social. See Frankenburg and Dick, 1975; Frankenburg et al, 1973.

[6] See Saxena, 2003

[7] Moldavsky et al, 2001

[8] See Siegel et al, 1992

[9] See Beitchman et al, 2001

[10] See Paul, 1996

[11] Refer to anxiety disorders chapter

[12] See Dunn and Dunn, 1981

[13] See Black and Uhde, 1994

[14] See Kovacs, 1996; Emslie et al, 1997

[15] See Akiskal, 1985

[16] See Emslie et al, 1997. Depression is frequent in patients with pervasive developmental disorder and mental retardation. These patients , however, may present with behavioral problems in addition to withdrawal and sadness. Difficulty in communication, both verbal as well as nonverbal, results in inability to show appropriate emotional reaction. Assessment of depression in these patients should focus on vegetative signs of depression instead of depressed mood (see Ghaziuddin et al, 2002), psychotropics including ECT are helpful in these populations (see Campbell and Malone 1991; van Waardse et al, 2001).

[17] See Weller et al, 1996

[18] See Emslie et al, 1998

[19] See Ryan et al, 2003

[20] See Tomb, 1996

[21] See Emslie et al, 1998

[22] See Livingston, 1996

[23] See Masi et al, 2001; Popper, 1993

[24] See Eisenberg 1958

[25] See Masi et al, 2001

[26] See Kotimaa et al, 2003

[27] See Aylward and Brager, 2002

[28] CPT, Continuous Performance Tests, are computer-based tests designed to assess simple and complex reaction time, divided attention, auditory and visual vigilance and impulsivity. These tests yield scores on errors of omission and commission, and serve as measures of sustained attention. Attentional dysfunction is associated with a greater number of such errors in auditory and visual testing.

[29] See Castellanos et al, 2003

[30] See Pelham et al, 1985

[31] See Dulcan et al, 1998; Pliszka, 2003

[32] See McCracken, 1998

[33] See Rubia et al, 1999

[34] See Stahl, 2003

[35] See Weiss, 1996.

[36] See Geller et al, 1994

[37] See Horrigan and Barnhill, 1999

[38] See Leibenluft et al, 2003

[39] See Kowatch and DelBello, 2003

[40] See Kowatch et al, 2003

[41] See Kowatch et al, 2000

469

[42] Physicians Desk Reference, 57th Edition, Thomson PDR, Montvale, New Jersey, 2003, page 415.

[43] See Kowatch et al, 2003

[44] See Leckman and Cohen, 1999.

[45] Although these drugs are better tolerated, the FDA has not yet approved them for Tourette's.

[46] See Stewart et al, 2003

[47] See Shprintzen et al, 1978

[48] See Leckman and Cohen, 1996